LEGAL AND ETHICAL ISSUES *for the* IBCLC

ELIZABETH C. BROOKS, JD, IBCLC, FILCA

IBCLC in Private Practice
Wyndmoor, Pennsylvania

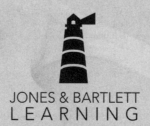

JONES & BARTLETT
LEARNING

World Headquarters
Jones & Bartlett Learning
5 Wall Street
Burlington, MA 01803
978-443-5000
info@jblearning.com
www.jblearning.com

Jones & Bartlett Learning books and products are available through most bookstores and online booksellers. To contact Jones & Bartlett Learning directly, call 800-832-0034, fax 978-443-8000, or visit our website, www.jblearning.com.

Substantial discounts on bulk quantities of Jones & Bartlett Learning publications are available to corporations, professional associations, and other qualified organizations. For details and specific discount information, contact the special sales department at Jones & Bartlett Learning via the above contact information or send an email to specialsales@jblearning.com.

Legal and Ethical Issues for the IBCLC is an independent publication and has not been authorized, sponsored, endorsed, or otherwise approved by IBLCE, ILCA, or owners of the trademarks or service marks referenced in this publication. The statements and opinions expressed herein are solely those of the author and do not represent the views or opinions of IBLCE, ILCA, or any person or party other than the author.

The author, editor, and publisher have made every effort to provide accurate information. However, they are not responsible for errors, omissions, or for any outcomes related to the use of the contents of this book and take no responsibility for the use of the products and procedures described. Treatments and side effects described in this book may not be applicable to all people; likewise, some people may require a dose or experience a side effect that is not described herein. Drugs and medical devices are discussed that may have limited availability controlled by the Food and Drug Administration (FDA) for use only in a research study or clinical trial. Research, clinical practice, and government regulations often change the accepted standard in this field. When consideration is being given to use of any drug in the clinical setting, the health care provider or reader is responsible for determining FDA status of the drug, reading the package insert, and reviewing prescribing information for the most up-to-date recommendations on dose, precautions, and contraindications, and determining the appropriate usage for the product. This is especially important in the case of drugs that are new or seldom used.

Production Credits
Publisher: Kevin Sullivan
Acquisitions Editor: Amanda Harvey
Editorial Assistant: Sara Bempkins
Editorial Assistant: Rebecca Myrick
Production Manager: Carolyn Rogers Pershouse
Marketing Communications Manager: Katie Hennessy
V.P., Manufacturing and Inventory Control: Therese Connell
Composition: Paw Print Media
Cover Design: Scott Moden
Cover Images: (top) U.S. Supreme Court columns © Lee Prince/ShutterStock, Inc.; (bottom) mother breastfeeding child © Igor Stepovik/ShutterStock, Inc.
Printing and Binding: Edwards Brothers Malloy
Cover Printing: Edwards Brothers Malloy

Library of Congress Cataloging-in-Publication Data
Brooks, Elizabeth C.
  Legal and ethical issues for the IBCLC / Elizabeth C. Brooks.
      p. ; cm.
  Legal and ethical issues for the international board certified lactation consultant
  Includes bibliographical references and index.
  ISBN 978-1-4496-1503-1 (pbk.)
1. Breastfeeding. 2. Consultants—Legal status, laws, etc. 3. Professional ethics. I. Title. II. Title: Legal and ethical issues for the international board certified lactation consultant.
  [DNLM: 1. Breast Feeding. 2. Consultants—legislation & jurisprudence. 3. Ethics, Professional. 4. Lactation. WS 125]
  RJ216.B87 2012
  174.2'9892—dc23
                                2011014353

6048

Printed in the United States of America
16 15 14 13 12   10 9 8 7 6 5 4 3 2 1

Dedication

I lovingly dedicate this book to:

My parents, who raised a girl born in the 1950s in a home where gender was deemed irrelevant to competence and accomplishment;

My children, who taught me that a competent woman can have it all if she accepts sequential rather than concurrent accomplishments;

My husband, who supported me through the transitions.

Contents

Introduction

Fine print first: The contents of this book represent the individual views of the author, as a licensed attorney who is also a certified IBCLC. I do not write on behalf of any of the organizations whose practice-guiding documents are cited in this work.

Does an International Board Certified Lactation Consultant (IBCLC) *really* have to worry about legal or ethical issues?

Well, I don't know. While I am a lawyer, I am not *your* lawyer.

Though that tidy disclaimer seemingly skirts the issue, the universal answer has to be: Of course these issues concern the IBCLC. We have a certification that enjoys an international range and reputation, but it must blend with laws that may differ from country-to-country (or state-to-state). We face common legal and ethical challenges everyday in the workplace—no matter what our work or geopolitical setting. Lactation consultants are often frustrated in that it is so difficult to find out how, simply, to "do the right thing." As a practicing IBCLC with a law degree, my training gives me perspective to offer guidance on struggling through the options, to devise an appropriate, safe, legal, and ethical plan of action in the consultation of a breastfeeding dyad.

Many practitioners fret about these issues because they fear they will be sued, or lose their job or certification, because of some action they took (or failed to take) when providing breastfeeding care. The goal of this book is to explain and demystify, using plain language, the grand and scary legal notions we hear about, but may not fully understand. Lactation management crosses many disciplines in the healthcare arena. Many IBCLCs carry other titles and licenses. This affects what we can, and cannot, do while "wearing the IBCLC hat." IBCLCs want guidance on proper, legal, and ethical behavior, and this book will explain those boundaries.

It is relatively easy to initiate legal action, in all jurisdictions. The allegations may be unfounded, but once the suit has been started, it requires a prompt and serious response. If you find yourself on the wrong end of a lawsuit or job-related inquiry, this book will not replace the advocacy that *your* lawyer can provide. Most IBCLCs will never find themselves in that unhappy position. But if you are, immediately notify your professional liability (a.k.a. malpractice) insurance carrier, since their role is to provide you with a good attorney. If you do not have such insurance, hire a good lawyer on your own. By the same token, if something you read here makes you think about how you might need to change your own practice, don't take my word for it. Ask your lawyer, accountant, or other advisor. The ethics of their professions require them to give advice specific to you and your situation.

This book raises general awareness of the legal and ethical issues faced by IBCLCs who counsel breastfeeding mothers and children. While there are excellent chapters in other publications that discuss legal issues for the IBCLC, and there is plenty of published writing about legal issues faced by the breastfeeding mother, no single book focuses solely on the ethics and legal tensions for the IBCLC. Our professional ethical code is aligned in many ways with those of other healthcare professions (e.g., nurses, midwives, family practice doctors), but our work as IBCLCs transcends the neater boundaries of those other professions.

Let's take an easy example. Imagine the infant whose short lingual frenulum makes breastfeeding a challenge. Baby tires quickly and ends feeding sessions too soon, ultimately losing weight. Mom has traumatized, bleeding nipples, and she is in agonizing pain:

- The pediatrician will be concerned about the baby who is not gaining well. One swift and sure way to increase baby weight: offer formula supplements to baby via bottle.
- The obstetrician or midwife will want to heal that patient's nipple injury. One swift and sure way to promote healing: avoid using the injured body part.

Where does the IBCLC, with her legal and ethical duties to the mother, to the baby, and to the breastfeeding relationship (International Board of Lactation Consultant Examiners [IBLCE] Scope of Practice, 2008), fit in with the care plans just described, both of which would have a profoundly negative effect on lactation?

Through my "legal-lactation lens" I hope to offer basic facts and explanations about these kinds of situations. I tend to be blunt and cut to the chase, which is a form of communication that works best when the reader happens to agree with me. But I prefer not to obfuscate. You can decide for yourself whether you agree with my conclusions, but you will not close this book wondering where I stand.

Some parts of this book offer quiz questions, drawn from actual experiences of IBCLCs serving breastfeeding families. Options for different answers are provided, and you are truly encouraged to make a choice. What would *you* do? I offer what I consider to be the best answer, and why, but your choice may be different and equally valid. Interestingly, the ethics problems that trouble IBCLCs the most do not involve our own behaviors, but rather those of colleagues whom we perceive to be acting unethically or illegally (Noel-Weiss, 2009). What are we supposed to do with this disconcerting information? IBCLCs are not immune to these uncomfortable scenarios, and this books hopes to offer some guidance.

One last caution: professional responsibilities can change for IBCLCs. They may move to new jobs where different policies and procedures are in place. The laws and regulations in their jurisdiction may be changed, affecting how they must document their consultations or seek reimbursements. The certification organization (the International Board of Lactation Consultant Examiners, www.iblce.org) and the separate and distinct professional association (the International Lactation Consultant Association, www.ilca.org) may amend the practice-guiding documents under their authority. The prudent reader will double-check at those websites to determine if changes have been made to the basic documents since publication of this book.

Please note that I tend to use the feminine form in these pages, both to doff my hat to women, who overwhelmingly make up the IBCLC profession, and to simplify the prose with one gender.

Think of this book as a resource, simply, to help you "do the right thing."

REFERENCES

International Board of Lactation Consultant Examiners. (2008). *Scope of practice for International Board Certified Lactation Consultants.* Retrieved from http://www.iblce.org/upload/downloads/ScopeOf Practice.pdf

Noel-Weiss, J. (2009, July 24). *Ethics and lactation consultants: A needs assessment.* Lecture presented at ILCA Annual Conference, Orlando, FL.

DISCLAIMER

Chapter 1

Who Is Who, and
Why Does It Matter?

L et's call her Millennial Mom—a member of the Net Generation who was born sometime after 1982. She is technologically savvy, a multi-tasker communicating frequently with family, friends, and colleagues, using an assortment of computers, phones, handheld devices, and Internet services. Indeed, her daily life is saturated with technology and media: By the time she reached 21 years of age, she had logged 20,000 hours of television, 10,000 hours of video games, 10,000 hours on a cell phone (not counting text messages), and 200,000 emails (Barnes, Marateo, & Ferris, 2007). In the same period, she spent less than 5000 hours reading print media—one-tenth the time spent learning and communicating using her electronic media (Bonamici, Hutto, Smith, & Ward, 2005). She likes immediate answers to her questions or concerns, and is adept at mining the information available to her in her complex electronic network of formal and informal resources. She'll quickly divert to another course of action if the present one does not seem to be working; she values the opinions and experiences of her peers (Oblinger & Oblinger, 2005).

And she has sore nipples from breastfeeding her 10-day-old infant.

How does she handle this problem? She hops onto the computer at 3:00 a.m. and enters the phrase *breastfeeding help sore nipples* into the popular search engine at Google. com. Over 107,000 options are provided: websites, blogs, chat rooms, and member forums. Some are sponsored by commercial interests with a product to sell. Other sites provide member responses describing personal experiences of what did and didn't work and guessing at what the cause for those sore nipples might be. Columns and blogs, written by people with mysterious strings of letters after their names, offer information and sympathy. Millennial Mom surfs quickly—scanning the pages, moving to new sites, looking for something to jump out. The words *lactation consultant* pop up on many of these pages, so Millennial Mom tries a Google search using *sore nipples lactation consultant*. Now she has 177,000 options to explore, including a "sponsored site" (a paid advertiser on Google) telling her about something called a *doula*. And someplace else mentions a lactation educator, and another site talks about peer counselors (is that anything like peer pressure?), and there is a meeting notice for a support group (don't addicts need support groups?), and here is one that claims formula now has the same ingredients as breastmilk.

1

So what's a sore mother to do? And why does it matter?

For the International Board Certified Lactation Consultant (IBCLC), Millennial Mom represents a true challenge. While an IBCLC is an allied healthcare provider who has "demonstrated specialized knowledge and clinical expertise in breastfeeding and human lactation" (International Board of Lactation Consultant Examiners [IBLCE], 2008, para. 1)—just the sort of expert help Millennial Mom can use—the role of the IBCLC is not well understood outside the confines of the profession. Even members in the healthcare field who regularly see mothers and babies (e.g., midwives, pediatricians, home healthcare or visiting nurses, obstetricians, neonatal intensive care professionals) may be unclear as to the IBCLC's training and expertise, and how that fits alongside their own roles of responsibility.

The first issue, of course, is whether Millennial Mom needs to see an IBCLC at all. For most mothers, their breastfeeding concerns can be soothingly addressed by a family member or friend who has "been there and done that." What is customarily at play is simply the new mother's quest for reassurance that whatever she is experiencing (good and bad) is a mere pothole on this fresh road to parenthood. If Millennial Mom does not have a social circle of breastfeeders (common today, given the drop in breastfeeding and surge in formula use starting in the mid-20th century [Hirschman & Butler, 1981]), there are in-person mother-to-mother support groups and website forums that serve the purpose. La Leche League International (LLLI) is perhaps the best known such group, providing these services (and more) for mothers all over the world (La Leche League International [LLLI], 2011b).

For purposes of this scenario, and for purposes of this book, let us assume that Millennial Mom really does have a lactation problem that cannot adequately be addressed by an experienced family member or volunteer. Why does it matter that our mother has turned up 177,000 hits on her Internet search about sore nipples and lactation consultants?

Confusing and Overlapping Job Titles in the Marketplace

It matters to IBCLCs who provide "safe, competent and evidence-based" lactation care (IBLCE, 2008), because while we offer precisely the sort of education, support, and care Millennial Mom needs, she may not even know we exist. While she is doing a "scan-and-cram" on the computer to find out who (or what) can give her some relief, we IBCLCs continually run the risk of "confusion in the marketplace" because our clinical role and expertise is not well known or understood. Our marketplace is composed of the mothers we serve and the public health and medical professionals with whom we interact because they are the people who will seek out (or refer to) an IBCLC. If Millennial Mom makes an appointment with someone she found on a list on some website for new mothers, she may assume she is getting an IBCLC when she is not. Conversely, the very real clinical contribution an IBCLC can make to the care of a breastfeeding mother may be discounted by those who think we are "just volunteers." Families may think we offer our services for free, just like volunteer mother-to-mother support groups. We do not; unless there is a prior arrangement to offer IBCLCs services on a reduced fee or pro bono publico basis, the services of an IBCLC are entitled to fair compensation. This is a reflection of the skill and expertise we bring to the mother, and ought also to be covered/reimbursable to the mother by her healthcare ministry/health insurance provider (a reflection of the value the system places on specialized care for human lactation).

Indeed, the profession as a whole may be tarred and feathered, should the mother who *thought* she was getting the specialized skill of an IBCLC instead have a very unsatisfactory experience interacting with someone lacking the training and accountability of an IBCLC. Because off she will go, to write on her blog or update her Facebook page or send her 140-character tweet, reducing to permanent cyber history her disappointment with the IBCLC profession. And the next day at 3:00 a.m., Millennial Mom No. 2 will come along, start surfing the Web for information about *her* sore nipples. She will stumble upon a blog post blasting all lactation consultants and their profession because of Millennial Mom No. 1's disappointing encounter. Ouch.

As IBCLCs, our own excellent and ethical professional behaviors will secure our personal reputations, but it is incumbent upon *each* of us to help educate those in the marketplace (the mothers, and the public health and medical professionals with whom we interact) about what it takes to be an IBCLC, and why that is different from any other sort of lactation helper. And so, prompted as we are under our IBLCE Code of Professional Conduct (IBLCE CPC) to "protect the health, welfare and safety of the public by providing the internationally recognized measure of knowledge in lactation and breastfeeding care" (IBLCE, 2011e, p.1), we begin by describing many of the various players in the arena of breastfeeding support, in addition to the IBCLC, whose role and impact stands apart from other helpers (International Lactation Consultant Association [ILCA] & Henderson, 2011).

Primary Healthcare Provider

First, a statement of the obvious: Millennial Mom may not make any phone calls whatsoever to find lactation support. She may just throw up her hands and wean, without talking to a soul.

Or, she may call her own (or her baby's) primary healthcare provider. It may be the family practice doctor, the pediatrician, the midwife, the obstetrician, the physician, or the nurse answering the phone triage line at any of these offices. Training and education focused on human lactation varies widely in each of these disciplines. It is safe to say that human lactation is *not* a part of the required curricula for most healthcare disciplines (though that trend is changing). Fortunate students will get one lecture on the topic in their many years of classroom study. They may be lucky enough to do rounds during their clinical training under the tutelage of someone who has taken the time, as a practicing healthcare provider, to acquire evidence-based expertise in the topic of breastfeeding. Millennial Mom may get excellent breastfeeding advice using these options.

Quite simply, other mothers will not. Indeed, the level of misinformation about breastfeeding given to women by trusted healthcare providers about a very basic human function is astonishing. One physician told a mother that one breast makes all the fat, one makes all the protein, and plugged ducts are caused by blood clots in the breast (Smith, 1999). One would hope such egregiously erroneous statements are extremely rare, but for Millennial Mom, this may be the only advice she gets, and she has no reason to doubt its validity as it comes from her primary healthcare provider.

IBCLCs' knowledge runs very narrow, but very deep. We know an awful lot about one particular biologic function, whether viewed from the baby's perspective, the mother's perspective, or the "relationship's" perspective (since breastfeeding, by its very nature, requires the mother and baby dyad to work together). We cannot expect all other healthcare providers to be as immersed in the minutiae of the field of human lactation as are we. But while IBCLCs are members of the healthcare team required by the IBLCE Code of Professional Conduct and IBLCE Scope of Practice to share pertinent information about a lactation consultation with everyone else providing care for the mother and baby, the reverse is not true. The midwife, for example, does not need to alert an IBCLC if Millennial Mom has had an office visit to address sore nipples. So the IBCLC will not have an opportunity to educate Millennial Mom (and the midwife) if the care plan contains erroneous or outdated advice, even if that advice was given with the very best of intentions.

International Board Certified Lactation Consultant (IBCLC)

IBCLCs are the premier providers of care for breastfeeding and human lactation. IBCLCs are members of a stand-alone, allied healthcare profession concentrating on human lactation.[1] IBCLCs are to human lactation and breastfeeding what speech-language pathologists are to human communication and swallowing (Ad Hoc Committee on the Scope of Practice in Speech-Language Pathology, 2007) or what physiotherapists are to human function and movement (The Physiotherapy Site, 2011).

In New Zealand,

> [the] allied health professions have a distinct, specialised body of knowledge and skills and actively work with people accessing health and disability services across a range of settings. Allied health professionals . . . have a professional association, an appropriate code of ethics and standards of practice, and a recognised system for monitoring ongoing competence. (Allied Health Professional Associations' Forum, 2011, para. 2)

---

[1] Sometimes called "allied health professionals" or "allied health practitioners," the Joint Commission (formerly the Joint Commission on Accreditation of Healthcare Organizations, although its old acronym of JCAHO [pronounced *jay-coh*] is still used by many) defines this very broad category of workers as "health professionals qualified by training and frequently by licensure to assist, facilitate, or complement the work of physicians, dentists, podiatrists, nurses, pharmacists, and other specialists in the healthcare system" (Joint Commission, 2002, Introduction).

Rigorous defined eligibility requirements must be met in order to take the once-yearly certification exam conducted by the International Board of Lactation Consultant Examiners. Scores of hours of classroom-style instruction, and hundreds or thousands of hours of supervised clinical work *solely* in human lactation must be completed before one can take the exam. IBCLCs have "demonstrated specialized knowledge and clinical expertise in breastfeeding and human lactation and are certified by the International Board of Lactation Consultant Examiners (IBLCE)" (IBLCE, 2008, para. 1). Thereafter, IBCLCs must recertify every 5 years (IBLCE, 2012d). Certification as an IBCLC is voluntary, but it is conditional, and revocable for cause, under a defined disciplinary procedure. The certification is an internationally recognized credential: Every IBCLC around the world must meet the same criteria to take the exam; every IBCLC around the world takes the same exam in any given year (although it may be translated into one of nineteen languages) (IBLCE, 2012a).

Once certified as an IBCLC, the professional *must* adhere to the mandatory IBLCE Code of Professional Conduct (IBLCE CPC) and mandatory IBLCE Scope of Practice for IBCLCs (IBLCE SOP), and is *encouraged* to follow the voluntary Standards of Practice for IBCLCs promulgated by the professional association, the International Lactation Consultant Association (ILCA Standards). An IBCLC does not operate in a vacuum: She is a member of the healthcare team working with the mother, baby, and family (IBLCE, 2011e, 2008; International Lactation Consultant Association [ILCA], 2006b).

The IBLCE has registered the acronym *IBCLC* and the phrase *Registered Lactation Consultant* (RLC) with the U.S. Patent and Trademark Office, as certification marks. Only those who have been designated as IBCLC by the IBLCE are entitled to use those initials, as "the certification mark, as used by persons authorized [by IBLCE], certifies the quality of the services performed by those approved by the certifier" (IBLCE, 1997 [renewed 2007]). Similarly, "Registered Lactation Consultant . . . as used by authorized persons, certifies that persons performing lactation consulting have met the standards, qualifications and testing of the certifier" (IBLCE, 2003b). Some countries do not, however, recognize RLC. In Germany, the term *lactation consultant, IBCLC* is similarly trademark-protected through the Patent Office, by the German Lactation Consultants' Association, which permits its use only by IBCLCs (von der Ohe, 1998).

Lactation Consultant Intern or Student

Qualification to take the IBLCE exam for IBCLCs may take years to acquire. Those in active training or mentorship programs may devise and use a term like "lactation consultant intern" to signify their status as serious, aspiring IBCLCs. While it is tempting to use a phrase like "IBCLC-in-training" or "IBCLC Candidate" or even "IBCLC Designee," the use of those five special initials is available only to those who already have been so certified (IBLCE, 2011e). Clearly, someone in training is not there yet, although it is fitting to be labeled in a fashion indicating a course of instruction intended to culminate in certification.

Lactation Consultant

IBCLCs are frequently called, simply, "lactation consultants." That is understandable. It is a mouthful to say "International Board Certified Lactation Consultant" or even "I-B-C-L-C" in everyday communication, especially in a clinical consult with a mother. Similarly, it is easier to say "I am a cardiac surgeon" than "I am an American Board of Thoracic Surgery Diplomate," which an excellent cardiac surgeon may well be (American Board of Thoracic Surgery, 2011; Society of Thoracic Surgeons, 2012).

The two-word phrase *lactation consultant* does *not* have any trademark or certification mark protection. So anyone can call themselves a lactation consultant and hang out a shingle (or construct a website) and begin to discuss breastfeeding matters with individual mothers—even charging them for the service. This self-labeled lactation consultant is not required to uphold the ethical and professional standards required of IBCLCs, because she isn't an IBCLC. And she can't be disciplined by IBLCE, either, since their jurisdictional reach is only to current IBCLC certificants (IBLCE, 2011d, 2011e). She probably is not carrying professional liability insurance, designed to protect against negligent practice, because such insurance is designed for members of a recognized healthcare profession (CM&F Group, 2011b). Note that while she may carry liability insurance for her clinical work in another role or profession (e.g., registered dietitian or nurse), that is no guarantee that she'd be covered for this lactation consulting on the side. Indeed, this is just the sort of exclusion insurers love to use to negate their obligation to defend (CM&F Group, 2011a).

To demonstrate just how attractive that phrase *lactation consultant* is considered to be, ponder the following. One of the largest artificial baby milk (or formula) manufacturers in the United States is the subject of frequent reports of violations of the World Health Organization's (WHO) *International Code of Marketing of Breast-milk Substitutes* (WHO Code; sometimes referred to as the International Code) for directly marketing formula to the public (Walker, 2007). In 2010 the formula manufacturer started a heavily promoted campaign encouraging mothers to call a toll-free number to talk to a "lactation consultant" about breastfeeding issues. This rather begs the question of why anyone would rely on breastfeeding advice from a company whose profits depend on mothers *not* breastfeeding. Be that as it may, none of the "lactation consultants" answering the toll-free number is an IBCLC. Indeed, an effort to hire IBCLCs for this work backfired when they all refused for ethical reasons grounded in Principle 24 of the then-governing IBLCE Code of Ethics (since replaced by the IBLCE Code of Professional Conduct), mandating IBCLC support for the WHO Code (Penchuk, 2010). But the formula company got their program up and running anyway, hiring non-IBCLCs (whose ethical constraints differ from those of IBCLCs), while insisting that the phone-answerers be termed "lactation consultants" in the marketing materials.

It is ironic that it is IBCLCs who commonly use the term "lactation consultant" to loosely describe their work, perpetuating confusion in the marketplace, when they have gone to extraordinary effort to earn the distinguished IBCLC certification.

Graduate of Accredited Course or Curriculum in Human Lactation

Coming to your college or university soon! As IBCLCs have only been around since 1985 (IBLCE, 2011c) not many children scream out "IBCLC!" when asked by a doting grandparent what they want to be when they grow up. Most children will suggest career choices for which (perhaps unknown to them at the moment) an educational and training path are well-established. The IBCLC is fairly new, barely 26 years on the scene at the time of this writing. Recognized university-level curricula for a course of instruction and clinical training, lasting at least 1 year and culminating in a degree in human lactation, is in the formative stages.

The Lactation Education Accreditation and Approval Review Committee (LEAARC) was established in July 2008 (using the former cumbersome moniker of Accreditation and Approval Review Committee on Education in Human Lactation and Breastfeeding, or AARC) as a joint effort by ILCA and IBLCE, under the auspices of the Commission on Accreditation of Allied Health Education Programs (CAAHEP). It is designed "to establish, maintain, and promote appropriate standards of quality for educational programs in Lactation and Breastfeeding and to provide recognition for educational programs that meet or exceed the minimum standards" (LEAARC, 2012a, para. 3).

By February 2012 LEAARC had approved several short-term courses on lactation (LEAARC, 2012b) (see more below), but the process of accreditation of university-level academic curricula is not yet finalized. A multi-year effort involving international lactation and education experts created a model curriculum framework, intended to be adaptable for various international postsecondary teaching settings. The goal is that LEAARC will make recommendations to CAAHEP for accreditation of academic programs sponsored by accredited postsecondary institutions (LEAARC, 2010). One day soon, perhaps when Millennial Mom's infant grows up clamoring to become an IBCLC, her parents will easily find a university or college offering the education she needs to attain the certification and profession of her dreams.

Attendee at Lactation Education Accreditation and Approval Review Committee (LEAARC)-Approved Course

By February 2012, LEAARC had approved 22 short-term courses in human lactation and breastfeeding, by educators based in the United States, Canada, Australia, Denmark, and the United Kingdom. The LEAARC approval is a "reliable indicator of educational quality to employers, insurers, counselors, educators, governmental officials, and the public, based on the fact that the education program adheres to established criteria and standards of the profession" (LEAARC, 2012b, p. 1). These courses must be taught by an IBCLC certified at least 5 years, and offer at least 45 hours of the classroom instruction needed to meet IBLCE requirements to sit the IBCLC exam. The idea is that any of these courses can be a stepping stone toward IBCLC certification, or excellent instruction if one has a passing or professional interest in the subject matter. But as all of the providers clearly indicate, completing their course(s) does not create an IBCLC. Some, but not all, of the LEAARC-approved courses offer up titles or certificates upon successful completion of the course.

It is these *titles*, so similar-sounding to "International Board Certified Lactation Consultant," that create marketplace confusion. While Millennial Mom (or a hospital administrator, for that matter) may easily appreciate the difference between a "student" at a school and a "graduate" of a school, she may not be so clear on the difference between an International Board Certified Lactation Consultant and a Certified Lactation Counselor® or Certified Lactation Specialist. It is not a stretch to see that confusion might arise were Millennial Mom to stumble upon one of these similarly named short-term course attendees during her late-night surf for expert help. What follows is not an exhaustive list of terms describing successful attendees at such LEAARC-approved courses, but does offer examples of the most similarly-named programs.

Certified Lactation Counselor® (CLC®)
This 5-day, 45-hour program offered in the United States is "designed to provide a solid, up-to-date, research-based body of information regarding lactation as well [as] the art of counseling" (Healthy Children Center for Breastfeeding, n.d., para. 13), although "completion of this course does not expand the practice parameters of any health professional" (Healthy Children Center for Breastfeeding, n.d., para. 19). At the end of the program, a test may voluntarily be taken. If successfully completed, the student receives the designation Certified Lactation Counselor® or CLC® (the former registered as a certification mark; the latter having filed for same) (Healthy Children Project, 2010, 2011). The certification is awarded by a testing authority, the Academy of Lactation Policy and Practice (ALPP) (Academy of Lactation Policy and Practice [ALPP], 2011). The credential "identifies a specialist in lactation counseling" (ALPP, 2011, para. 1). It is valid for 3 years; recertification requires 18 hours of continuing education (Healthy Children's Center for Breastfeeding, n.d.). A disciplinary process may be initiated against any certificant for violation of CLC program requirements (ALPP, 2009), and CLCs have a scope of practice focusing on "safe, evidence-based counseling for pregnant, lactating and breastfeeding women" (ALPP, 2011, para. 2). The CLC is an accredited competency course recognized by the American Nurses Credentialing Center (American Nurses Credentialing Center, 2012a), "verifying that [CLCs] have this valuable competency based nursing skill, even if they are not nurses" (Healthy Children Center for Breastfeeding, n.d., para. 16).

Certified Lactation Specialist (CLS)
This 45-hour, 5-day course, offered in the United States by Lactation Education Consultants, "is a stepping stone to the IBCLC credential" where "participants will be taught how to use appropriate counseling skills, how to teach mothers and families, and most importantly, how to function hands-on as a clinician" (Lactation Education Consultants, n.d., para. 3). There is no requirement to recertify, nor is a disciplinary or grievance process associated with this program.

Certified Breastfeeding Specialist (CBS)

A 45-hour online course through Lactation Education Resources (LER) is part of their training in preparation for the IBLCE exam, and is for "students wanting a Certified Breastfeeding Specialist credential while they are accumulating clinical practice hours in order to qualify to take the IBLCE certification exam" (Lactation Education Resources, n.d., para. 2). Those who complete the 45-hour class are entitled to take a CBS test administered by LER, but the training counts toward IBLCE qualification regardless. There is no requirement to recertify, nor is a disciplinary or grievance process associated with this program.

Certificate for Lactation Consultant

The University of California San Diego Extension (UCSD) has a three-part classroom and clinical training program that is something of a hybrid: It *does* provide all eligibility requirements for a student to take the IBLCE exam (Baker, n.d.b).

Lactation Educator-Counselor

This course is also offered by UCSD, although no LEAARC approval was sought for this course offering. It is a 45-hour class; the successful student "is a 'certificated' Lactation Educator Counselor," an entry level practitioner who deals "primarily with the **normal** process of lactation" (Baker, n.d.a, para. 1) (emphasis in original).

Attendee at Non-LEAARC–Approved Course

As LEAARC was established in 2008, there are many courses offered around the world that have not yet undergone its review process. And, not all courses (whether submitted for LEAARC approval or not) will award confusingly similar titles or certificates at their conclusion. Thus, the following is not an exhaustive list, but it describes some titles awarded at the end of the course which Millennial Mom may uncover during her Internet wanderings.

Certified Breastfeeding Counselor (CBC)

Requiring 30 hours' work with breastfeeding mothers (one-on-one, on the phone, and as a breastfeeding class teacher), and mandatory reading and assignments that can be flexibly acquired over approximately 12 months, the Certified Breastfeeding Counselor is "certification for life!" (Childbirth International, 2008, para. 2) that does not require continuing education or recertification. This course is offered by Childbirth International, Inc.

Certified Lactation Educator (CLE)

After 20 hours of classroom work, and required independent learning, the Childbirth and Postpartum Professional Association (CAPPA) awards the Certified Lactation Educator (CLE) credential, indicating qualification "to teach, support, and educate the public on breastfeeding and related issues" (Childbirth and Postpartum Professional Association, 2012a, para. 1). The CLE does not confer lactation consultant status, but those who have completed the course must abide by a code of conduct, grievance policy, and scope of practice focusing on education and teaching skills (Childbirth and Postpartum Professional Association, 2012b).

Community Breastfeeding Educator (CBE)
A 3-day, 20-hour course designed for community workers in maternal child health "to encourage the initiation and continuation of breastfeeding" is conducted by the same organization offering the LEAARC-approved CLC course (Healthy Children Center for Breastfeeding, 2011, p. 2), although this class does not provide for any testing or awarding of certificates or certifications.

Advanced Lactation Consultant (ALC) or Advanced Nurse Lactation Consultant (ANLC)

These two programs are accredited by the American Nurses Credentialing Center (ANCC) in the United States, as two (of many) nursing skills competency programs "validating skills or skill sets of nurses at all levels." (American Nurses Credentialing Center, 2012d, para. 4). The ALC and ANLC courses concentrate on breastfeeding and human lactation. The 5-day, 45-hour course is conducted as an "opportunity to earn advanced certification in lactation management" (Healthy Children Center for Breastfeeding, 2011, p. 3).

Recall that IBLCE is the only entity that can award certification as an IBCLC. IBCLCs are required to recertify each 5 years with IBLCE, although this requirement can be met by retaking the test, or acquiring sufficient continuing education recognition points (CERPs) through classroom-style learning (IBLCE, 2012d). IBLCE does not offer recertification based upon evaluation of *clinical* competence.

Compare that with these two certifications through ANCC, that evaluate clinical (hands-on) skills in lactation, for both the Advanced Lactation Consultant (ALC) course (marketed to IBCLCs and CLCs®) and the Advanced Nurse Lactation Consultant (ANLC) course (marketed to registered nurses [RNs]). This is appealing to RNs in the United States, many of whom work in institutions seeking Magnet recognition from ANCC, a separate U.S.-based program that "recognizes healthcare organizations for quality patient care, nursing excellence and innovations in professional nursing practice " (ANCC, 2012b, p. 1). Clinical competency evaluations, conducted by a certified credentialing agency like ANCC, are a highly valued measure of quality nursing care, especially (but not exclusively) for an institution seeking Magnet recognition.

Similarly, it may be appealing to the non-nurse IBCLC to complete the ALC course, because (as we'll explore later) it is a sad, true, and frustrating fact that many hospitals in the United States will not hire an IBCLC to provide dedicated lactation care unless she is also an RN. Why would a hospital have such a requirement? Training as a nurse is *not* a prerequisite for certification as an IBCLC, but having employees with several licenses or certifications facilitates the hospital administrators' need to staff many departments. Also, the ability of an IBCLC to be "recognized" by the hospital's extraordinarily complex reimbursement system is greatly enhanced if she carries either licensure or an ANCC certification. The Byzantine system that approves insurance payments (either for the mother, who carries health insurance, or the hospital, to reimburse for providing skilled lactation care) looks for a healthcare provider who has a license (as RNs do) or certification by a huge, long-standing, and well-recognized entity (as ANCC is).[2] As we'll see later, IBCLCs do not have independent licensure in the United States from state-based boards; instead, they have worldwide-recognized certification from IBLCE. The behemoth health-insurance-driven system of reimbursement in the United States looks for round pegs to fit into round holes, and ANCC certification is a recognized round peg—whether it is issued to a nurse or a lactation consultant. So, if the non-RN IBCLC now carries the ALC credential from ANCC, she may be more readily reimbursed for the services she provides. This makes her an attractive candidate for employment at a hospital or birthing center.

These two programs may, however, erode the pool of potential IBCLC candidates or recertificants. A CLC who has completed a 5-day course and exam can now take another 5-day course and sit for the ALC certification exam (Healthy Children Center for Breastfeeding, 2011). That is a considerably shorter investment of time (both classroom and supervised clinical hours) than is required of an IBCLC applicant or recertifier. Similarly, an RN with an intense interest in specializing in breastfeeding and human lactation may find the ANLC route significantly cheaper and easier to accomplish. In the end, both the CLC and the RN will have a certification as something that includes the phrase *lactation consultant*. Thus the stepping stone toward IBCLC certification through IBLCE has been effectively detoured to another certifying agency, offering a confusingly similar title.

Attendee of Short-Term Class or Conference on Breastfeeding Management

That's a very long string of words that is an umbrella for a huge—and growing—group of educational offerings.

Each year, there are hundreds (probably thousands) of classes and conferences, all over the globe, devoted to issues of breastfeeding and human lactation. It may be a mandatory in-service given at a hospital for its employees. It may be a course of instruction requiring the student or attendee to pay a fee. It could be a class (or series of classes) hosted by a public health agency or a commercial entity and advertised to the public at large. They may last a day; they may last several days. Attendees may receive

---

[2] ANCC, since 1991, has certified over 250,000 nurses in the United States alone (ANCC, 2012c). IBLCE, since 1985, has certified over 30,000 IBCLCs worldwide; 22,000 hold current certification (IBLCE, 2011a).

a certificate of attendance or certificate of completion. Some of these venues offer the continuing education credits required by many healthcare professions.

Instruction may be intended for a healthcare practitioner audience, or a mother audience, or a public health agency administrative audience. Attendees may be members of other healthcare professions (e.g., nurses, doctors, midwives) who are intrigued by this field and want to learn something applicable to their current area of practice. They may be current or recently lactating women, interested in volunteering as mother-to-mother counselors who can offer encouragement and support to other new mothers. Perhaps they are students acquiring necessary hours of didactic instruction to qualify for the IBLCE exam. Course content may be dense and scientific (highlighting the latest research); it may be warm and fuzzy (games to play with your toddler while you breastfeed your infant). Attendees may take a short quiz at the end to test their new knowledge; they may spend the entire time reading emails on their laptops or working Sudoku puzzles.

And therein lies the problem. There is such a thirst for general breastfeeding knowledge, and so many courses and conferences claiming to quench it, that the world is awash with classes. They teach a lot (or a little) to attendees who learn a lot (or a little). The graduates may then go forth into the marketplace, believing or asserting they are trained to address complex clinical lactation situations. Further, they may be hired (by mothers or hospitals or clinics) with the expectation they can deliver on that promise, when they cannot.

Mother-to-Mother Counselor

Many of the issues a new mother faces can be easily and appropriately addressed by another experienced mother. New parents have all kinds of questions about every aspect of infant care: the umbilical cord, bathing the baby, how to change diapers (and how to clean a baby girl bottom vs. a baby boy bottom), how much sunshine and fresh air is okay, how many layers of clothing to put on the baby, when germ-laden though well-intended friends get to hold the baby—the list goes on. Breastfeeding is certainly a big part of any baby's day, and as such is a subject of just as much concern and pride by the new parents as any other aspect of babydom.

Society and culture have changed dramatically since 1800, when just about everyone in the world lived a buggy ride or footpath away from their mothers, grandmothers, sisters, aunts, and best friends—all of whom breastfed, because that was (and still is) the biologic norm. To be sure, there were circumstances where a mother could not breastfeed her child; childbearing still has a high mortality rate today in many countries of the world (UNICEF, 2010). But the notion of buying factory-made food to give to the baby was just not an option until the late 1800s (Wolf, 2001). If the mother was not there to directly feed the infant, the baby was breastfed by another woman (a practice variously termed wet-nursing, shared nursing, cross-nursing, or cross-feeding) (Thorley, 2009), or received milk that the mother or another lactating woman had earlier hand-expressed. And certainly there were moments of desperation, where the motherless infant received milk from the family cow or goat or coconut tree.

By the mid-1900s there was a huge societal and cultural shift away from breast-feeding in the United States and other industrialized cultures, and toward use of artificial baby formula dispensed in bottles (thanks, in part, to pervasive marketing campaigns by the formula and bottle makers [Wolf, 2001]). Thus, it was no longer feasible for a new breastfeeding mother to simply ask her mother or sister or best friend her common, everyday, run-of-the-mill new-mother-breastfeeding question. The mother's traditional circle of support couldn't reassure her about breastfeeding frequency, or the appearance of a breastfed baby's stool, or whether waking to feed at night is normal—because they simply did not know. Their children had been raised on formula from a bottle, not breastfeeding.

Out of this huge need, La Leche League International (LLLI) was born in 1956. A group of seven breastfeeding mothers met at a kitchen table in Chicago, Illinois (when the breastfeeding rate in the United States hovered at 20%), because they recognized the need "to help mothers worldwide to breastfeed through mother-to-mother support, encouragement, information, and education, and to promote a better understanding of breastfeeding as an important element in the healthy development of the baby and mother" (LLLI, 2011a, 2011b, opening para.). Today, a La Leche League leader (LLLL) is recognized worldwide as a one-to-one breastfeeding supporter for the mother who needs basic information and cheerleading. Building on the LLLI model, the Australian Breastfeeding Association (ABA) was started in 1964, though called the Nursing Mothers' Association at the time (Australian Breastfeeding Association, 2010); the Association of Breastfeeding Mothers (ABM) was founded in the United Kingdom in 1979 (Association of Breastfeeding Mothers, 2011).

All of these groups (and others like them, serving smaller regions throughout the world) have the simple mission to support breastfeeding mothers. Using a grassroots system of neighborly assistance, counselors are volunteers who have breastfed their child(ren) and have completed a short training course about lactation basics and counseling techniques. Support may be offered in person or over the phone by a specific counselor assigned to the mother; new mothers may utilize a "warm line" for help over the phone by whomever answers that day. These organizations schedule support group meetings (weekly, bi-weekly, or monthly) where families and babies can gather together for the common purpose of sharing the ins and outs of being a breastfeeding parent. LLLI, ABA, and ABM all have extensive websites providing answers to "frequently asked questions," materials to be downloaded, and links to find local counselors.

Peer Counselor (e.g., WIC Program, United States)

Expanding on the mother-to-mother counselor model pioneered by LLLI, some public health agencies charged with providing nutrition and public health education have a "peer counselor" program for breastfeeding support.

In the United States, the Food and Nutrition Service of the U.S. Department of Agriculture funds and administers the Special Supplemental Nutrition Program for Women, Infants and Children (referred to in thankful shorthand as WIC) (Food and Nutrition Service of U.S. Dept. of Agriculture, 2011). WIC "provides nutritious food, nutrition education (including breastfeeding promotion and support), and referrals to health and other social services to participants at no charge. [WIC] is a Federal grant program . . . which . . . provides these funds to WIC State agencies to pay for WIC foods, nutrition education, breastfeeding promotion and support, and administrative costs" (Food and Nutrition Service of U.S. Dept. of Agriculture, 2011, p. 1). In addition, a comprehensive program provides evidence-based training to establish peer counselor programs (Loving Support, 2012). Each state (or even county within a state) may use their funding for education and counseling differently; some peer counselors will work as volunteers; others will be paid staff members at their local WIC offices. Similarly, some WIC offices employ IBCLCs on staff; others do not (Food and Nutrition Service of U.S. Dept. of Agriculture, 2012). A scope of practice focuses on providing counseling and support, and recognizing when referral to a healthcare provider (such as an IBCLC) may be required (Loving Support, 2004).

La Leche League does not itself use peer counselors; they provide La Leche League Leaders to assist breastfeeding families. But they do offer a training curriculum for peer counselors that may be used by agencies looking to establish such a program (Baker, K. [LLLI], 2011). In Great Britain, using the LLLI program, a peer counselor program was established in 1990 and has grown significantly (La Leche League GB [Great Britain], n.d.).

Doula

> The word *doula* comes from the ancient Greek meaning "a woman who serves" and is now used to refer to a trained and experienced professional who provides continuous physical, emotional, and informational support to the mother before, during, and just after birth; or who provides emotional and practical support during the postpartum period. (DONA International, 2005b, para. 1)

An international organization provides a certification program for birth doulas and postpartum doulas. There are standards of practice and a code of ethics for each designation, recertification every 3 years, and a grievance procedure (DONA International, 2005a).

Doulas may be hired to help during the pregnancy and childbirth stages, assisting a mother through these milestone life events, or they may be employed after the birth of the baby, assisting the family at home. Breastfeeding assistance is often described as part of the doula's service.

If your head is spinning by now, imagine Millennial Mom.

Different Job Titles Carry Different Legal and Ethical Responsibilities

So back to square one. Let us put on the IBCLC hat now and view the forthcoming matters through the IBCLC lens, as this book is written for the very specific niche audience of IBCLCs (if 25,000+ lactation professionals can be considered a niche). We presume Millennial Mom is confused about the menu of available breastfeeding helpers. How does this impact the competent IBCLC, who is well aware of (and stays within) her professional boundaries?

Each and every one of the breastfeeding helpers described in the previous section—which is not an exclusive listing—has come to her title or certification using a different route. Different roles carry different responsibilities, and an IBCLC ought to be able to credibly describe the variations between breastfeeding helper training and expertise. The time will come when she will be asked to explain who is who, and why it matters. An IBCLC may find herself in the position of explaining to her boss (or prospective boss) why hiring a graduate from a short-term class is simply not the same as hiring an IBCLC certificant. She may have to go to bat for a client, who is fighting her insurance company's decision to deny coverage of the IBCLC consult as "education" rather than "health care." The IBCLC may find that her ability to serve mothers and babies is cramped by colleagues or supervisors claiming she has no clinical role to play, despite 10 years' certification. Lest you think this is all philosophical, these are real-life scenarios three IBCLCs had to face in 2010. Thus, it makes sense that the IBCLC—who has the most to gain by adequately explaining her legitimate role in the collaborative care of a breastfeeding dyad—should shoulder the responsibility of articulating kind (and constant) reminders of the IBCLC's rights and responsibilities.

So let's compare how legal and ethical responsibilities differ for the IBCLC and her compatriots with training for different titles.

Training Differs for Various Titles

What is mentioned in the preceding pages bears repeating: Different programs require different education and training before one is declared "done" and ready to serve the public on a paid or volunteer basis. Some classes offer classroom and homework only; the course might be completed in a matter of days, or require several months or years. Other instructional programs prescribe a range of topics that must be learned, over a range of child ages (as the human child self-weans somewhere between 2.5–7 years of age—much older than the typical breastfeeding baby in the United States) (Dettwyler, 1995). Some programs require hands-on clinical training (which starts out heavily monitored, and gradually moves to less over-the-shoulder supervision as the student acquires more skill and experience). Other programs require time spent in patient/client education or counseling, but with no hands-on clinical interaction.

The IBCLC certainly "gets" that a weekend class about breastfeeding management for mothers of full-term babies cannot begin to provide the rich and detailed skill a clinician specialized in human lactation must bring to bear. We never know what kind of mother will walk in our door, or be lying in the postpartum bed, as we do our daily work. We need to be prepared to consider (and explain) anything affecting breastfeeding, whether baby- or mother-related: infertility or breast surgery history; prematurity; milk synthesis; insufficient glandular tissue; interventions and medications of birth; physical or congenital anomalies; neurologic or musculoskeletal syndromes; insufficient milk transfer and drainage with their complications of engorgement, reduced milk supply, and mastitis, to name a few.

The IBCLC's never-ending chore is to know who brings what kind of breastfeeding training to this mother–baby dyad, and whether it is appropriate to meet the needs of that family. Mastering some diplomatic skills will be very helpful, because (sadly) the discovery that the mother has been given poor advice by another caregiver can create a contentious atmosphere. When the IBCLC learns the mother has been seen by someone who has insufficient training for the issues at hand (or by someone who instead has very specialized skill in one profession, but not much in the field of human lactation) she is placed in the extremely uncomfortable role of explaining why the care plan she is crafting with the mother is at odds with what the other breastfeeding helper suggested. And understandably, the mother's first set of questions will be, "Why is this care plan different from the person I saw last week? They told me *ABC*, and you're suggesting *XYZ*. Who is right? Whom do I believe?" Practice hint: If you find yourself in this situation, remember that there are always two sides to a story. What the mother *reports* was the instruction from the other helper may not have been the actual instruction. The salient fact is that the mother *thinks* this is what the other caregiver said. Don't devote a lot a time in forensic reconstruction of her other appointment. Instead, validate your client's concern, and steer her back to the situation (and expert) right there in front of her ("It *is* frustrating when you get different advice from different professionals! Your baby makes amazing strides every day, so the picture changes very quickly. Let's review your new care plan, based on what we saw today, which is designed to boost your supply from here on out.")

It may be easiest simply to remember (and be able to articulate) the training and certification *for the IBCLC*, as she is the premiere allied healthcare professional for breastfeeding and human lactation. All healthcare providers working with mothers and babies are supposed to be promoting breastfeeding as the biologic norm and public health imperative—that is what their professional associations and medical societies are advising them to do as a standard of practice (ILCA, 2006a). If you find yourself in the position of having to defend your job and qualifications (especially when you are being compared to someone else with similar passion, but less training, about breastfeeding), list out your own training and certification requirements, focused as they are solely on human lactation and ask whether the other caregiver can document similar hours of concentrated instruction.

Scope of Practice Generally

A scope of practice (SOP) describes everything that a practitioner is entitled to do as part of her clinical and instructional interactions with clients or patients. The IBLCE Scope of Practice for IBCLCs, issued and enforced by IBLCE, "encompasses the activities for which IBCLCs are educated and in which they are authorized to engage" (IBLCE, 2008, para. 2). This primary practice-guiding document for IBCLCs will be described in greater detail in another chapter.

"Scope of practice" is a very loaded term, and decades of battling have been known to ensue when one healthcare profession perceives that a different group of practitioners is invading their clinical territory (Reiger, 2008). If you want to put a fright into any healthcare provider, suggest that something she is doing is "outside her scope of practice." The implication is that if you are "outside" your SOP, you are doing something you should not be doing, and sanctions will follow.

The SOP may be enforced by an independent governing authority (a state or national board, for example) that issues a mandatory license to someone wishing to practice a craft or profession within the geographical reach of that governing authority. By issuing the license, the governing authority is making a very basic quality assurance to the public: This person met the educational and training requirements to have this license and is practicing within the scope of practice associated with it (Rooney & van Ostenberg, 1999). The practitioner usually pays an annual license fee in order to practice. If there is any infraction or malfeasance, a disciplinary process ensues: A complaint can be filed, investigation commenced, and sanctions imposed (including revocation of the license). Licensing boards keep records of all licenses within their jurisdiction, including those that are current, expired, or revoked.

Crudely put, a scope of practice is all about turf, and turf is green—and green means money. Professions seeking a lock on certain kinds of procedures or patients will proclaim that others attempting to do similar work are "outside their scope of practice." The (usually longer-established) profession is aiming to keep the patients, the work, and the remuneration (Rogers, 2001). Authorities issuing the license receive a fee (every year), or the practitioner is not allowed to practice at all. This can be a substantial source of annual revenue for the government: These boards issue annual licenses for everything from barbers to brain surgeons. For example, the Commonwealth of Pennsylvania has 29 professional and occupational licensing boards falling under the authority of the Pennsylvania Department of State (Pennsylvania Dept. of State, 2011a). Each of those administer several kinds of licenses for different subcategories of their profession (e.g., dentist, dental hygienist, and dental assistants are three distinct licenses, with three distinct scopes of practice [Pennsylvania Dept. of State, 2011b]). Inactive or volunteer members of the profession have their own categories of licensure, SOP, and annual fee. Each category of practitioner, under each board, pays an annual fee into the state treasury. A portion of the fees are used to fund the work of the boards themselves. Someone has to be paid, for example, to conduct those disciplinary investigations. But it still generates a lot of revenue: Active dentists in Pennsylvania pay $250 for their license each year; there were 7520 dentist licenses registered in Pennsylvania in 2010 (with active, inactive, expired, and deceased status) (Pennsylvania Dept. of State, n.d.).

The SOP for professions governed by a license-issuing agency may be described in regulations issued by the same governmental authority. Those regulations carry the weight of law. Those regulations about scope of practice can be extremely detailed. In Pennsylvania, an entire chapter of the State Code is devoted to the State Board of Nurses, and contains sections defining nurses, license and renewal fees, nursing scope of practice (and interpretations thereof), even down to specific clinical procedures (venipuncture, resuscitation, anesthesia) (State Board of Nursing, 2010).

While customarily an SOP is associated with a license, this is not universal. A prime example is our own IBLCE Scope of Practice for IBCLCs (IBLCE SOP), which is associated with our international certification rather than licensure. The enforcement mechanism for the IBLCE SOP is through the IBLCE Discipline Committee's complaint process. The preambles of both the IBLCE SOP and IBLCE CPC are built upon the notion of protecting public safety (IBLCE, 2008, 2011e). The complaint process is clearly designed to address issues of IBCLC violations of the IBLCE Code of Professional Conduct (IBLCE, n.d., 2011d, 2012c), but it is the very last line of the IBLCE Scope of Practice that indicates how the SOP may be used by members of the profession to ensure enforcement: "IBCLCs have the duty to act with reasonable diligence by . . . reporting to IBLCE any other IBCLC who is functioning outside this Scope of Practice" (IBLCE, 2008, p. 4). While the face of the IBLCE SOP does not indicate that members of the public may also file a complaint, the IBLCE complaints procedure discusses "individuals bringing complaints" (IBLCE, 2011d, p. 1) who are required to prepare and sign complaints on a form provided by IBLCE (IBLCE, n.d.).

Some breastfeeding peer counselor groups have a defined scope of practice even though a license is not required to provide their level of support (Loving Support, 2004). This can be an effective means to teach everyone, up front, the level of assistance this peer counselor can give, and to reinforce when referrals to other allied healthcare providers (like IBCLCs!) may be needed. Bear in mind, under this peer counselor SOP, there is no formal complaint or sanctions process, with the threat of licensure forfeiture, to keep the counselor in line.

Licensure vs. Credentials vs. Certification vs. Accreditation

There are hundreds of different healthcare professions, each with varied training and specialization. Practitioners are given authority to practice by their home state, province, or country. Within any profession, practitioners may acquire additional recognition for mastering specific practice areas. The following describes general categories of importance; each carries different rights and responsibilities for the title bearer.

Licensure

Many IBCLCs also carry another title, such as registered nurse, and the concept of licensure is quite familiar in other healthcare fields. Here are two definitions to compare:

> Licensure is always conferred by a governmental entity or its designated agent, such as a licensing or regulatory board (e.g. a state, provincial, or national medical or nursing board), and addresses the minimum legal requirements for a health care organization or practitioner to operate, care for patients, or function. Unlike accreditation or certification approaches that are based on optimal and achievable standards or a demonstration of special knowledge or capability, the purpose of licensure requirements is to protect basic public health and safety. (Rooney & van Ostenberg, 1999, p. 12)

> Licensing of individual health care providers is usually intended to assure that only qualified people are engaged in health care practice. The primary purpose is to protect the public health by helping the public identify qualified providers and by prohibiting unqualified persons from providing services that require expertise. (Miller, 2006, p. 122)

Thus, we see that a "license" is:

- Mandatory
- Issued by a government authority, which maintains records of license holders (current, expired, revoked, etc.)
- Renewed annually, for a fee
- Issued upon proof of minimum educational or competence requirements
- A definition of the occupation or profession of the license holder
- Supported by a scope of practice describing with specificity the means and manner of the practitioner's work
- Designed to protect individual and public health and welfare
- Supported by a disciplinary procedure for those practicing without a valid license, or beyond the scope of practice for that license

In early 2012, there was not one state in the United States that had issued a license to an IBCLC. Obtaining licensure by any new profession happens state by state, requiring work (often for years) with state legislative bodies, and the existing executive branch that oversees professional boards within the state. The group seeking licensure has to establish the need for a new category of healthcare provider; there may be existing professions that resist the legitimization of "the new kids on the block." The practitioners themselves have to be convinced that it is worthwhile for them to now pay a fee, every year, to the state board, in addition to fees they already incur for continuing education, recertification with IBLCE, and professional development. Though the barriers to entry are real, the trend is for recognition of more disciplines for licensure (Miller, 2006).

The United States Lactation Consultant Association states, "licensing forms the basis of autonomous practice, provides a stronger voice in health care delivery, improves the process of reimbursement for services, and is the framework upon which the US health care system bases the structure of its workforce" (United States Lactation Consultant Association, 2011, p. 1). The motivation is simple: reimbursement. Or, money. The worldwide-recognized hallmark certification in human lactation (which IBCLC represents) just does not currently fit into the reimbursement system in the United States, whose infrastructure is built upon licensure. Most reimbursement schema look for licensure because that is the round peg fitting into the round hole that permits the insurance companies to approve payments either to the mother (who carries health insurance) or the institution (which seeks reimbursement for the clinical care its employees provide). It is difficult for IBCLCs to argue that they bring "value" to the employing institutions (in the long term) if the very work they do fails to generate reimbursements (in the short term). Of course, "value" can be measured in many ways. Perhaps the pregnant woman wavering between two delivery hospitals will choose the one with IBCLCs on staff, because breastfeeding success is one of her primary goals after the birth of this baby. The obstetrical patient can generate years of future business ("downstream revenue capture") for the institution: Her satisfactory birth experience is a measure of assurance that her extended family members will receive similar high-quality care for their broken bones, appendectomies, routine screenings, or complex surgeries (Phillips, 2007). Recognizing the critical role licensure plays in triggering reimbursement, the professional association for U.S.-based IBCLCs has made it a priority to provide its members the training and tools needed to seek licensure in each state.

Credentials

The IBCLC proudly displays her framed credential on her wall; the initials are on her identification badge at work; she wears them on her lapel in the form of a pin. What exactly does it mean to earn a credential? The answer is fairly simple: If we can keep several similar-sounding terms distinct in our minds. One expert managed to cram our four key concepts all into one sentence:

> In addition to the individual *licensing* by governmental agencies, there are many private methods of *credentialing*, including *accreditation* of educational programs, *certification* of individuals, and credentialing by institutions. (Miller, 2006, p. 137, emphasis added)

A credential, which some literature interchanges with the word certification, is a voluntary means of establishing expertise in a certain practice area. Here is another definition:

> The collection, verification, and use of a practitioner's credentials is often a quality mechanism defined by an individual health care organization. . . . Professional credentials usually include training, education, experience, and licensure. The process of obtaining, verifying, and assessing the qualifications of the health care practitioner to

provide specific patient services is frequently referred to as "credentialing." . . . Credentials review is an ongoing process for rechecking the individual's qualifications and competence. Advantages to the credentials review approach are that it is typically based on self-regulation within the profession and health care organization, and can promote continuous improvement, education, and professional accountability. (Rooney & van Ostenberg, 1999, p. 14–15)

Indeed, the International Board of Lactation Consultant Examiners follows this model (with the exception of the licensure element) in awarding the credential for which it tests, our very own International Board Certified Lactation Consultant. It states:

The International Board Certified Lactation Consultant (IBCLC) credential identifies a knowledgeable and experienced member of the maternal-child health team who has specialized skills in breastfeeding management and care. The IBLCE certification program offers the only international certification in lactation consulting. IBCLCs have passed a rigorous examination that demonstrates the ability to provide competent, comprehensive lactation and breastfeeding care. (IBLCE, 2012e, paras. 1–2)

Thus, we see that a "credential" is:

- Voluntary
- Issued by a private organization, which may maintain records of current credential holders
- Awarded upon demonstration, by examination, of specialized knowledge and skill in one practice area
- Subject to ongoing education or improvement requirements
- Earned separately from a license
- Designed to demonstrate optimal and achievable standards, versus basic public health protection represented by the license

Certification

The term certification is often interchanged with credential, because the concepts behind them are so similar. One definition is

Certification of individuals. Private professional organizations sponsor programs to certify that individuals meet certain criteria and are considered prepared to practice in the discipline. Individual certification is generally related to performance, usually including passing a test. (Miller, 2006, p. 138)

The very fine distinction is this: A practitioner may decide to acquire the training and education that demonstrate the special skill (become certified), without going to the trouble of actually (paying for and) taking a test to obtain the credential from the private testing authority (become credentialed).

Why not get credentialed? Perhaps a practitioner is just looking for better job security or clinical assignments, and her supervisor will be satisfied upon completion of coursework or mentored workshops to provide those adjustments without going through the formalities of credentialing. Perhaps working under the tutelage of a skilled mentor is incentive enough for assuming extra training. Some states require the taking of a test to demonstrate certification in certain specialties and to consequently allow the practitioner to work in that field. Other states do not (recall that licensure and scope of practice are determined by the parochial interests of the government board issuing them). And the reality is that healthcare providers move. They may want to demonstrate to a new regulatory board the skills acquired elsewhere. Thus, clinical privileges for the specialty may be recognized or awarded at the new venue for "board certification *or equivalent training and experience*" (Miller, 2006, p. 138, emphasis added). Allowing the practitioner to have her cake and eat it too.

Another fine distinction for credential holders and those who have certification is that any practitioner may simply choose not to renew the distinction, and this is not to be seen as reflecting poorly on the standards of care or performance these clinicians can offer. Perhaps they have since moved on to a different practice area, or they didn't take the required continuing education courses necessary for recertification. Certification and credentialing are distinctions that are voluntarily sought and voluntarily maintained. You still have the right to practice even without a specialized distinction. For example, an applicant for certification as a clinical nurse specialist (CNS) in Pennsylvania must first demonstrate that she has a current, unrestricted license as a professional nurse, also issued by Pennsylvania (Pennsylvania Dept. of State, 2011c). Even if she fails to meet the criteria for CNS, that nurse can still do whatever work is permitted by her "regular" nurse's license. Because a license is mandatory, however, this nurse will not practice at all unless she has one.

In summary, certification is:

- Voluntary
- Issued by a private organization, which usually maintains records of those with current certification
- Given upon demonstration, by examination, or other clinical and educational training, of specialized knowledge and skill in one practice area
- Subject to ongoing education or improvement requirements
- Earned separately from a license
- Designed to demonstrate optimal and achievable standards versus basic public health protection represented by the license

Accreditation

Accreditation addresses organizational rather than individual practitioner capability or performance. Unlike licensure, accreditation focuses on continuous improvement strategies and achievement of optimal quality standards rather than adherence to minimal standards intended to assure public safety. (Rooney & van Ostenburg, 1999, p. 15)

Accreditation affects institutions, primarily educational and healthcare facilities. Using postsecondary education as an example, it is the formalized process by which an educational institution (think college or university) proves that it can produce top-notch graduates, capable of going forth to intelligently practice in their field after didactic and clinical education. Independent, private professional organizations establish criteria that are used to evaluate educational programs. They will review the programs being offered by the institution to see if they align with the criteria and therefore pass muster. Accreditation is a voluntary process, but most institutions seek it because excellent students wisely demand it. Their degrees, coming as they do from an accredited institution, confer the quality assurance necessary to allow the graduates to take a licensing exam (Miller, 2006). The most pertinent example is the Lactation Education Accreditation and Approval Review Committee (LEAARC), the joint effort by ILCA and IBLCE, under the auspices of the Commission on Accreditation of Allied Health Education Programs (CAAHEP), "to establish, maintain and promote appropriate standards of quality for educational programs in Lactation and Breastfeeding and to provide recognition for educational programs that meet or exceed the minimum standards" (LEAARC, 2012a, para. 2).

Some healthcare facilities (think hospitals) also seek accreditation, whereby trained external peer reviewers evaluate facility compliance with preestablished performance standards, visiting on-site to do so. They look at such areas such as infection control or privacy protection. The standards are typically developed by consensus of healthcare experts; they are published, reviewed, and updated as policy and treatment options evolve (Rooney & van Ostenburg, 1999). In the United States, one well-known accreditation and certification authority is the Joint Commission:

> An independent, not-for-profit organization, The Joint Commission accredits and certifies more than 19,000 healthcare organizations and programs in the United States. Joint Commission accreditation and certification is recognized nationwide as a symbol of quality that reflects an organization's commitment to meeting certain performance standards. (Joint Commission, 2012, para. 1)

Ask any employee whose hospital is about to undergo inspection by the Joint Commission just how seriously the administrators take their responsibilities for "continuous improvement strategies and achievement of optimal quality standards" (Rooney & van Ostenburg, 1999, p. 15).

To sum it up, accreditation is:

- Voluntary
- Issued by a private organization
- Based on preestablished performance/quality standards that are developed by industry experts
- Based on standards that may also be periodically reviewed and revised, in light of advances in technology and treatment
- A measure of organizational (versus individual) performance
- An optimal measure of excellence

Professional Liability Insurance

Returning to the theme of different rights and responsibilities for different titles: The ability to procure professional liability insurance is dependent upon your title. Especially in the litigation-prone United States, healthcare professionals of all stripes—not just IBCLCs—are leery of the day when they think they will, inevitably, be sued. While the imagined number of lawsuits is greater than the actual number, it is undeniable that healthcare providers, and the institutions for which they work, practice under policies and procedures that assume lawsuits (both valid and specious) are simply an unavoidable part of the landscape (Carrier, Reschovsky, Mello, Mayrell, & Katz, 2010).

Professional liability insurance was devised to remedy very real-life injuries, to compensate patients/clients who suffered because their practitioners should have done a better job. This is one of our basic civil rights: to be able to seek redress for wrongs against us. As such, it is unwise for any healthcare provider to "go bare": to practice without having a valid professional liability (a.k.a. malpractice) insurance policy. If nothing else, the legal experts the policy provides for are worth the price of the premiums. If you get slapped with a lawsuit, your first call should be to your insurers, so they can immediately assign a lawyer to your case. While a lawsuit is a stressful and frightful experience, it will bring you immeasurable peace of mind to know that someone who is trained in litigation (versus you, trained in your field of health care) is handling the case. Even unfounded and outrageous lawsuits must be defended.

It is impossible to summarize the insurance industry in a few paragraphs. But some basic notions are easy to understand. Insurance companies, like any company, exist to make more money than they spend. They work with "risk," and make very exacting calculations, looking at a tremendous amount of data, to figure out how likely it is that they will have to pay out on a claim brought against you. You pay higher premiums if, by their calculations, they will be more likely to pay out a claim on you. That is why teenage boys pay higher car insurance premiums than 50-year-old mothers. Statistics do not lie: Teenage boys are more likely than gray-templed mothers to get into a serious car accident, and so it is more likely the insurance company will have to pay out on a claim for an accident caused by one of their teenaged policy holders.

Insurance companies have devised many ways to stay in business; that is, to take more money in than they pay out. One way is the insurance policy itself: It very clearly and specifically spells out who is covered, and for what kinds of claims. The definitions section of an insurance policy is critically important; it describes (among other things) just who this policy covers and for what sorts of risks. The exclusions section is equally important: It describes what risks are *not* covered by the policy, even if you are, without a shadow of a doubt, the defined insured. In health care, the insurance policy is designed to protect against lawsuits grounded in the tort of negligence (which means an honest mistake that resulted, however unwittingly, in injury to the patient/client), and the costs for the premium are based on the analysis of how likely it is the insurance company will have to defend (or pay out on) your lawsuit.

But intentional torts are a whole different matter. Those are committed by someone who actually, truly wanted to go out and create harm. It is the difference between mistakenly giving the wrong medicine to the wrong patient (perhaps for failure to double-check labels), and intentionally swapping out the aspirin pill intended for the patient with a cyanide pill. Most insurers will say, "Forget it. Honest mistakes we will defend, but we will *exclude* you if you are accused of an intentional tort. You are on your own to defend against that one."

Here is where is gets interesting for IBCLCs and other breastfeeding helpers. There is a large market offering professional liability insurance, from many different vendors, to healthcare providers. But it is offered to *healthcare providers*, who are defined (there's that pesky requirement again) by standards that are easy-to-measure for all applicants. And the easiest way for the insurance company to verify a practitioner's line of work is to look for valid licensure or certification (CM&F Group, 2011b).

And so the issue is Of all the different kinds of breastfeeding helpers that are out there, who is entitled to carry professional liability insurance? Are the institutions that are hiring these helpers, to have clinical contact with their patients inside their hallowed institutional halls, aware that some of these practitioners are "going bare"? For, if it is wise as a matter of personal protection that the individual practitioner carry insurance, it is doubly certain that any employer (with their "deep pockets") will want to be sure the individual practitioner has that malpractice insurance. If the hospital gets sued, and facts reveal that someone who had clinical contact with the patient is not licensed, or certified, or carrying any insurance of any kind, the institution's culpability soars.

This is not just an academic inquiry. Budget constraints at some hospitals in the United States have caused them to lay off the IBCLC staff, and hire at reduced salary, or on a per diem basis, breastfeeding helpers who have taken a short-term class (or no class at all). This can result in "unintended consequences" both for the breastfeeding mothers (who are not given the specialized health care they expected from the hospital, with unfavorable maternal-child health consequences), and the risk managers at the institution (who must now explain to their insurance provider how they ever allowed noninsured, noncertified/licensed practitioners near the patients) (Clegg, Francis, & Walker, 2010).

You Should Get What You Think You Paid For

We've all heard the saying, "You get what you pay for." Would that it were so, for lactation assistance. Remember Millennial Mom? She is looking for help and willing to pay for it. She ought to be able to rely on this adage, and actually get the kind of help she thinks she is paying for. In the fairly new field of lactation consultation, this sadly is not a universal truth.

As alluded to at the start of this chapter, there is nothing to stop any person who has completed any of the levels of breastfeeding education and training described (or none, for that matter) from "hanging out a shingle" and charging mothers for advice and consultation on breastfeeding. Some such practitioners will stay, ethically and professionally, within the rigid confines of the training and limited scope of practice their particular course provided. Presumably such helpers will charge less for their help than those who have taken years (like the IBCLC) to acquire their specialized skills. Of, course, what the market will bear differs from place to place (a New York City IBCLC can charge $250 for a home visit; an IBCLC in Kansas can charge $90 for the same 1.5–2.0 hour consultation) (International Lactation Consultant Association, 2012). Some practitioners are not so scrupulous, and the unwary mother may find she has paid a hefty fee to see someone who couldn't help, or worse, exacerbated the problem with non-evidence-based suggestions of care.

Discipline Options Vary with the Title

And that's the kicker. There is not much that unhappy, still-sore Millennial Mom can do if it turns out she was confused by the ads on the Web and corralled into paying for an expensive consult by someone who was overstepping her bounds. If the overstepper is not licensed or certified, there is no board or agency with whom Millennial Mom can file her complaint. Overstepper will not be subjected to a disciplinary procedure or sanctions. Millennial Mom instead must go to the extraordinary time, stress, and expense of filing some kind of lawsuit against the overstepper in hopes of getting redress. A lawsuit is a far more onerous and time-consuming venture than going to a state licensing board and filling out a complaint form. The board has it as their purpose to protect the public health safety, and hence they make the filing of complaints fairly simple (Pennsylvania Dept. of State, 2010). It is an aggravating fact of life that the oversteppers of the world—those most in need of being reined in for infractions against safe professional practice—are so difficult to bridle.

The IBCLC Is the Full Package

Summing all of this up, how can we support the premise that the IBCLC credential is (dare it be said?) the cream that has risen to the top of the milk? A review, of all the IBCLC had to master, and what she now is entitled to do:

1. The IBLCE Exam Blueprint defines the 13 discipline areas and 12 chronologic (or age-of-baby) periods, all focused on human lactation and breastfeeding, of which the exam taker must be competent. This is everything an entry-level IBCLC needs to know: The IBCLC exam covers all these topics (IBLCE, 2011b). It is a well-defined, highly-specific, and comprehensive listing of subjects, covering aspects of human lactation both from the mother's and the baby's perspectives.

2. The Clinical Competencies for the Practice of IBCLCs describe the responsibilities and activities that are part of IBCLC practice. Even a newly certified IBCLC is expected to be able to plunge, from day one, into her practice. This document describes with specificity the skills needed to interact with clients/patients, and other healthcare providers, applying all that information one had to master from the IBLCE Exam Blueprint (IBLCE, 2010).

3. To take the exam (which costs several hundred dollars), the candidate must provide proof that lactation-specific classroom work has been completed. A minimum of 90 hours is required starting with the 2012 exam (IBLCE, 2012a, 2012b).

   Course providers charge various fees for their programs. Many have gone through the voluntary process of having their curriculum approved by LEAARC, a "seal of approval" of the educational quality of the short-term course (LEAARC, 2012b). The IBCLC applicant has several other general educational requirements (amounting to about two years of college- or university-level classes, all of which require tuition) in health disciplines deemed pertinent (e.g., medical terminology, biology, and human anatomy) (IBLCE, 2012a).

4. Hands-on training is required. Lactation-specific clinical hours must be accrued (the minimum ranges from 300–1000 hours, depending on the IBLCE pathway), with intensive supervision and evaluation along the way. That is 300–1000 clinical hours *focused just on breastfeeding*. Teaching mothers how to bathe a baby, change a diaper, or care for an umbilical cord does not count (IBLCE, 2012a). Put into simple mathematical perspective: A lactation consultation with a mother may take 20 minutes (not counting preliminary paperwork); a complex consultation may take 1.5–2.0 hours. This means the applicant—who is not yet even an IBCLC—must *minimally* be involved in supervised clinical training involving at least 300 mother–baby dyads, and she may see as many as 3000 dyads. This is a significant commitment of time and training, in one very specialized area, before one is entitled to fly solo.

   Acquiring these clinical hours can be the toughest hurdle to jump on the way to IBCLC certification, especially if the applicant is not currently employed where she has regular access to mothers and babies (for example, in a postpartum unit of a birthing center). Many nonteaching institutions are reluctant to take on student clinicians. Teaching facilities are better equipped (and funded) to take on the administrative burden of supervising students. While IBLCE Pathway 3 (mentorship) was developed to allow students to cobble together clinical training under a mentor's tutelage, as a practical matter in 2012 there are not enough mentors offering supervised hours in varied clinical settings to meet the demand of IBCLC applicants. The IBCLC applicant must be prepared to pay fees and/or tuition for this phase of her education, just as she did for the classroom requirements.

5. The IBCLC exam is given once a year (on the last Monday in July), lasts about 5 hours, and uses multiple-choice options to answer analytical and photograph-based questions. It is given around the world, and is translated into nearly two dozen languages. Exam content, translation, and administration are protected by the highest of security standards. The test is proctored on site by independent monitors. On the day of the exam, test takers are allowed to indicate, with explanation, those questions they felt were ambiguous or erroneous. Confirmed "lemons" are thrown out, for every test that year. This complex post-examination, pre-scoring review process takes time; exam results are sent out in October of each year.

6. To be allowed to offer the exam at all, IBLCE first had to have its certification program (i.e., the IBCLC exam) recognized by the National Commission for Certifying Agencies (NCCA), which is the accrediting arm of the Institute for Credentialing Excellence (ICE) (IBLCE, 2011c; Institute for Credentialing Excellence, 2009). To pass muster with NCCA, IBLCE had to demonstrate that the test content, test methods, and test reliability all meet the rigorous NCCA Standards for the Accreditation of Certification Programs. IBLCE must periodically be reviewed by NCCA to assure standards (which may be revised) are continuing to be met (Institute for Credentialing Excellence, 2009). The statistical report that IBLCE issues each year, a psychometric explanation of the annual exam results, is a part of this complex process of establishing that the test is, and remains, the global standard of competence assessment in lactation consultation (Gross, 2009).

7. The successful test taker is the IBCLC, or "certificant," using the vernacular of certifying agencies like IBLCE. The IBCLC receives a certificate from IBLCE, indicating she has successfully completed all requirements for certification and is thus awarded the right to use the title "IBCLC." She is also encouraged to join ILCA, the independent professional association for IBCLCs, as a means of nurturing her professional education and development.

8. The IBCLC must practice within the IBLCE Scope of Practice for IBCLCs and abide by the IBLCE Code of Professional Conduct. These mandatory practice-guiding documents are reminders of the IBCLC's responsibility to protect public health and safety in the administration of care to breastfeeding dyads. Failure to do so can subject the certificant to review under a defined, due-process-protecting disciplinary process administered

by IBLCE; sanctions can be as severe as revocation of IBCLC certification. The IBCLC is also encouraged to follow the voluntary ILCA Standards of Practice (ILCA, 2006b), although as a model of professional conduct there is no formal sanctions process to enforce them.

9. While there is no universal licensure for IBCLCs, the IBLCE Scope of Practice for IBCLCs, the disciplinary process established by IBLCE for its certificants, and the registry of currently certified IBCLCs that IBLCE maintains on its website, *all* provide the same minimum public safeguards, on an international scale, that licensure purports to offer on a state-by-state basis. Like a licensing board, IBLCE maintains a roster of currently certified IBCLCs on its website, searchable by name. Like a complaints process through a licensing board, IBLCE has a defined disciplinary procedure. Like a license, certification is premised on the notion of protecting public health and safety.

10. IBCLCs must recertify every 5 years. This can be accomplished by retaking the examination or by acquiring lactation-specific continuing education credits (continuing education recognition points, or CERPs) (IBLCE, 2012d). The exam is considered entry level, but the questions evolve with each examination to reflect the newest research and evidence-based practice. Thus, the recertifying IBCLC must stay on top of her game, whether she chooses to recertify by exam or CERPs.

Summary

For Millennial Mom, the IBCLC represents an allied healthcare provider highly trained in the evidence-based care of a breastfeeding mother, her baby, and their breastfeeding relationship. The IBCLC passed a certification exam that covered a tremendous amount of material: a test given by an accredited organization, a test that must be regularly evaluated to demonstrate that it measures knowledge of lactation. Once certified with her credential recognized around the world, the IBCLC must stay on top of current research and clinical practice, as she must recertify every 5 years. She is held accountable under her IBLCE Code of Professional Conduct and IBLCE Scope of Practice for IBCLCs, and encouraged to use best practices according to the ILCA Standards of Practice. If she cannot meet her mandatory professional obligations, she is subject to disciplinary action. If she chooses not to recertify, she forfeits her right to continued use of the title "International Board Certified Lactation Consultant." To repeat: The IBCLC's knowledge runs narrow but deep. See **Table 1-1** to compare the IBCLC with other breastfeeding helpers.

Table 1-1   Comparison of Education and Training: IBCLCs and Other Breastfeeding Helpers

	Short-Term Class/Course	College-Level Class Prerequisites	Supervised Clinical Training Prerequisites	Certificate of Completion Given	LEAARC Approval	Credential Awarded by Independently Accredited Organization	Mandatory License	Defined Scope of Practice	Code of Ethics (or) Professional Conduct	Defined Complaint/ Disciplinary Procedure	Registry of currently licensed/certified practitioners	Professional Liability Insurance Coverage	Easy Payment or Insurance Reimbursement for Care?
IBCLC	X (as prerequisite to exam)	X	X			X (IBLCE)		X	X	X	X	X	
IBCLC student/intern in IBLCE pathway	X (as prerequisite to exam)	X	X					X	X	X	X	X	
"Lactation consultant" Healthcare professional (MD, RN, etc.)	?	X (not necessarily in lactation)	? / X	?		(X) (for certain clinical specialties)	X	? / X	? / X	? / X	? / X	? / X	? / X
Midwife		(X) (varies by state/country)	X			(X) (varies by state/country)	(X) (varies by state/country)	X	X	X	(X) (varies by state/country)	X	(X) (varies by state/country)
Postpartum doula	X							X	X	X			
LLL Leader								X	X	X		X (X) (insurance as a volunteer, not HCP)	
Mother-to-mother counselor	X			X									
WIC peer counselor (USA)	X			X				X					
CLC (HC/ALPP/ANCC)	X			X	X	X (ANCC)		X	X	X			
CLS (LEC)	X			X	X								
CBS (LER)	X			X	X								
CBC (CI)	X			X									
CBE (HC)	X			X									
LC (UCSD)		X		X	X								
LE-C (UCSD)	X		X	X									
ALC (HC/ALPP/ANCC)	X		X			X (ANCC)				(X) (re: eligibility only)		X	(X)
ANLC (HC/ALPP/ANCC)	X	X	X			X (ANCC)	X	X		(X) (re: eligibility only)		X	X
CLE (CAPPA)	X			X				X					
Class/in-service attendee	X			X									

Abbreviations used:

ALC	Advanced Lactation Consultant
ALPP	Academy of Lactation Policy and Practice
ANCC	American Nurses Credentialing Center
ANLC	Advanced Nurse Lactation Consultant
CAPPA	Childbirth and Postpartum Professional Association
CBC	Certified Breastfeeding Counselor
CBE	Community Breastfeeding Educator
CBS	Certified Breastfeeding Specialist
CI	Childbirth International
CLC	Lactation Counselor Certificate, also called Certified Lactation Counselor
CLE	Certified Lactation Educator
CLS	Certified Lactation Specialist
HC	Healthy Children's Center for Breastfeeding
HCP	Healthcare Provider
IBCLC	International Board Certified Lactation Consultant
IBLCE	International Board of Lactation Consultant Examiners
LC	Lactation Consultant (certificate program, UCSD)
LEAARC	Lactation Education Accreditation and Approval Review Committee
LE-C	Lactation Educator-Counselor
LEC	Lactation Education Consultants
LER	Lactation Education Resources
LLL	La Leche League
MD	Doctor of Medicine
RN	Registered Nurse
UCSD	University of California San Diego Extension
WIC	Special Supplemental Nutrition Program for Women, Infants, and Children (U.S. Dept. of Agriculture)

REFERENCES

Academy of Lactation Policy and Practice (ALPP). (2009). *ALPP candidate handbook certified lactation counselor (CLC) certification*. Retrieved from http://www.talpp.org/CLC_Candidate_Handbook_2010S.pdf

Academy of Lactation Policy and Practice (ALPP). (2011). *The CLC: Certified lactation counselor*. Retrieved from http://www.talpp.org/certification.html

Ad Hoc Committee on the Scope of Practice in Speech-Language Pathology. (2007). Introduction. In *Scope of practice in speech-language pathology*. Retrieved from http://www.asha.org/docs/html/SP2007-00283.html

Allied Health Professional Associations' Forum. (2011, July 3). *Allied health*. Retrieved from http://alliedhealth.org.nz/index.php?page=contact-us-2

American Board of Thoracic Surgery. (2011). *About the board*. Retrieved from https://www.abts.org/sections/About_Us/index.aspx

American Nurses Credentialing Center (ANCC). (2012a). *Accredited competency courses*. Retrieved from http://www.nursecredentialing.org/Accreditation/NursingSkillsCompetencyProgram/AccreditedCompetencyCourses.aspx

American Nurses Credentialing Center (ANCC). (2012b). *ANCC magnet recognition program*. Retrieved from http://www.nursecredentialing.org/Magnet.aspx

American Nurses Credentialing Center (ANCC). (2012c). *Certification FAQs*. Retrieved from http://www.nursecredentialing.org/FunctionalCategory/FAQs/CertiticationFAQs.aspx#2

American Nurses Credentialing Center (ANCC). (2012d). *Nursing skills competency program*. Retrieved from http://nursecredentialing.org/Accreditation/NursingSkillsCompetencyProgram.aspx

Association of Breastfeeding Mothers (ABM; United Kingdom). (2011). *About the ABM*. Retrieved from http://abm.me.uk/sites/default/files/About%20the%20ABM%20(web)%20(1)_0.pdf

Australian Breastfeeding Association. (2010). *ABA constitution*. Retrieved from https://www.breastfeeding.asn.au/aboutaba/ABA_Constitution.pdf

Baker, G. (n.d.a). *Lactation educator counselor*. Retrieved from http://breastfeeding-education.com/home/clec-2/

Baker, G. (n.d.b). LC pathways and schedules. In *Lactation consultant*. Retrieved from http://breastfeeding-education.com/wp-content/uploads/2012/01/LC-Pathways-Schedules.pdf

Baker, K. (2011). *Peer counselor programs: Who, what and why?* [originally published in Leaven (LLLI), Aug 1999]. Retrieved from http://www.llli.org/llleaderweb/lv/lvaugsep99p92.html

Barnes, K., Marateo, R., & Ferris, S. P. (2007, April/May). Teaching and learning with the net generation. *Innovate, 3*(4). Retrieved from http://www.innovateonline.info/pdf/vol3_issue4/Teaching_and_Learning_with_the_Net_Generation.pdf

Bonamici, A., Hutto, D., Smith, D., & Ward, J. (2005, October 13). *The "net generation": Implications for libraries and higher education*. PowerPoint lecture presented at Orbis-Cascade Consortium, http://www.orbiscascade.org/council/c0510/Frye/ppt

Carrier, E., Reschovsky, J., Mello, M., Mayrell, R., & Katz, D. (2010, September). Physicians' fears of malpractice lawsuits are not assuaged by tort reforms. *Health Affairs, 29*(9), 1585–1592. Retrieved from http://content.healthaffairs.org/content/29/9/1585.abstract

Childbirth and Postpartum Professional Association (CAPPA). (2012a). *Become a certified lactation educator*. Retrieved from http://www.cappa.net/get-certified.php?lactation-educator

Childbirth and Postpartum Professional Association (CAPPA). (2012b). *Scope of practice*. Retrieved from http://www.cappa.net/about-cappa.php?scope-of-practice

Childbirth International. (2008). *Breastfeeding counselor—certification requirements.* Retrieved from http://www.childbirthinternational.com/lactation/certification.htm

Clegg, S., Francis, D., & Walker, M. (2010, July). *Five steps to improving job security for the hospital-based IBCLC* (Monograph). Morrisville, NC: United States Lactation Consultant Association.

CM&F Group (malpractice insurers). (2011a). *Insurance Policy Reference* [General healthcare provider professional liability policy]. Retrieved from http://www.cmfgroup.com/top_nav/policy_reference.html

CM&F Group (malpractice insurers). (2011b). *Malpractice insurance for internatoinal board certified lactation consultants* [professional liability insurance offered through USLCA]. Retrieved from http://www.cmfgroup.com/insurance_products/professional_liability_individual/ibclc_lactation_consultant.html

Dettwyler, K. A. (1995). A time to wean: The hominid blueprint for the natural age of weaning in modern human populations. In P. Stuart-Macadam & K. A. Dettwyler, *Breastfeeding: Biocultural Perspectives* (pp. 39–74). New York, NY: Aldine De Gruyter.

DONA International. (2005a). *DONA international certification.* Retrieved from http://www.dona.org/develop/certification.php

DONA International. (2005b). *What is a doula?* Retrieved from http://www.dona.org/mothers/index.php

Food and Nutrition Service. (2011, August). *WIC the special supplemental nutrition program for women, infants and children* [Fact sheet]. Retrieved from http://www.fns.usda.gov/wic/WIC-Fact-Sheet.pdf

Food and Nutrition Service. (2012, February 17). Program delivery. In *About WIC.* Retrieved from http://www.fns.usda.gov/wic/aboutwic/wicataglance.htm

Gross, L. (2009). *Statistical report of the 2009 IBLCE exmination.* Retrieved from http://www.iblce.org/upload/downloads/2009StatisticalReport.pdf

Healthy Children Center for Breastfeeding. (n.d.). *The center for breastfeeding's certified lactation counselor (CLC) training program.* Retrieved from http://www.healthychildren.cc

Healthy Children Center for Breastfeeding. (2011). *Course catalogue fall 2011-spring 2012.* Retrieved from http://www.healthychildren.cc/Flyer12S.pdf

Healthy Children Project. (February 18, 2010 [filing date]). *U.S. Certification Mark Serial No. 77938432 [CLC].* Washington, DC: U.S. Patent and Trademark Office.

Healthy Children Project. (April 5, 2011 [registration date]). *U.S. Certification Mark 3939681 [Certified Lactation Counselor].* Washington, DC: U.S. Patent and Trademark Office.

Hirschman, C., & Butler, M. (1981, February). Trends and differentials in breast feeding: An update. *Demography, 18*(1), 39–54. Retrieved from http://www.jstor.org/stable/2061048

Institute for Credentialing Excellence. (2009). *National commission for certifying agencies standards.* Retrieved from Institute for Credentialing Excellence website: http://www.credentialingexcellence.org/AccreditationServices/CertificationAccreditation/StandardsInterpretations/tabid/93/Default.aspx

International Board of Lactation Consultant Examiners. (n.d.). *Confidential IBLCE CPC complaint form.* Retrieved from http://www.iblce.org/upload/downloads/ComplaintForm.pdf

International Board of Lactation Consultant Examiners. (1997, March 11; renewed 2007). *U.S. Certification Mark 2042667 [IBCLC].* Washington, DC: U.S. Patent and Trademark Office.

International Board of Lactation Consultant Examiners. (2003a). *Code of ethics for international board certified lactation consultants.* Retrieved from http://www.iblce.org/upload/downloads/CodeOfEthics.pdf

International Board of Lactation Consultant Examiners. (2003b, August 5). *U.S. Certification Mark 2749041 [Registered Lactation Consultant].* Washington, DC: U.S. Patent and Trademark Office.

International Board of Lactation Consultant Examiners. (2008, March 8). *Scope of practice for international board certified lactation consultants.* Retrieved from http://www.iblce.org/upload/downloads/ScopeOfPractice.pdf

International Board of Lactation Consultant Examiners. (2010, December 6). *Clinical competencies for the IBCLCs practice*. Retrieved from http://www.iblce.org/upload/downloads/ClinicalCompetencies.pdf

International Board of Lactation Consultant Examiners. (2011a, January). *Number of IBCLCs in the world*. Retrieved from http://www.iblce.org/upload/downloads/NumberIBCLCsWorld.pdf

International Board of Lactation Consultant Examiners. (2011b, July 5). *IBLCE exam blueprint* [Fact sheet]. Retrieved from http://www.iblce.org/upload/downloads/IBLCEExamBlueprint.pdf

International Board of Lactation Consultant Examiners. (2011c, July 27). *About us*. Retrieved from http://www.americas.iblce.org/about-us

International Board of Lactation Consultant Examiners. (2011d, September 24). *Disciplinary procedures for the code of professional conduct for IBCLCs for the IBLCE*. Retrieved from http://www.iblce.org/upload/downloads/IBLCEDisciplinaryProcedures.pdf

International Board of Lactation Consultant Examiners. (2011e, November 1). *Code of professional conduct for IBCLCs*. Retrieved from http://iblce.org/upload/downloads/CodeOfProfessionalConduct.pdf

International Board of Lactation Consultant Examiners. (2012a). *Exam requirements overview*. Retrieved from http://www.americas.iblce.org/exam-requirements-overview

International Board of Lactation Consultant Examiners. (2012b). *IBCLC: Global certification for lactation consultants*. Retrieved from http://americas.iblce.org/about-the-ibclc-credential

International Board of Lactation Consultant Examiners. (2012c). *Professional ethics [disciplinary forms and procedures]*. Retrieved from http://www.iblce.org/professional-ethics

International Board of Lactation Consultant Examiners. (2012d). *Recertification requirements*. Retrieved from http://americas.iblce.org/recertification-requirements

International Board of Lactation Consultant Examiners. (2012e). *What is an IBCLC?* Retrieved from http://americas.iblce.org/what-is-an-ibclc

International Lactation Consultant Association. (2006a, November). *Position statements on breastfeeding: November 2006* [List/links to position statements of 46 international healthcare organization]. Retrieved from http://www.ilca.org/files/resources/international_regional_documetns/PositionStatementson BreastfeedingonWeb.pdf

International Lactation Consultant Association. (2006b). *Standards of practice for international board certified lactation consultants*. Retrieved from http://www.ilca.org/files/resources/Standards-of-Practice-web.pdf

International Lactation Consultant Association. (2012). *Find a lactation consultant*. Retrieved from http://www.ilca.org/i4a/pages/index.cfm?pageid=3432

International Lactation Consultant Association, & Henderson, S. (2011, June). *Position paper on the role and impact of the IBCLC* (Monograph). Retrieved from http://www.ilca.org/files/resources/ilca_publications/Role%20%20Impact%20of%20the%20IBCLC-webFINAL_08-15-11.pdf

Joint Commission. (2002). Introduction. In *Joint commission guide to allied health professionals*. Retrieved from http://www.jcrinc.com/Books-and-E-books/joint-commission-guide-to-allied-health-professionals/333

Joint Commission. (2012). *About the joint commission*. Retrieved from http://www.jointcommission.org/about_us/about_the_joint_commission_main.aspx

Lactation Education Accreditation and Approval Review Committee (LEAARC). (2010, October). *Accreditation procedures for lactation consultant education programs*. Retrieved from http://www.leaarc.org/download/LEAARC_Procedures.pdf

Lactation Education Accreditation and Approval Review Committee (LEAARC). (2012a). *Home page*. Retrieved from http://www.leaarc.org

Lactation Education Accreditation and Approval Review Committee (LEAARC). (2012b, March 8). *LEAARC approved courses*. Retrieved from http://www.leaarc.org/download/LEAARC_ApprovedCourses.pdf

Lactation Education Consultants. (n.d.). *Certified lactation specialist course.* Retrieved from http://www.lactationeducationconsultants.com/course_clsc.html

Lactation Education Resources (LER). (n.d.). *The lactation consultant training program—core.* Retrieved from http://www.leron-line.com/LC_Training_online/Lactation_Consultant_Training_online.htm

La Leche League GB (Great Britain). (n.d.). *Major independent evaluation shows effectiveness of La Leche League GB peer counsellor programme.* Retrieved from http://www.laleche.org.uk/pdfs/LLLGB%20PCP%20EVALUATION%20SUMMARY%20JAN%2008.pdf

La Leche League International. (2011a). *A brief history of La Leche League International.* Retrieved from http://www.llli.org/lllihistory.html

La Leche League International. (2011b). *Mission* [Home page]. Retrieved from http://www.llli.org

Loving Support. (2004). *Section 6 scope of practice [WIC peer counselors]* [PowerPoint slides]. Retrieved from http://www.nal.usda.gov/wicworks/Learning_Center/LS_training/2004/Presentations/ppt1/Section_06.ppt

Loving Support. (2012, March). *Using loving support to implement best practices in peer counseling.* Retrieved from http://www.nal.usda.gov/wicworks/Learning_Center/support_peer.html

Miller, R. D. (2006). Individual providers and caregivers. In *Problems in health care law* (9th ed., pp. 121–212). Sudbury, MA: Jones & Bartlett.

Oblinger, D. G., & Oblinger, J. L. (Eds.). (2005). *Educating the net generation.* Retrieved from http://www.educause.edu/educatingthenetgen

Penchuk, E. (2010, June 7). Latest help from Similac [Online forum message]. Retrieved from http://community.lsoft.com/archives/LACTNET.html

Pennsylvania Dept. of State. (n.d.). *Search for a license.* Retrieved from http://www.licensepa.state.pa.us/Search.aspx

Pennsylvania Dept. of State. (2010, August 23). *Facts you should know when submitting a complaint.* Retrieved from http://www.portal.state.pa.us/portal/server.pt/community/general_information/12501/how_complaints_are_handled/571973

Pennsylvania Dept. of State. (2011a, January 14). Licensing. In *Bureau of professional and occupational affairs.* Retrieved from http://www.recovery.pa.gov/portal/server.pt/community/licensing/12483

Pennsylvania Dept. of State. (2011b, January 18). *State board of dentistry licensure information.* Retrieved from http://www.portal.state.pa.us/portal/server.pt/community/state_board_of_dentistry/12509/licensure_information/613687

Pennsylvania Dept. of State. (2011c, March 29). Application for clinical nurse specialist (July 2010). In *Pennsylvania state board of nursing licensure information.* Retrieved from http://www.portal.state.pa.us/portal/server.pt/community/state_board_of_nursing/12515/licensure_information/572048

Phillips, C. R. (2007, June 18). *Family centered maternity care: The business case* [Monograph]. Retrieved from http://www.pandf.com/resources/WhitePaperPandf.pdf

Reiger, K. (2008, May). Domination or mutual recognition? Professional subjectivity in midwifery and obstetrics [Abstract]. *Social Theory and Health, 6*(2), 132–147. Retrieved from http://www.palgrave-journals.com/sth/journal/v6/n2/abs/sth200712a.html

Rogers, C. (2001, September). Comment: Nonphysician providers and limited-license practitioners: Scope-of-practice issues [Abstract]. *Bulletin of the American College of Surgeons, 86*(9), 43. Retrieved from http://www.ncbi.nlm.nih.gov/pubmed/10136595

Rooney, A. L., & van Ostenberg, P. R. (1999). Licensure, accreditation, and certification: Approaches to health services quality [Monograph]. *Quality assurance methodology refinement series of U.S. Agency for International Development.* Retrieved from http://www.hciproject.org/node/894

Smith, L. J. (1999). *Absurd advice: Ridiculous reasons to wean* (2nd ed.) [Monograph]. Dayton, OH: Bright Future Lactation Resource Centre.

Society of Thoracic Surgeons. (2012). *What is a thoracic surgeon?* Retrieved from http://www.sts.org/patient -information/what-thoracic-surgeon

State Board of Nursing, Pa. Code ch. 21, § 21.1 et. seq. (2010).

The Physiotherapy Site. (2011). *What is physiotherapy?* Retrieved from http://www.thephysiotherapysite .co.uk/physiotherapy/physiotherapists/what-is-physiotherapy

Thorley, V. (2009). Mothers' experiences of sharing breastfeeding or breastmilk: co-feeding in Australia 1978–2008. *Breastfeeding Review, 17*(1), 9–18. Retrieved from http://www.waba.org.my/pdf/BFR _Mar_09_Thorley.pdf

UNICEF: United Nation's Children's Fund. (2010, September). *WHO/UNICEF/UNFPA/The World Bank estimates of maternal mortality 2008* [Statistical table]. Retrieved from http://www.childinfo.org /maternal_mortality_countrydata.php

United States Lactation Consultant Association. (2011, July). *Licensure for IBCLCs frequently asked questions (FAQs).* Retrieved from http://www.ilca.org/files/USLCA/Resources/Publications/Licensure_FAQs_for _IBCLCs.pdf

von der Ohe, G. (1998, December). *IBCLC lactation consultant: A relatively new professional group in medicine* [Newsletter reprint (with updated numbers for 2007)]. Retrieved from http://www.velb.org/english/docs /job-description-ibclc.pdf

Walker, M. (2007). *Still selling out mothers and babies: Marketing of breast milk substitutes in the USA* (Monograph). Weston, MA: National Alliance for Breastfeeding Advocacy Research, Education and Legal Branch (NABA REAL).

Wolf, J. H. (2001). Introduction. In *Don't kill your baby: Public health and the decline of breastfeeding in the nineteenth and twentieth centuries* (pp. 1–8). Columbus, OH: Ohio State University Press.

Chapter 2

In a Nutshell: Who Is the Patient (or) Client, and What Is the IBCLC's Responsibility?

International Board Certified Lactation Consultants (IBCLCs) wake up, put on their working clothes for the day, and are immediately faced with a legal and ethical quandary that most healthcare providers (HCPs) will never face: Who is the patient (or) client? Is it:

- Mother, whose lactating breasts provide the human milk the child needs?
- Baby, who so clearly benefits from the human milk his biology demands?
- Breastfeeding itself, with the babe lovingly cradled in mother's arms for each feed, a reflection of an integral component of child-rearing cultures?

The tensions are obvious, and they happen every day. If the mother must return to work in a setting several miles from her home, in order to earn income to shelter and feed her entire family, it is difficult to feed the baby at breast throughout the day. If the baby comes from a family with a history of allergy (or diabetes or heart disease), sustained exclusive breastfeeding is a known protection from those health risks (Horta, Bahl, Martines, & Victora, 2007; Ip et al., 2007). What if the mother isn't interested in exclusive breastfeeding—or in breastfeeding at all? Or, imagine the mother who has been regularly using a breast pump, providing wonderful amounts of milk for her very premature baby in the neonatal intensive care unit (NICU). If she tells the IBCLC she plans to continue this regimen upon discharge, should the IBCLC be pressing the mother instead to feed the baby at breast? It can be vexing for the IBCLC trying to figure out when to push, and when to pull, as she discusses care plans involving a "patient/client" that can manifest as a mother, or a baby, or the dyad.

Let us back up even further. The obvious starting point is: Which term (*patient* or *client*) should we even use? One medical dictionary uses these definitions for those words:

Client. The patient of a healthcare professional (Client, 2001)
Patient. 1. One who is sick with, or being treated for, an illness or injury. 2. An individual receiving medical care. (Patient, 2001)

These definitions would turn human lactation, an inherently natural biologic function of the mammary glands, into an "illness or injury" that clearly it is not. Surely we don't consider perspiration an "illness or injury" of the sudoriferous glands, because secretions of sweat from the sweat glands is considered a normal, everyday human biologic function. Nonetheless, the lactation consultant profession uses the terms "client" and "patient" fairly consistently by IBCLCs who are describing their work, even though breastfeeding is a very normal human process. Those who are hospital- or birthing center–based favor *patient*, while those who are in private practice or public health/educational settings use *client*. As a practical matter, there is no penalty or privilege accorded the use of either term.

Each of the IBCLC's three major practice-guiding documents provide support for the notion that the IBCLC must juggle all three balls of mother, baby, and the breastfeeding relationship as her "patient/client." **Table 2-1** indicates those sections of the mandatory IBLCE Code of Professional Conduct (IBLCE CPC), the mandatory IBLCE Scope of Practice for IBCLCs (IBLCE SOP), and the voluntary ILCA Standards of Practice for IBCLCs (ILCA Standards) that address these IBCLC responsibilities, and there is plenty of overlap. We'll briefly examine the theories behind each designated "patient/client."

Sometimes the Mother Is the Patient/Client

This is probably the easiest notion to understand. After all, the IBCLC can talk to a mother, educate her, and consider her situation and goals for breastfeeding in the development of a care plan. And this is borne out by a swift scan of the practice-guiding documents for the IBCLC. We are instructed to act in the mother's best interests: Protect her privacy, learn her history, assess the lactation issues, teach her in a way that helps her learn, and work with her to fashion a care plan that takes into account everything from her language and culture to her economic means. IBCLCs are in a position to go to bat for the mother, whom we customarily see in the early postpartum days when she is exhausted, suffering hormonal mood swings, overwhelmed even if perfectly thrilled with her new role as mother, and often unable to concentrate on complex matters.

Here's a practice tip that will save the IBCLC a lot of heartache and sleepless nights: It is irrelevant if *you* want the mother to breastfeed her baby more than the *mother* wants to breastfeed her baby. After all, it is her baby, her body, and her family to raise, all in her familiar environment. Your role as the IBCLC is to provide evidence-based information to the mother (so she can make an informed decision about her and her baby's care), and then support her and help to facilitate those informed decisions. It may well be that, as you provide teaching to the mother, she may come to realize that she can "do more breastfeeding" than she originally thought. But that is a serendipitous result. Nor will we explore here whether a new mother has attained the enlightenment

Table 2-1 Comparison of Practice-Guiding Document References to Person or Concept Under IBCLC Care

	IBLCE Code of Professional Conduct (2011)	IBLCE Scope of Practice for IBCLCs (2008)	ILCA Standards of Practice for IBCLCs (2006)
Mother as patient/client of IBCLC	Introduction, para. 3: "A crucial part of an IBCLC's duty to protect mothers and children is adherence to the principles and aim of the *International Code of Marketing of Breast-milk Substitutes* and subsequent relevant World Health Assembly's resolutions."	Duty to "uphold the standards of the IBCLC profession by: integrating knowledge and evidence when providing care for breastfeeding families" (para. 3).	Preface: IBCLC should adhere to practice-guiding documents "in all interactions with clients, families, and other healthcare professionals."
	Preamble, para. 1: "IBLCE endorses the broad human rights principles ... affirming that every human being has the right to the highest attainable standard of health. Moreover, IBLCE considers that every mother and every child has the right to breastfeed."	Duty to "protect, promote, and support breastfeeding by: educating women, families, health professionals and the community about breastfeeding and human lactation" (para. 4).	Standard 1.4: "Act as an advocate for breastfeeding women, infants, and children."
	Preamble, para. 2: "To guide their professional practice, it is in the best interest of all IBCLCs **and the public they serve** [emphasis added] that there is a Code of Professional Conduct which ... informs both IBCLCs and the public of the *minimum* [emphasis in original] standards of acceptable conduct."	Duty to "protect, promote, and support breastfeeding by: providing holistic, evidence-based breastfeeding support and care, from preconception to weaning, for women" (para. 4).	Standard 1.5: "Assist the mother in maintaining a breastfeeding relationship with her child."
	Definition 5: "IBCLCs may disclose such information to ... protect the client ... when the IBCLC reasonably believes that a client is unable to act adequately in her own or her child's best interest and there is thus risk of harm."	Duty to "protect, promote, and support breastfeeding by: using principles of adult education when teaching" clients (para. 4).	Standard 2.3: "Obtain informed consent from all clients prior to" assessing, making reports, taking photographs, or sharing information from the consultation.
	Principles Overview: "IBCLCs are personally accountable for acting consistently with the CPC to safeguard the interests of clients and justify public trust."	Duty to "provide competent services for mothers and families by: performing comprehensive maternal, child, and feeding assessments related to lactation" (para. 5).	Standard 2.4: "Protect client confidentiality at all times."
	Principle 1.1: "Fulfill professional commitments by working with mothers to meet their breastfeeding goals."	Duty to "provide competent services for mothers and families by: developing and implementing an individualized feeding plan in consultation with the mother" (para. 5).	Standard 3: Provide clinical care "through collaboration and problem solving with the client."

(continued)

Table 2-1 Comparison of Practice-Guiding Document References to Person or Concept Under IBCLC Care (continued)

IBLCE Code of Professional Conduct (2011)	IBLCE Scope of Practice for IBCLCs (2008)	ILCA Standards of Practice for IBCLCs (2006)
Principle 1.2: "Provide care to meet clients' individual needs that is culturally appropriate and informed by the best available evidence."	Duty to "provide competent services for mothers and families by: providing evidence-based information regarding a mother's use, during lactation, of medications (over-the-counter and prescription), alcohol, tobacco, and street drugs, and their potential impact on milk production and child safety" (para. 5).	Standard 3.1.1: "Obtain and document an appropriate history of the breastfeeding mother and child."
Principle 1.3: "Supply sufficient and accurate information to enable clients to make informed decisions."	Duty to "provide competent services for mothers and families by: providing evidence-based information regarding complementary therapies during lactation and their impact on a mother's milk production and the effect on her child" (para. 5).	Standard 3.1.3: "Discuss with the mother and document as appropriate all assessment information."
Principle 3.1: "Refrain from revealing any information acquired in the course of the professional relationship, except to another member of a client's healthcare team, or to other persons or entities for which the client has granted express permission. . . ."	Duty to "provide competent services for mothers and families by: providing support and encouragement to enable mothers to successfully meet their breastfeeding goals" (para. 5).	Standard 3.3.1: "Implement the plan of care in a manner appropriate to the situation and acceptable to the mother."
Principle 3.2: "Refrain from photographing, recording, or taping (audio or video) a mother or her child for any purpose unless the mother has given advance written consent on her behalf and that of her child."	Duty to "provide competent services for mothers and families by: using effective counseling skills when interacting with clients" (para. 5).	
Principle 4.1 "Receive a client's consent, before initiating a consultation, to share clinical information with other members of the client's healthcare team."	Duty to "provide competent services for mothers and families by: using the principles of family-centred care while maintaining a collaborative, supportive relationship with clients" (para. 5).	
Principle 4.2: "Inform an appropriate person or authority if it appears that the health or safety of a client or a colleague is at risk. . . ."	Duty to "report truthfully and fully to the mother and/or infant's primary health care provider and to the health care system by" accurate charting and record keeping (para. 6).	
Principle 5.3: "Withdraw voluntarily from professional practice if the IBCLC has a physical or mental disability that could be detrimental to clients."	Duty to "preserve client confidence by: respecting the privacy, dignity, and confidentiality of mothers and families" (para. 7).	

	Principle 6.3: "Treat all clients equitably without regard to age, ethnicity, national origin, marital status, religion, or sexual orientation."	Duty to "act with reasonable diligence by: functioning and contributing as a member of the health care team to deliver coordinated services to women and families" (para. 8).	
			Standard 1.4: "Act as an advocate for breastfeeding women, infants, and children."
Infant (or) child as patient/client of IBCLC	Introduction, para. 3: "A crucial part of an IBCLC's duty to protect mothers and children is adherence to the principles and aim of the *International Code of Marketing of Breast-milk Substitutes* and subsequent relevant World Health Assembly's resolutions."	Duty to "uphold the standards of the IBCLC profession by: integrating knowledge and evidence when providing care for breastfeeding families" (para. 3).	
	Preamble, para. 1: "IBLCE endorses the broad human rights principles . . . affirming that every human being has the right to the highest attainable standard of health. Moreover, IBLCE considers that every mother and every child has the right to breastfeed."	Duty to "protect, promote, and support breastfeeding by: educating women, families, health professionals, and the community about breastfeeding and human lactation" (para. 4).	Standard 1.5: "Assist the mother in maintaining a breastfeeding relationship with her child."
	Preamble, para. 2: "To guide their professional practice, it is in the best interest of all IBCLCs **and the public they serve** [emphasis added] that there is a Code of Professional Conduct which . . . informs both IBCLCs and the public of the *minimum* [emphasis in original] standards of acceptable conduct."	Duty to "provide competent services for mothers and families by: performing comprehensive maternal, child, and feeding assessments related to lactation" (para. 5).	Standard 4.1: "Educate parents and families to encourage informed decision making about infant and child feeding."
	Definition 5: "IBCLCs may disclose such information to . . . protect the client . . . when the IBCLC reasonably believes that a client is unable to act adequately in her own or her child's best interest and there is thus risk of harm."	Duty to "provide competent services for mothers and families by: providing evidence-based information regarding a mother's use, during lactation, of medications (over-the-counter and prescription), alcohol, tobacco, and street drugs, and their potential impact on milk production and *child safety*" (para. 5) (emphasis added).	
	Principles Overview: "IBCLCs are personally accountable for acting consistently with the CPC to safeguard the interests of clients and justify public trust."	Duty to "provide competent services for mothers and families by: providing evidence-based information regarding complementary therapies during lactation and their impact on a mother's milk production and the *effect on her child*" (para. 5) (emphasis added).	
	Principle 1.2: "Provide care to meet clients' individual needs that is culturally appropriate and informed by the best available evidence."	Duty to "provide competent services for mothers and families by: using the principles of family-centred care while maintaining a collaborative, supportive relationship with clients" (para. 5).	

(continued)

Table 2-1   Comparison of Practice-Guiding Document References to Person or Concept Under IBCLC Care (continued)

	IBLCE Code of Professional Conduct (2011)	IBLCE Scope of Practice for IBCLCs (2008)	ILCA Standards of Practice for IBCLCs (2006)
	Principle 3.1: "Refrain from revealing any information acquired in the course of the professional relationship, except to another member of a client's healthcare team, or to other persons or entities for which the client has granted express permission. . . ."	Duty to "report truthfully and fully to the mother and/or infant's primary health care provider and to the health care system by" accurate charting and record keeping (para. 6).	
	Principle 3.2: "Refrain from photographing, recording, or taping (audio or video) a mother or her child for any purpose unless the mother has given advance written consent on her behalf and that of her child."	Duty to "preserve client confidence by: respecting the privacy, dignity, and confidentiality of mothers and families" (para. 7).	
	Principle 4.2: "Inform an appropriate person or authority if it appears that the health or safety of a client or a colleague is at risk. . . ."	Duty to "act with reasonable diligence by: assisting families with decisions regarding the feeding of children by providing information that is evidence-based and free of conflict of interest" (para. 8).	
	Principle 5.3: "Withdraw voluntarily from professional practice if the IBCLC has a physical or mental disability that could be detrimental to clients."	Duty to "act with reasonable diligence by: functioning and contributing as a member of the health care team to deliver coordinated services to women and families" (para. 8).	
	Principle 6.3: "Treat all clients equitably without regard to age, ethnicity, national origin, marital status, religion, or sexual orientation."		
Breastfeeding relationship as concept protected by IBCLC	Introduction, para. 3: "A crucial part of an IBCLC's duty to protect mothers and children is adherence to the principles and aim of the *International Code of Marketing of Breast-milk Substitutes* and subsequent relevant World Health Assembly's resolutions."	Duty to "uphold the standards of the IBCLC profession by: integrating knowledge and evidence when providing care for breastfeeding families" (para. 3).	Standard 1.5: "Assist the mother in maintaining a breastfeeding relationship with her child."
	Preamble, para. 1: "IBLCE endorses the broad human rights principles . . . affirming that every human being has the right to the highest attainable standard of health. Moreover, IBLCE considers that every mother and every child has the right to breastfeed."	Duty to "protect, promote, and support breastfeeding by: educating women, families, health professionals and the community about breastfeeding" (para. 4).	Standard 1.8: "Support and promote well-designed research in human lactation and breastfeeding, and base clinical practice, whenever possible, on such research."

Principles Overview: "Provide services that protect, promote and support breastfeeding."	Duty to "protect, promote, and support breastfeeding by: facilitating the development of policies which protect, promote and support breastfeeding" (para. 4).	Standard 3.3.5: "Facilitate referral to other healthcare professionals, community services, and support groups as needed."
	Duty to "protect, promote, and support breastfeeding by: acting as an advocate for breastfeeding as the child-feeding norm" (para. 4).	Standard 4: "Breastfeeding education and counseling are integral parts of the care provided by the IBCLC."
	Duty to "protect, promote, and support breastfeeding by: providing holistic, evidence-based breastfeeding support and care, from preconception to weaning, for women" (para. 4).	Standard 4.1: "Educate parents and families to encourage informed decision making about infant and child feeding."
		Standard 4.2: "Utilize a pragmatic problem solving approach, sensitive to the learner's culture, questions, and concerns."
	Duty to "protect, promote, and support breastfeeding by: complying with the *International Code of Marketing of Breast-milk Substitutes* and subsequent relevant World Health Assembly resolutions [the WHO Code against unethical marketing of infant formula, bottles, teats and infant foods]" (para. 4).	Standard 4.4: "Provide positive feedback and emotional support for continued breastfeeding, especially in difficult or complicated circumstances."
	Duty to "provide competent services for mothers and families by: integrating cultural, psychosocial, and nutritional aspects of breastfeeding" (para. 5).	Standard 4.5: "Share current evidence-based information and clinical skills in collaboration with other healthcare providers."
	Duty to "provide competent services for mothers and families by: using the principles of family-centred care while maintaining a collaborative, supportive relationship with clients" (para. 5).	
	Duty to "act with reasonable diligence by: assisting families with decisions regarding the feeding of children by providing information that is evidence-based and free of conflict of interest" (para. 8).	
	Duty to "act with reasonable diligence by: functioning and contributing as a member of the health care team to deliver coordinated services to women and families" (para. 8).	

necessary to be "truly informed" in her "decision-making." Many of life's lessons are learned by experience and appreciated in hindsight, and mothering is no different. The first-time mother who carefully balances the teeter-totter of risks and benefits of a parenting issue (perhaps even one involving breastfeeding) may come to a different "informed decision" with her subsequent children, even given the identical risks and benefits to ponder. Why? Her mothering, breastfeeding, and life experience will now be different. Each mother will make decisions that fit her age and stage in life; the IBCLC merely provides the evidence-based input.

One of the great skills to master as an IBCLC is the ability to *listen* to the mother. Respond in a manner meaningful to the mother, to let her know that you have heard her concerns and haven't simply "put in the teaching tape" when you are having a discussion with her. IBCLCs are full of fascinating facts and research, but *in the moment*, the mother does not care one whit about the latest *Journal of Human Lactation* article. Instead, a mother wants to sense that you are her ally. That makes her far more receptive to your advice and suggestions. It may be the 20th time this week you have talked about the normalcy of frequent night feeds, but it is the first time *this* mother is sharing her nervousness and concern about all that breastfeeding at night. If she senses that you are offering a standard response, rather than an answer directed to *her* about *her* baby, she may well tune you out (Cadwell, 2010).

Sometimes the Infant Is the Patient/Client

By its very nature, breastfeeding requires the mother and the baby to be together. The newborn is utterly incapable of "getting himself there" if he is not proximate to the mother at the time the urge to feed strikes. English psychoanalyst and pediatrician D. W. Winnicott wrote in the early 1960s that the infant simply cannot exist "apart from someone" (ideally the mother) to care for and nurture it (Winnicott, 2001). Who better than an IBCLC, well-trained in the matters of breastfeeding and lactation, to "speak" for the child? Much of our work is teaching infant basics to new parents, who are often unaware of the subtle movements and cues that signal the baby's desire to suckle. Parents may unwittingly hinder the process: Baby mittens do prevent scratches on the baby's face, but they are an incredible hindrance to the infant who is trying so hard to taste, smell and feel his hands as a primary means to communicate. By discussing lactation from the baby's standpoint, the IBCLC can be a powerful advocate for the person in the room who can't speak up for himself.

The baby is a human mammal, and mammals survive and thrive on their species-specific milk. The urge to be protected in the warm arms of his mother, suckling often to receive nutritious and protective colostrum, is something the newborn is inherently capable (using instinct and reflexes) of accomplishing (Colson, 2010; Colson, Meek, & Hawdon, 2008). The infant is unaware, however, that his mother comes to this process encumbered by years of cultural and social training. While the mother has equally capable instincts and reflexes to nurture her newborn (Colson, 2010), she may not have spent much time around newborn babies. Her preparation during pregnancy may have involved reading or Internet surfing or going to a class, but it is unlikely she spent 24 hours a day with a newborn until the midwife plopped her own on her chest and said "Congratulations!" Nonetheless, a new mother is eager to learn what her baby is trying to communicate. When the IBCLC uses *the mother's* baby as the model, pointing out different infant behaviors, it has an immediate and powerful impact on the mother's ability to absorb the teaching (Cadwell, 2010). The IBCLC can capitalize on this by emphasizing in her teaching and care the primary need of the baby: to breastfeed.

Sometimes Breastfeeding Is the Patient/Client

As IBCLCs, we are members of the healthcare team (International Board of Lactation Consultant Examiners [IBLCE], 2011, 2008; International Lactation Consultant Association [ILCA], 2006). Other healthcare providers with whom we interact may only see a part of our whole, and as IBCLCs we have a responsibility to protect the unique dynamic of breastfeeding, requiring as it does a lactating mother and actively suckling infant working as a dyad. IBCLCs may be the only ones who recognize that the care being offered *today* can either support, or sabotage, exclusive (or even partial) breastfeeding down the road. And with less breastfeeding, there is more sickness—for both mother and child (Horta et al., 2007; Ip et al., 2007).

Many common birthing practices and interventions can profoundly negatively impact the baby's ability to breastfeed and impair the mother's sense that she can competently nurture her baby (Smith & Kroeger, 2010). Yet, most childbirth preparation classes will spend several sessions discussing birth options and procedures (for an event that occurs on one day), without a peep about the impact on breastfeeding (a process that should, by rights, occur for years [Dettwyler, 1995]). Indeed, many mothers are led to believe that medical and surgical interventions are harmless to birthing and breastfeeding, when the evidence screams otherwise (Smith & Kroeger, 2010; Wilf, 2010).

After delivery, mothers may be given advice that is not currently accepted practice by IBCLCs in the field of human lactation. This puts the IBCLC in the position, as an allied healthcare provider (translation: lower on the ladder) of "correcting" medical advice offered by the primary healthcare provider (HCP) (translation: higher on the ladder). Indeed, this may be the most omnipresent legal/ethical issue the IBCLC faces in her day-to-day practice, no matter her country or work setting. Delicate personality and political issues come into play, as the IBCLC weighs, in a very time-sensitive situation, how she can effectively get her point across without being dismissed, battled, or worst, ignored altogether. Fortunately, this is not the universal reaction when an IBCLC suggests an alternate, breastfeeding-protective option for the HCP to consider. Some of our colleagues are thrilled to have the IBCLC's expertise to shed light on matters hitherto unconsidered. As explored in another chapter, our profession is relatively young, and it should not come as a surprise that our clinical role and expertise is not well understood by some colleagues.

The medical model, based on treating illness or caring for sick persons, does not offer an ideal environment for teaching normal breastfeeding. And yet, many mothers are learning about breastfeeding from a postpartum hospital bed. The IBCLC may be a voice of reason, reminding everyone from the attending physician to the mother, that breastfeeding is a safe biologic process perfected by Mother Nature long before any of us came along.

Breastmilk vs. Breastfeeding

The advent of the modern age has brought with it the invention of modern technology that can be put to good use . . . including machines intended to assist breastfeeding. Before we leap to the ubiquitous breast pump, think for a minute about the washing machine or wash board, bicycle or automobile, telephone, computer, propane gas stove or microwave, heating pad, or refrigerator. Don't they all, in some small way, make the hectic life of a new mother a little bit easier, allowing her to take 15 minutes to sit and nurse the baby? Imagine our grandmothers, who had to rise from the rocking chair to walk over and manually change the television channel, before the advent of the remote control. The point is that technology or labor-saving devices as such aren't to be scorned. It can be tempting to use an argument that since breastfeeding is "natural" and "biologic" that one doesn't need any more "equipment" than lactating breasts and a willing healthy infant. But this doesn't take into account the totality of circumstances and options available to the mother, which an IBCLC must consider during a lactation consultation.

A later chapter will discuss real and perceived conflicts of interest, a genuine legal/ethical issue of which the IBCLC must be cognizant as she discusses use of name-brand products and gadgets (Lo & Field, 2009). At the very least, an IBCLC is required to become familiar with the research behind, and utility of, the many products peddled each year to breastfeeding mothers; her client (the mother) is very likely to ask the IBCLC to offer an opinion about pump A or cream B or gadget C. Often the research touting a product is funded by the manufacturer, raising a legitimate suspicion that the results are biased. Fortunately, there are excellent resources available to the IBCLC, where analysis of breastfeeding tools has been done for us by researchers without a commercial conflict of interest (Genna, 2009).

All of which brings us to the salient point for this chapter: Should the IBCLC's professional goal be the provision of breastmilk, or breastfeeding at breast? With improvements in breast pump effectiveness (especially when combined with hand-expression) (Genna, 2009; Morton et al., 2009; Morton, 2010), the increased survival rate of very premature babies (Stoll et al., 2010), the increasing birth rates for mothers who used medically assisted fertility (Filicori et al., 2005), and short paid maternity leaves in many "modern" countries (United Nations Statistics Division, 2011), there is a phenomenon in the 21st century of mothers exclusively expressing their milk, for weeks and even months on end. Some do it for the entire time of their lactation cycle, with their child(ren) getting all that milk via a supplemental device, customarily a bottle (MOBI Motherhood International, 2007). The phrase *breastmilk-fed* has joined the vernacular, to differentiate the child who gets his breastmilk by some means other than mother's breast, versus the breastfed playmate who received his breastmilk the good old-fashioned way, by suckling at breast. As an IBCLC, one must be aware that there are mothers for whom this is their path; temporarily or permanently, it is one they have chosen outright, or one they have come to after exhausting every other avenue. Non-judgmental information and support from the IBCLC will serve such mothers well.

The Root of IBCLC Responsibility: Provide Information and Support

Were Millennial Mom to use her Twitter account to reduce this entire book to a tweet, her 137-character message would read: *The IBCLC's legal and ethical responsibility is to provide evidence-based information and support so the mother can make an informed decision about lactation.*

This is compatible with the notions just discussed (of having the mother or the baby as a client, or the act of breastfeeding as a client) since the IBCLC in her consultant role interacts *with* the mother. The information she provides, the teaching she offers, the physical adjustments she suggests, will all be given to the mother. The IBCLC's motivation may be that she is promoting and protecting the right of the infant/client/patient to have his mother's milk, but the conversation will be conducted with the mother. Similarly, if the IBCLC is brought in to consult with other HCPs (such as a neonatologist seeking a consultation to discuss with the IBCLC about a mother protecting her supply with hand-expression or pumping, so as to plan for the premature infant's enteral feeds [Wight, Morton, & Kim, 2008]), the IBCLC's input will involve a discussion of what information has been or will be shared with the mother.

We will explore in subsequent chapters how IBCLC consultations play out in day-to-day practice; there are very different routes an IBCLC will choose to take as the facts of a situation change ever so slightly. Nonetheless, it is useful to describe here the foundation of an IBCLC's responsibility to the patient/client. **Table 2-2** indicates those sections of the mandatory IBLCE Code of Professional Responsibility, the mandatory IBLCE Scope of Practice for IBCLCs, and the voluntary ILCA Standards of Practice for IBCLCs that address the core IBCLC responsibilities of providing evidence-based information and support, to allow for informed decision making by the mother.

We start from the very basic human premise that a loving mother wants to do the best for herself and her child. We acknowledge that the IBCLC doesn't decide *for* the mother what course of action is to take place. That is the mother's job, though she will

Table 2-2   Comparison of Practice-Guiding Document References to IBCLC Core Responsibilities

The IBCLC's legal and ethical responsibility is to provide evidence-based information and support so the mother can make an informed decision about lactation.

	IBLCE Code of Professional Conduct (2011)	IBLCE Scope of Practice for IBCLCs (2008)	ILCA Standards of Practice for IBCLCs (2006)
IBCLC to provide evidence-based information	Introduction, para. 2: "IBLCE was founded to protect the health, welfare and safety of the public by providing the internationally recognized measure of knowledge [emphasis added] in lactation and breastfeeding care through the IBLCE exam."	Preface: "The aim of this Scope of Practice is to protect the public by ensuring that all IBCLCs provide safe, competent, and evidence-based care" (para. 2).	Standard 1.6: "Maintain and expand knowledge and skills for lactation consultant practice by participating in continuing education."
	Principle 1.2: "Provide care to meet clients' individual needs that is culturally appropriate and informed by the best available evidence."	Duty to "uphold the standards of the IBCLC profession by: integrating knowledge and evidence when providing care for breastfeeding families" (para. 3).	Standard 1.7: "Undertake periodic and systematic evaluation of one's clinical practice."
	Principle 1.4: "Convey accurate, complete and objective information about commercial products (see Principle [5.1])."	Duty to "maintai[n] knowledge and skills through regular continuing education" (para. 3).	Standard 1.8: "Support and promote well-designed research in human lactation and breastfeeding, and base clinical practice, whenever possible, on such research."
	Principle 1.5: "Present information without personal bias."	Duty to "protect, promote, and support breastfeeding by: providing holistic, evidence-based breastfeeding support and care, from preconception to weaning, for women" (para. 4).	Standard 4.5: "Share current evidence-based information and clinical skills in collaboration with other health care providers."
	Principle 2.3: "Be responsible and accountable for personal conduct and practice."	Duty to "provide competent services for mothers and families by: providing evidence-based information regarding a mother's use, during lactation, of medications (over-the-counter and prescription), alcohol, tobacco, and street drugs, and their potential impact on milk production and child safety" (para. 5).	
	Principle 5.1: "Disclose any actual or apparent conflict of interest, including a financial interest in relevant goods or services, or in organizations which provide relevant goods or services."	Duty to "provide competent services for mothers and families by: providing evidence-based information regarding complementary therapies during lactation and their impact on a mother's milk production and the effect on her child" (para. 5).	

Principle 5.2: "Ensure that commercial considerations do not influence professional judgment."	Duty to "report truthfully and fully to the mother and/or infant's primary health care provider and to the health care system by" accurate charting and record keeping (para. 6).	
	Duty to "act with reasonable diligence by: assisting families with decisions regarding the feeding of children by providing information that is evidence-based and free of conflict of interest" (para. 8).	Standard 1.4: "Act as an advocate for breastfeeding women, infants, and children."
IBCLC to provide support to patient/client	Preamble, para. 1: "[E]very human being has the right to the highest attainable standard of health. Moreover, IBLCE considers that every mother and every child has the right to breastfeed."	Duty to "protect, promote and support breastfeeding by: educating women, families, health professionals, and the community about breastfeeding and human lactation" (para. 4).
	Principle 1.1: "Fulfill professional commitments by working with mothers to meet their breastfeeding goals."	Duty to "protect, promote, and support breastfeeding by: acting as an advocate for breastfeeding as the child-feeding norm" (para. 4).	Standard 1.5: "Assist the mother in maintaining a breastfeeding relationship with her child."
	Principle 1.2: "Provide care to meet clients' individual needs that is culturally appropriate and informed by the best available evidence."	Duty to "protect, promote, and support breastfeeding by: providing holistic, evidence-based breastfeeding support and care, from preconception to weaning, for women" (para. 4).	Standard 2: "The IBCLC must practice with consideration for rights of privacy and with respect for matters of a confidential nature."
	Principle 4.1: "Receive a client's consent, before initiating a consultation, to share clinical information with other members of the client's healthcare team."	Duty to "provide competent services for mothers and families by: developing and implementing an individualized feeding plan in consultation with the mother" (para. 5).	Standard 3.3.1: "Implement the plan of care in a manner appropriate to the situation and acceptable to the mother."
	Principle 6.3: "Treat all clients equitably without regard to age, ethnicity, national origin, marital status, religion, or sexual orientation."	Duty to "provide competent services for mothers and families by: providing evidence-based information regarding a mother's use, during lactation, of medications (over-the-counter and prescription), alcohol, tobacco, and street drugs, and their potential impact on milk production and child safety" (para. 5).	Standard 3.3.4: "Provide appropriate oral and written instructions and/or demonstration of interventions, procedures, and techniques."
		Duty to "provide competent services for mothers and families by: providing evidence-based information regarding complementary therapies during lactation and their impact on a mother's milk production and the effect on her child" (para. 5).	Standard 4.1: "Educate parents and families to encourage informed decision making about infant and child feeding."

(continued)

Table 2-2   Comparison of Practice-Guiding Document References to IBCLC Core Responsibilities (continued)

	IBLCE Code of Professional Conduct (2011)	IBLCE Scope of Practice for IBCLCs (2008)	ILCA Standards of Practice for IBCLCs (2006)
		Duty to "provide competent services for mothers and families by: providing support and encouragement to enable mothers to successfully meet their breastfeeding goals" (para. 5).	Standard 4.2: "Utilize a pragmatic problem-solving approach, sensitive to the learner's culture, questions, and concerns."
		Duty to "provide competent services for mothers and families by: using effective counseling skills when interacting with clients" (para. 5).	Standard 4.3: "Provide anticipatory guidance (teaching) to promote optimal breastfeeding practices [and] minimize the potential for breastfeeding problems or complications."
		Duty to "provide competent services for mothers and families by: using the principles of family-centred care while maintaining a collaborative, supportive relationship with clients" (para. 5).	Standard 4.4: "Provide positive feedback and emotional support for continued breastfeeding, especially in difficult or complicated circumstances."
		Duty to "preserve client confidence by: respecting the privacy, dignity, and confidentiality of mothers and families" (para. 7).	
		Duty to "act with reasonable diligence by: functioning and contributing as a member of the health care team to deliver coordinated services to women and families" (para. 8).	
		Duty to "act with reasonable diligence by: working collaboratively and interdependently with other members of the health care team" (para. 8).	Standard 1.5: "Assist the mother in maintaining a breastfeeding relationship with her child."
Patient/client responsible for informed decision making	Principle 1.3: "Supply sufficient and accurate information to enable clients to make informed decisions."	Duty to "protect, promote, and support breastfeeding by: using principles of adult education when teaching clients" (para. 4).	Standard 2.3: "Obtain informed consent from all clients prior to" assessing, making reports, taking photographs, or sharing information from the consultation.
	Principle 1.5: "Present information without personal bias."	Duty to "provide competent services for mothers and families by: developing and implementing an individualized feeding plan in consultation with the mother" (para. 5).	Standard 3: "The clinical practice of the IBCLC focuses on providing clinical lactation care and management. This is best accomplished by promoting optimal health, through collaboration and problem solving with" the client.
	Principle 4.1: "Receive a client's consent, before initiating a consultation, to share clinical information with other members of the client's healthcare team."	Duty to "provide competent services for mothers and families by: providing evidence-based information regarding a mother's use, during lactation, of medications (over-the-counter and prescription), alcohol, tobacco, and street drugs, and their potential impact on milk production and child safety" (para. 5).	

Duty to "provide competent services for mothers and families by: providing evidence-based information regarding complementary therapies during lactation and their impact on a mother's milk production and the effect on her child" (para. 5).	Standard 3: "The role of the IBCLC includes: anticipatory guidance and prevention of problems."
Duty to "provide competent services for mothers and families by: using effective counseling skills when interacting with clients" (para. 5).	Standard 3.1.3: "Discuss with the mother and document as appropriate all assessment information."
Duty to "provide competent services for mothers and families by: using the principles of family-centred care while maintaining a collaborative, supportive relationship with clients" (para. 5).	Standard 3.3.1: "Implement the plan of care in a manner appropriate to the situation and acceptable to the mother."
Duty to "report truthfully and fully to the mother and/or infant's primary health care provider and to the health care system by" accurate charting and record keeping (para. 6).	Standard 3.3.4: "Provide appropriate oral and written instructions and/or demonstration of interventions, procedures, and techniques."
Duty to "preserve client confidence by: respecting the privacy, dignity, and confidentiality of mothers and families" (para. 7).	Standard 4.1: "Educate parents and families to encourage informed decision making about infant and child feeding."
Duty to "act with reasonable diligence by: assisting families with decisions regarding the feeding of children by providing information that is evidence-based and free of conflict of interest" (para. 8).	
Duty to "act with reasonable diligence by: functioning and contributing as a member of the health care team to deliver coordinated services to women and families" (para. 8).	
Duty to "act with reasonable diligence by: working collaboratively and interdependently with other members of the health care team" (para. 8).	

benefit from accurate information from the IBCLC to assist her decision making. We don't make arrogant or paternalistic assumptions about what the mother can "handle," selectively filtering the information and options we share with her. Parenting is a time-consuming, energy-intensive, and emotionally see-sawing process—but only the mother knows her limits. To circumscribe the lactating mother's right to decide for herself how she will handle her situation does her a great disservice, and cuts against the very premise of informed decision making.

There is not much published research or writing on the topic of ethics for lactation consultants. Much has had to be extrapolated from literature about nurses and the nursing profession. Comparing the professions of nursing and lactation consultation makes a certain amount of sense, as

> Both are part of self-regulated specialties with members accountable to a registering/certifying body. In both cases, practitioners are predominantly female professionals providing "bedside" or "hands-on" care. The members of both specialties rarely work as primary healthcare providers and report to or take their directives from primary medical supervisors (Noel-Weiss & Walters, 2006, p. 205).

The notion of patient autonomy is well documented in the nursing literature "especially with regard to informed consent" (Noel-Weiss & Walters, 2006, p. 205). The ethics principle of autonomy revolves around the idea that the patient/client is, and should be, self-governing and self-determining. The patient/client decides which course of action to take after receiving information and recommendations; the HCP respects this right of self-determination. As such, the HCP (e.g., an IBCLC) is expected to be truthful, to respect privacy, to offer full disclosure of information, and "to support a patient/client's decision making needs" (Noel-Weiss & Walters, 2006, p. 208). To be sure, the IBCLC may find herself personally disappointed if she provides compelling reasons to exclusively breastfeed, and the mother chooses another course. If the IBCLC has given the full menu of information and options, in an unbiased fashion, she can at least take solace in knowing she has met her basic responsibilities to the patient/client.

Summary

The IBCLC has a unique cross-disciplinary role. While she serves in a consultative role to the mother, she has a professional obligation to (1) the lactating mother, (2) the child, and (3) the breastfeeding relationship as her "patient/client." The IBCLC role requires, at its root, that the mother be given evidence-based information and support so she is able to make informed decisions about lactation issues.

REFERENCES

Cadwell, K. (2010, July 22). *What women want: Adapting practices to meet the real needs of mothers.* Plenary presentation at 2010 conference of the International Lactation Consultant Association, San Antonio, TX.

Client. (2001). In D. Venes (Ed.), *Taber's cyclopedic medical dictionary* (19th ed., p. 433). Philadelphia, PA: F. A. Davis Co.

Colson, S. (2010, July 22). *Biological nurturing: A new neurobehavioral approach to breastfeeding.* Plenary presentation at 2010 conference of the International Lactation Consultant Association, San Antonio, TX.

Colson, S., Meek, J., & Hawdon, J. (2008, July). Optimal positions for the release of primitive neonatal reflexes stimulating breastfeeding [Abstract]. *Early Human Development, 84*(7), 441–449. Retrieved from http://www.earlyhumandevelopment.com/article/S0378-3782(07)00242-3/abstract

Dettwyler, K. A. (1995). A time to wean: The hominid blueprint for the natural age of weaning in modern human populations. In P. Stuart-Macadam & K. A. Dettwyler, *Breastfeeding: Biocultural perspectives* (pp. 39–74). New York, NY: Aldine De Gruyter.

Filicori, M., Cognigni, G. E., Gamberini, E., Troilo, E., Parmegiani, L., & Bernardi, S. (2005, March). Impact of medically assisted fertility on preterm birth. *BJOG: An International Journal of Obstetrics & Gynaecology, 12*, 113–117. Retrieved from http://onlinelibrary.wiley.com/doi/10.1111/j.1471-0528.2005.00598.x/full

Genna, C. W. (2009). *Selecting and using breastfeeding tools.* Amarillo, TX: Hale Publishing.

Horta, B. L., Bahl, R., Martines, J. C., & Victora, C. G. (2007). *Evidence on the long-term effects of breastfeeding: Systematic reviews and meta-analyses.* Retrieved from http://whqlibdoc.who.int/publications /2007/9789241595230_eng.pdf

International Board of Lactation Consultant Examiners. (2008, March 8). *Scope of practice for international board certified lactation consultants.* Retrieved from http://www.iblce.org/upload/downloads/ScopeOf Practice.pdf

International Board of Lactation Consultant Examiners. (2011, November 1). *Code of professional conduct for IBCLCs.* Retrieved from http://iblce.org/upload/downloads/CodeOfProfessionalConduct.pdf

International Lactation Consultant Association. (2006). *Standards of practice for international board certified lactation consultants.* Retrieved from http://www.ilca.org/files/resources/Standards-of-Practice-web.pdf

Ip, S., Chung, M., Raman, G., Chew, P., Magula, N., DeVine, D., . . . Lau, J. (2007, April). *Breastfeeding and maternal and infant health outcomes in developed countries* (Rep. No. 153). Rockville, MD: U.S. Agency for Healthcare Research and Quality.

Lo, B., & Field, M. (Eds.). (2009). *Conflict of interest in medical research, education, and practice.* Retrieved from http://www.ncbi.nlm.nih.gov/bookshelf/br.fcgi?book=nap12598

MOBI Motherhood International. (2007). *About us.* Retrieved from http://www.mobimotherhood.org/MM /Default.aspx

Morton, J. (2010). *Maximizing milk production with hands-on pumping* [Streaming video]. Retrieved from http://newborns.stanford.edu/Breastfeeding/MaxProduction.html

Morton, J., Hall, J. Y., Wong, R. J., Thairu, L., Benitz, W. E., & Rhine, W. D. (2009, July 2). Combining hand techniques with electric pumping increases milk production in mothers of preterm infants [Abstract]. *Journal of Perinatology, 29*, 757–764. Retrieved from http://www.nature.com/jp/journal/v29/n11/abs /jp200987a.html

Noel-Weiss, J., & Walters, G. (2006). Ethics and lactation consultants: Developing knowledge, skills, and tools. *Journal of Human Lactation, 22*(2), 203–212. Retrieved from http://jhl.sagepub.com/content /22/2/203.full.pdf+html

Patient. (2001). In D. Venes (Ed.), *Taber's cyclopedic medical dictionary* (19th ed., p. 1594). Philadelphia, PA: F. A. Davis Co.

Smith, L. J., & Kroeger, M. (2010). *Impact of birthing practices on breastfeeding* (2nd ed.). Sudbury, MA: Jones & Bartlett.

Stoll, B. J., Hansen, N. I., Bell, E. F., Shankaran, S., Laptook, A. R., Walsh, M. C., . . . Newman, N. S. (2010, September). Neonatal outcomes of extremely preterm infants from the NICHD neonatal research network [Abstract]. *Pediatrics, 126*(3), 443–456. Retrieved from http://www.ncbi.nlm.nih.gov/pubmed /20732945

United Nations Statistics Division. (2011, December). Statistics and indicators on women and men. In *Work: Maternity leave benefits* [Statistical table]. Retrieved http://unstats.un.org/unsd/demographic/products /indwm/tab5g.htm#tech

Wight, N. E., Morton, J. A., & Kim, J. H. (2008). *Best medicine: Human milk in the NICU.* Amarillo, TX: Hale.

Wilf, R. (2010, September 20). *The elephant in the room: How maternity care practices affect breastfeeding and what you can do about it.* Lecture presented at Pennsylvania Resource Organization for Lactation Consultants meeting, Philadelphia, PA.

Winnicott, D. W. (2001). *Family and individual development* (6th ed.). East Sussex, UK: Brunner-Routledge.

Chapter 3

IBCLC Practice Guidelines:
The Rules of the Road

Just what, exactly, are the "rules of the road" for the International Board Certified Lactation Consultant (IBCLC)? To what can she refer if she wants guidelines about what she can do (or not do), or what she can say (or not say)? And what happens if she disagrees with those guidelines?

There is no way to avoid just slogging through the guidelines themselves, point by point. Many IBCLCs, if they are honest with themselves, will admit they haven't done this since they studied to take their certification examination with the International Board of Lactation Consultant Examiners (IBLCE). Some of you may bravely admit you didn't even review the practice-guiding documents at all, favoring the odds that you'd only get a handful of questions on the topic, and could afford to get them wrong and still pass the overall exam because of your mastery of the other topics. That is perfectly fine (and legal and ethical, by the way).

Note that we use the term *guideline*. While some of the discussion below will involve *mandatory* professional behaviors, there is always a little wiggle room to take into account the facts of the case at hand; to look at the mother and baby who are there, right now, with the IBCLC. Ethics and legal principles allow for extenuating or unusual circumstances to be taken into account. Nothing is written in stone, immutable and inflexible forever. In fact, the same guideline may offer several different interpretations, depending on the facts involved.

Here's an easy example. You are seeing a mother with low milk supply because baby, who had been ill, was not feeding frequently or effectively. You know that increasing the number of times per day that milk is removed from the breasts will recalibrate supply upward (the supply–demand response) (Riordan & Wambach, 2010). You will tell the mother about the supply–demand response, and then explore how she can achieve this (International Board of Lactation Consultant Examiners [IBLCE] Code of Professional Conduct [CPC], 2011e, Principles 1.2, 1.3, 1.4). As you begin to tell her of the option to rent a hospital-grade breast pump, she informs you there is no electricity at home, because of her religion. You think to yourself, "That's just plain crazy. I couldn't live without my electric blanket, electric coffee maker, and television." But you keep these thoughts to yourself (IBLCE, 2011e, CPC Principle 1.5). Instead, you immediately start teaching about the use of hand-expression to move the milk, and techniques to use during breastfeeding (i.e., breast compression) that can coax baby to suckle effectively (IBLCE, 2011e, CPC Principles 1.1, 1.2, 1.3, 1.5; Riordan & Wambach, 2010).

But didn't we just learn that a required role for the IBCLC is to tell the mother all of her options, so she can make "informed decisions" (IBLCE, 2011e, CPC Principle 1.3)? Doesn't the IBCLC also have to talk about electric breast pumps, so that mother is fully informed of her options? Of course not. Because equally compelling is the IBCLC's responsibility to "provide care to meet clients' individual needs that is culturally appropriate" (IBLCE, 2011e, CPC Principle 1.2). The IBCLC will disregard her own love of electric appliances, respect the mother's circumstances that do not permit for use of electricity, and simply meet the mother where *she* is.

Table 3-1 offers a helpful comparison of the requirements of the major practice-guiding documents, but do read what follows for a translation into plain English of what those requirements mean.

For All IBCLCs, Everywhere

Certification as an IBCLC is an *international* distinction, conferred on those who have completed the rigorous requirements to sit for the exam, and have successfully passed it. Every IBCLC everywhere met the same didactic and clinical training requirements; every IBCLC everywhere must recertify every 5 years (IBLCE, 2012).

Similarly, every IBCLC everywhere has the same requirement to practice under the guidelines we're about to explore. If she was certified while living in the United States, then moved to France, subsequently took a short-term post in Malaysia, and has now returned to the United States, her training and certification and practice methodology are the same in all of those locations. Local cultural and social practices may influence the consultation (for example, food customs for the brand new mother differ in North America, Europe, and Asia), but what makes an IBCLC an IBCLC does not change, and she is held to the same professional standard in each venue.

The IBLCE Code of Professional Conduct: A "Must"

All IBCLCs everywhere are required to adhere to the IBLCE Code of Professional Conduct. This document is the practice-guiding mother of them all. "To guide their professional practice, it is in the best interest of all IBCLCs and the public they serve that there is a Code of Professional Conduct" that describes minimum standards of acceptable conduct, laid out in eight broad principles that identify professional practices the IBCLC is *required* to follow (IBLCE, 2011e, CPC Preamble para. 2). But first . . . a bit of history.

The IBLCE Code of Professional Conduct is a complete revision and rewrite of the earlier IBLCE Code of Ethics (IBLCE COE). The original IBLCE COE was

Table 3-1   Comparison of Key Concepts in Practice-Guiding Documents for IBCLCs

Task or Role for IBCLC	IBLCE Code of Professional Conduct (2011): "Must"	IBLCE Scope of Practice for IBCLCs (2008): "Must"	ILCA Standards of Practice for IBCLCs (2006): "Should"	Int'l [WHO] Code of Marketing of Breast-milk Substitutes, as it applies to health workers: "Should," Unless It Is a "Must"
Protection of public health safety and welfare	Introduction Preamble	Para. 2	Standard 3, introduction Standard 3.3.3	Preamble Article 1 Article 2 Article 10
Respect individual needs/values of client/patient	Principle 1.2	Para. 5 Para. 6	Preface Standard 3.2 Standard 3.3.1 Standard 3.3.2 Standard 4.2	
Avoid discrimination	Principle 6.3	Para. 3 Para. 7	Preface Standard 2, introduction Standard 4.2	
Act with good faith, honesty, integrity, fairness	Principle 2.3 Principle 6.1 Principle 7.3 Principle 7.4	Para. 3 Para. 6	Preface Standard 2, introduction Standard 2.1 Standard 2.5	
Avoid conflicts of interest, especially regarding commercial products	Principle 1.4 Principle 5.1 Principle 5.2 Principle 6.1	Para. 8	Standard 1.3 Standard 3.3.6	Preamble Article 4 Article 5 Article 6 Article 7
Use equipment/tools appropriately	Principle 5.1 Principle 5.2	Para. 4	Standard 1.3 Standard 3.3.6	Preamble Article 1 Article 6
Maintain confidentiality; obtain consent	Principle 3.1 Principle 3.2 Principle 4.1	Para. 6 Para. 7	Standard 2, introduction Standard 2.3 Standard 2.4	
Use evidence-based practice	Principle 1.2 Principle 1.5	Para. 3 Para. 4 Para. 5	Standard 1.8 Standard 4.5	Article 4
Maintain competence in specialty; know when to refer	Principle 2.1 Principle 2.3	Para. 1 Para. 3 Para. 5 Para. 6	Standard 1.6 Standard 1.7 Standard 3.3.5	

(continued)

Table 3-1   Comparison of Key Concepts in Practice-Guiding Documents for IBCLCs (continued)

Task or Role for IBCLC	IBLCE Code of Professional Conduct (2011): "Must"	IBLCE Scope of Practice for IBCLCs (2008): "Must"	ILCA Standards of Practice for IBCLCs (2006): "Should"	Int'l [WHO] Code of Marketing of Breast-milk Substitutes, as it applies to health workers: "Should," Unless It Is a "Must"
Be factual and truthful in providing services and advertising of IBCLC, and product information	Principle 5.2 Principle 7.1 Principle 7.2 Principle 7.3 Principle 7.4	Para. 3 Para. 5 Para. 6	Standard 2.2 Standard 3	Article 1 Article 2 Article 4 Article 5 Article 6 Article 7 Article 9 Article 10
Provide information to permit informed decision making	Principle 1.3 Principle 1.5 Principle 4.1	Para. 3 Para. 4 Para. 5 Para. 6 Para. 8	Standard 2.3 Standard 3, introduction Standard 3.2 Standard 3.4.2 Standard 4.1	Preamble Article 1 Article 2 Article 4 Article 5 Article 6 Article 7 Article 9
Provide information without bias; recognize different opinions exist	Principle 1.5 Principle 2.2	Para. 3 Para. 4 Para. 5 Para. 8	Standard 3, introduction Standard 3.3 Standard 4.2 Standard 4.4 Standard 4.5	Article 1 Article 2 Article 4 Article 5 Article 6 Article 7 Article 9
Provide education on human lactation; share information with other HCPs	Principle 1.1 Principle 2.2 Principle 3.1 Principle 4.1	Para. 3 Para. 4 Para. 5 Para. 6 Para. 8	Standard 3, introduction Standard 3.3.7 Standard 4.5	Preamble Article 4 Article 6
Provide support to client/patient	Principle 1.1 Principle 1.2 Principle 1.3	Para. 4 Para. 5 Para. 7 Para. 8	Standard 1.4 Standard 1.5 Standard 3.3.1 Standard 3.3.2 Standard 3.3.4 Standard 4.3 Standard 4.4	Preamble

Withdraw if impaired; be disciplined if convicted of a crime	Principle 2.4 Principle 5.3 Principle 6.2 Principle 8.1 Principle 8.2	Para. 8	Standard 2, introduction	
Report violations of law or practice-guiding documents	Principle 2.4 Principle 4.2 Principle 8.1	Para. 8	Standard 1, introduction	
Follow *Int'l* [WHO] *Code of Marketing of Breast-milk Substitutes* section for health workers	Introduction	Para. 4	Standard 1.2	Article 7
Respect intellectual property law, specifically	Principle 2.5			
Respect policies and laws, generally	Preamble Definitions Principle 2.1 Principle 2.4 Principle 6.1 Principle 6.3 Principle 7.1	Para. 2 Para. 3 Para. 4 Para. 6 Para. 8	Preface Standard 1, introduction Standard 2, introduction Standard 2.1 Standard 2.5	Preamble Article 10 Article 11
Maintain and update charts/files/consents according to policies and laws	Principle 2.4 Principle 3.1 Principle 3.2 Principle 4.1	Para. 3 Para. 4 Para. 6 Para. 8	Standard 2, introduction Standard 2.3 Standard 3.1 Standard 3.3.4 Standard 3.3.7	
Advocate for mothers, babies, and breastfeeding	Introduction Preamble Principle 1.1	Para. 3 Para. 4 Para. 5 Para. 8	Standard 1.4 Standard 1.5	Preamble Article 1 Article 2 Article 4 Article 5 Article 6 Article 7 Article 10

first implemented March 1, 1997, when the profession was barely 10 years old (Scott, 1996). The IBLCE COE applied to all IBCLCs, who were "personally accountable for [their] practice and, in the exercise of professional accountability," were required to adhere to the enumerated principles (also called tenets) (IBLCE, 2003b, COE para. 3). The inaugural IBLCE COE had 23 principles (Scott, 1996); the 24th principle was added in 1999 (IBLCE, 1999) and the 25th and final principle was made effective as of December 1, 2004 (IBLCE, 2003b).

IBLCE replaced the IBLCE COE, in its entirety, with the IBLCE CPC, explaining simply that "it is a best practice for credentialing bodies [to] periodically review . . . policies and procedures" (IBLCE, 2011d, p. 1). The IBLCE CPC was earlier made available for a brief review and comment period; after revising the language in light of comments received, the final IBLCE CPC was approved by the IBLCE Board and issued with an effective date of November 1, 2011.

IBCLCs tested or recertified through July 2011 will have learned, and practiced under, the guidance offered by the IBLCE COE. From November 1, 2011, onward, all current IBCLCs, and all initial or recertification candidates, will be required to practice under the IBLCE CPC. It is important for those certified under the preexisting schema to understand how the new mandate for professional behavior compares to what they knew and followed under the earlier ethical code.

Fortunately, most of the concepts from the old IBLCE COE were retained, and are a part of the new IBLCE CPC (though with slightly different wording and changed enumeration). IBLCE explained the name change for its penultimate practice-guiding document for IBCLC ethics by simply stating, "Professional conduct encompasses ethical behavior, and is a broader and stronger term" (IBLCE, 2011d, p. 1). **Table 3-2** compares the two documents.

To describe the IBLCE CPC, like its predecessor the IBLCE COE, as a "must" document, is to highlight a very powerful requirement. For if one *must* do something, then it stands to reason that failure to do so brings some sort of sanction. Recall the discussion of certification, which, like licensure, safeguards the public health and safety when there is a disciplinary process to enforce it. The IBLCE CPC has such a sanctions process: Principle 8.1 says "Every IBCLC shall comply fully with the IBLCE Ethics & Discipline process" (IBLCE, 2011e, CPC Principle 8.1).

The IBCLC is advised to become familiar with the procedures set out in the IBLCE Disciplinary Procedures. The document underwent substantial and substantive revision, and was made effective November 1, 2011, without prior notice to or input from certificants or other interested stakeholders. IBLCE's explanation for the overhaul is that "it is a best practice to periodically review policies and procedures. IBLCE reviewed its procedures with respect to ethics complaints and elected to streamline the same" (IBLCE, 2011d, p. 2). Streamlining was indeed accomplished; the earlier disciplinary procedures were described in 52 pages, while the new ones are described in 5.

Table 3-2 Comparison of 2011 IBLCE Code of Professional Conduct and 2003 IBLCE Code of Ethics

The CPC (left column) is compared with the closest-resembling section of the COE (right column). The CPC can be read in its entirety by scrolling down the left column. Sections of the COE appear out of order, to allow side-by-side comparison of the core elements.

2011 IBLCE Code of Professional Conduct (CPC) (effective Nov 1, 2011)	2003 IBLCE Code of Ethics (COE) (superseded by IBLCE CPC 2011 on Nov 1, 2011)
Introduction para. 1: The International Board of Lactation Consultant Examiners® (IBLCE®) is the global authority that certifies practitioners in lactation and breastfeeding care.	
Introduction para. 2: IBLCE was founded to protect the health, welfare and safety of the public by providing the internationally recognized measure of knowledge in lactation and breastfeeding care through the IBLCE exam. Successful candidates become International Board Certified Lactation Consultants (IBCLCs).	Preamble, para. 2: The purpose of the International Board of Lactation Consultant Examiners (IBLCE) is to assist in the protection of the health, safety, and welfare of the public by establishing and enforcing qualifications of certification and for issuing voluntary credentials to individuals who have attained those qualifications. The IBLCE has adopted this Code to apply to all individuals who hold the credential of International Board Certified Lactation Consultant (IBCLC), Registered Lactation Consultant (RLC).
Introduction para. 3: A crucial part of an IBCLC's duty to protect mothers and children is adherence to the principles and aim of the *International Code of Marketing of Breast-milk Substitutes* and subsequent relevant World Health Organization [*sic*] resolutions.	24. IBCLC, RLCs must adhere to those provisions of the *International Code of Marketing of Breast-milk Substitutes* and subsequent resolutions which pertain to health workers.
Preamble, para. 1: IBLCE endorses the broad human rights principles articulated in numerous international documents affirming that every human being has the right to the highest attainable standard of health. Moreover, IBLCE considers that every mother and every child has the right to breastfeed. Thus, IBLCE encourages IBCLCs to uphold the highest standards of ethical conduct as outlined in: • United Nations Convention on the Rights of the Child • United Nations Convention on the Elimination of All Forms of Discrimination Against Women (Article 12) • Council of Medical Specialty Societies *Code for Interactions with Companies*	
Preamble, para. 2: To guide their professional practice, it is in the best interest of all IBCLCs and the public they serve that there is a Code of Professional Conduct which: • Informs both IBCLCs and the public of the *minimum* standards of acceptable conduct; • Exemplifies the commitment expected of all holders of the IBCLC credential; • Provides IBCLCs with a framework for carrying out their essential duties; • Serves as a basis for decisions regarding alleged misconduct [emphasis in original].	Preamble, para. 1: It is in the best interests of the profession of lactation consultants and the public it serves that there be a Code of Ethics to provide guidance to lactation consultants in their professional practice and conduct. These ethical principles guide the profession and outline commitments and obligations of the lactation consultant to self, client, colleagues, society, and the profession.

(continued)

Table 3-2   Comparison of 2011 IBLCE Code of Professional Conduct and 2003 IBLCE Code of Ethics (continued)

2011 IBLCE Code of Professional Conduct (CPC) (effective Nov 1, 2011)	2003 IBLCE Code of Ethics (COE) (superseded by IBLCE CPC 2011 on Nov 1, 2011)
Definitions and Interpretations 1. For the purposes of this document, the Code of Professional Conduct for IBCLCs will be referred to as the "CPC."	
Definitions and Interpretations 2. IBCLCs will comply fully with the *IBLCE Disciplinary Procedures*.	[The IBCLC must . . .] 22. Accept the obligation to protect society and the profession by upholding the Code of Ethics for International Board Certified Lactation Consultants *and by reporting alleged violations of the Code through the defined review process of the IBLCE* [emphasis added]. [and] [The IBCLC must . . .] 14. Present professional qualifications and credentials accurately, using IBCLC, RLC only when certification is current and authorized by the IBLCE, and complying with all requirements when seeking initial or continued certification from the IBLCE. *The lactation consultant is subject to disciplinary action* for aiding another person in violating any IBLCE requirements or aiding another person in representing himself/herself as an IBCLC, RLC when he/she is not [emphasis added]. [and] [The IBCLC must . . .] 21. *Submit to disciplinary action* under the following circumstance: If convicted of a crime under the laws of the practitioner's country which is a felony or a misdemeanor, an essential element of which is dishonesty, and which is related to the practice of lactation consulting; if disciplined by a state, province, or other local government and at least one of the grounds for the discipline is the same or substantially equivalent to these principles; if committed an act of misfeasance or malfeasance which is directly related to the practice of the profession as determined by a court of competent jurisdiction, a licensing board, or an agency of a governmental body; or if violated a Principle set forth in the Code of Ethics for International Board Certified Lactation Consultants which was in force at the time of the violation [emphasis added].
Definitions and Interpretations 3. For the purposes of the CPC, "due diligence" refers to the obligation imposed on IBCLCs to adhere to a standard of reasonable care while performing any acts that could foreseeably harm others.	

Table 3-2   Comparison of 2011 IBLCE Code of Professional Conduct and 2003 IBLCE Code of Ethics (continued)

2011 IBLCE Code of Professional Conduct (CPC) (effective Nov 1, 2011)	2003 IBLCE Code of Ethics (COE) (superseded by IBLCE CPC 2011 on Nov 1, 2011)
Definitions and Interpretations 4. The term "intellectual property" (Principle 2.5) refers to copyrights (which apply to printed or electronic documents, manuscripts, photographs, slides and illustrations), trademarks, service and certification marks, and patents.	[The IBCLC must . . .] 25. Understand, recognize, respect, and acknowledge intellectual property rights, including but not limited to copyrights (which apply to written material, photographs, slides, illustrations, etc.), trademarks, service marks, and patents. 2
Definitions and Interpretations 5. The exception to the statement "refrain from revealing any information" (Principle 3.1) means that, to the extent required, IBCLCs may disclose such information to: (a) comply with a law, court or administrative order, or this CPC; (b) protect the client, in consultation with appropriate individuals or entities in a position to take suitable action, when the IBCLC reasonably believes that a client is unable to act adequately in her own and her child's best interest and there is thus risk of harm; (c) establish a claim or defense on behalf of the IBCLC and the client, or a defense against a criminal charge or civil claim against the IBCLC based upon conduct in which the client was involved; or (d) respond to allegations in any proceeding concerning the services the IBCLC has provided to the client.	
Definitions and Interpretations 6. "Misfeasance" describes an act that is legal but performed improperly, while "malfeasance" describes a wrongful act.	[The IBCLC must . . .] 21. Submit to disciplinary action under the following circumstance: If convicted of a crime under the laws of the practitioner's country which is a felony or a misdemeanor, an essential element of which is dishonesty, and which is related to the practice of lactation consulting; if disciplined by a state, province, or other local government and at least one of the grounds for the discipline is the same or substantially equivalent to these principles; if committed an act of *misfeasance or malfeasance which is directly related to the practice of the profession* as determined by a court of competent jurisdiction, a licensing board, or an agency of a governmental body; or if violated a Principle set forth in the Code of Ethics for International Board Certified Lactation Consultants which was in force at the time of the violation [emphasis added].
Introduction to CPC Principles: The CPC consists of eight principles, which require every IBCLC to: 1. Provide services that protect, promote and support breastfeeding 2. Act with due diligence 3. Preserve the confidentiality of clients 4. Report accurately and completely to other members of the healthcare team 5. Exercise independent judgment and avoid conflicts of interest 6. Maintain personal integrity 7. Uphold the professional standards expected of an IBCLC	Introduction to all Principles: The International Board Certified Lactation Consultant, Registered Lactation Consultant shall act in a manner that safeguards the interests of individual clients, justifies public trust in her/his competence, and enhances the reputation of the profession. The International Board Certified Lactation Consultant, Registered Lactation Consultant is personally accountable for his/her practice and, in the exercise of professional accountability, must:

(continued)

Table 3-2   Comparison of 2011 IBLCE Code of Professional Conduct and 2003 IBLCE Code of Ethics (continued)

2011 IBLCE Code of Professional Conduct (CPC) (effective Nov 1, 2011)	2003 IBLCE Code of Ethics (COE) (superseded by IBLCE CPC 2011 on Nov 1, 2011)
8. Comply with the IBLCE Disciplinary Procedures IBCLCs are personally accountable for acting consistently with the CPC to safeguard the interests of clients and justify public trust.	
Principle 1: Provide services that protect, promote and support breastfeeding Every IBCLC shall: 1.1 Fulfill professional commitments by working with mothers to meet their breastfeeding goals.	
Principle 1: Provide services that protect, promote and support breastfeeding Every IBCLC shall: 1.2 Provide care to meet clients' individual needs that is culturally appropriate and informed by the best available evidence.	[The IBCLC must . . .] 1. Provide professional services with objectivity and with respect for the unique needs and values of individuals. [and] [The IBCLC must . . .] 7. Base her/his practice on scientific principles, current research, and information.
Principle 1: Provide services that protect, promote and support breastfeeding Every IBCLC shall: 1.3 Supply sufficient and accurate information to enable clients to make informed decisions.	[The IBCLC must . . .] 11. Provide sufficient information to enable clients to make informed decisions.
Principle 1: Provide services that protect, promote and support breastfeeding Every IBCLC shall: 1.4 Convey accurate, complete and objective information about commercial products (see Principle 7.1 [sic; probably meant 5.1]).	[The IBCLC must . . .] 5. Remain free of conflict of interest while fulfilling the objectives and maintaining the integrity of the lactation consultant profession.
Principle 1: Provide competent services Every IBCLC shall: 1.5 Present information without personal bias.	[The IBCLC must . . .] 18. Present substantiated information and interpret controversial information without personal bias, recognizing that legitimate differences of opinion exist.
Principle 2: Act with due diligence Every IBCLC shall: 2.1 Operate within the limits of the scope of practice.	[The IBCLC must . . .] 9. Recognize and exercise professional judgment within the limits of her/his qualifications. This principle includes seeking counsel and making referrals to appropriate providers.
Principle 2: Act with due diligence Every IBCLC shall: 2.2 Collaborate with other members of the healthcare team to provide unified and comprehensive care.	
Principle 2: Act with due diligence Every IBCLC shall: 2.3 Be responsible and accountable for personal conduct and practice.	[The IBCLC must . . .] 3. Fulfill professional commitments in good faith. [and] 8. Take responsibility and accept accountability for personal competence in practice.
Principle 2: Act with due diligence Every IBCLC shall: 2.4 Obey all applicable laws, including those regulating the activities of lactation consultants.	[The IBCLC must . . .] 21. Submit to disciplinary action under the following circumstance: If convicted of a crime under the laws of the practitioner's country which is a felony or a misdemeanor, an essential element of which is dishonesty, and which is *related to the practice of lactation*

Table 3-2   Comparison of 2011 IBLCE Code of Professional Conduct and 2003 IBLCE Code of Ethics (continued)

2011 IBLCE Code of Professional Conduct (CPC) (effective Nov 1, 2011)	2003 IBLCE Code of Ethics (COE) (superseded by IBLCE CPC 2011 on Nov 1, 2011)
	consulting; if disciplined by a state, province, or other local government and at least one of the grounds for the discipline is the same or substantially equivalent to these principles; if committed an act of misfeasance or malfeasance which is directly related to the practice of the profession as determined by a court of competent jurisdiction, a licensing board, or an agency of a governmental body; or if violated a Principle set forth in the Code of Ethics for International Board Certified Lactation Consultants which was in force at the time of the violation [emphasis added].
Principle 2: Act with due diligence Every IBCLC shall: 2.5 Respect intellectual property rights.	[The IBCLC must . . .] 25. Understand, recognize, respect, and acknowledge intellectual property rights, including but not limited to copyrights (which apply to written material, photographs, slides, illustrations, etc.), trademarks, service marks, and patents.
Principle 3: Preserve the confidentiality of clients Every IBCLC shall: 3.1 Refrain from revealing any information acquired in the course of the professional relationship, except to another member of a client's healthcare team, or to other persons or entities for which the client has granted express permission, except only as provided in the Definitions and Interpretations to the CPC.	[The IBCLC must . . .] 6. Maintain confidentiality.
Principle 3: Preserve the confidentiality of clients Every IBCLC shall: 3.2 Refrain from photographing, recording, or taping (audio or video) a mother or her child for any purpose unless the mother has given advance written consent on her behalf and that of her child.	[The IBCLC must . . .] 20. Obtain maternal consent to photograph, audiotape, or videotape a mother and/or her infant(s) for educational or professional purposes.
Principle 4: Report accurately and completely to other members of the healthcare team Every IBCLC shall: 4.1 Receive a client's consent, before initiating a consultation, to share clinical information with other members of the client's healthcare team.	[The IBCLC must . . .] 23. Require and obtain consent to share clinical concerns and information with the physician or other primary health care provider before initiating a consultation.
Principle 4: Report accurately and completely to other members of the healthcare team Every IBCLC shall: 4.2 Inform an appropriate person or authority if it appears that the health or safety of a client or a colleague is at risk, consistent with Principle 3.	[The IBCLC must . . .] 15. Report to an appropriate person or authority when it appears that the health or safety of colleagues is at risk, as such circumstances may compromise standards of practice and care.
Principle 5: Exercise independent judgment and avoid conflicts of interest Every IBCLC shall: 5.1 Disclose any actual or apparent conflict of interest, including a financial interest in relevant goods or services, or in organizations which provide relevant goods or services.	[The IBCLC must . . .] 17. *Disclose any financial or other conflicts of interest in relevant organizations providing goods or services.* Ensure that professional judgment is not influenced by any commercial considerations [emphasis added].

(continued)

Table 3-2   Comparison of 2011 IBLCE Code of Professional Conduct and 2003 IBLCE Code of Ethics (continued)

2011 IBLCE Code of Professional Conduct (CPC) (effective Nov 1, 2011)	2003 IBLCE Code of Ethics (COE) (superseded by IBLCE CPC 2011 on Nov 1, 2011)
Principle 5: Exercise independent judgment and avoid conflicts of interest Every IBCLC shall: 5.2 Ensure that commercial considerations do not influence professional judgment.	[The IBCLC must . . .] 17. Disclose any financial or other conflicts of interest in relevant organizations providing goods or services. *Ensure that professional judgment is not influenced by any commercial considerations* [emphasis added] [and] [The IBCLC must . . .] 12. Provide information about appropriate products in a manner that is neither false nor misleading.
Principle 5: Exercise independent judgment and avoid conflicts of interest Every IBCLC shall: 5.3 Withdraw voluntarily from professional practice if the IBCLC has a physical or mental disability that could be detrimental to clients.	[The IBCLC must . . .] 19. Withdraw voluntarily from professional practice if the lactation consultant has engaged in any substance abuse that could affect his/her practice; has been adjudged by a court to be mentally incompetent; or *has a physical, emotional or mental disability* that affects her/his practice in a manner that could harm the client [emphasis added].
Principle 6: Maintain personal integrity Every IBCLC shall: 6.1 Behave honestly and fairly as a health professional.	[The IBCLC must . . .] 4. Conduct herself/himself with honesty, integrity, and fairness. [and] [The IBCLC must . . .] 16. Refuse any gift, favor, or hospitality from patients or clients currently in her/his care which might be interpreted as seeking to exert influence to obtain preferential consideration.
Principle 6: Maintain personal integrity Every IBCLC shall: 6.2 Withdraw voluntarily from professional practice if the IBCLC has engaged in substance abuse that could affect the IBCLC's practice.	[The IBCLC must . . .] 19. Withdraw voluntarily from professional practice if the lactation consultant has engaged in any *substance abuse that could affect his/her practice*; has been adjudged by a court to be mentally incompetent; or has a physical, emotional or mental disability that affects her/his practice in a manner that could harm the client [emphasis added].
Principle 6: Maintain personal integrity Every IBCLC shall: 6.3 Treat all clients equitably without regard to age, ethnicity, national origin, marital status, religion, or sexual orientation.	[The IBCLC must . . .] 2. Avoid discrimination against other individuals on the basis of race, creed, religion, gender, sexual orientation, age, and national origin
Principle 7: Uphold the professional standards expected of an IBCLC Every IBCLC shall: 7.1 Operate within the framework defined by the CPC.	Preamble, para. 2: The purpose of the International Board of Lactation Consultant Examiners (IBLCE) is to assist in the protection of the health, safety, and welfare of the public by establishing and enforcing qualifications of certification and for issuing voluntary credentials to individuals who have attained those qualifications. *The IBLCE has adopted this Code to apply to all individuals who hold the credential of International Board Certified Lactation Consultant (IBCLC)*, Registered Lactation Consultant (RLC) [emphasis added].

Table 3-2 Comparison of 2011 IBLCE Code of Professional Conduct and 2003 IBLCE Code of Ethics (continued)

2011 IBLCE Code of Professional Conduct (CPC) (effective Nov 1, 2011)	2003 IBLCE Code of Ethics (COE) (superseded by IBLCE CPC 2011 on Nov 1, 2011)
Principle 7: Uphold the professional standards expected of an IBCLC Every IBCLC shall: 7.2 Provide only accurate information to the public and colleagues concerning lactation consultant services offered.	[The IBCLC must . . .] 10. Inform the public and colleagues of his/her services by using factual information. An International Board Certified Lactation Consultant, Registered Lactation Consultant will not advertise in a false or misleading manner.
Principle 7: Uphold the professional standards expected of an IBCLC Every IBCLC shall: 7.3 Permit use of the IBCLC's name for the purpose of certifying that lactation consultant services have been rendered only when the IBCLC provided those services.	[The IBCLC must . . .] 13. Permit use of her/his name for the purpose of certifying that lactation consultant services have been rendered only if she/he provided those services.
Principle 7: Uphold the professional standards expected of an IBCLC Every IBCLC shall: 7.4 Use the acronyms "IBCLC" and "RLC" or the titles "International Board Certified Lactation Consultant" and "Registered Lactation Consultant" only when certification is current and in the manner in which IBLCE authorizes their use.	[The IBCLC must . . .] 14. Present professional qualifications and credentials accurately, *using IBCLC, RLC only when certification is current and authorized by the IBLCE*, and complying with all requirements when seeking initial or continued certification from the IBLCE. The lactation consultant is subject to disciplinary action for aiding another person in violating any IBLCE requirements or aiding another person in representing himself/herself as an IBCLC, RLC when he/she is not [emphasis added].
Principle 8: Comply with the IBLCE Disciplinary Procedures Every IBCLC shall: 8.1 Comply fully with the IBLCE Ethics & Discipline process.	[The IBCLC must . . .] 21. *Submit to disciplinary action* under the following circumstance: If convicted of a crime under the laws of the practitioner's country which is a felony or a misdemeanor, an essential element of which is dishonesty, and which is related to the practice of lactation consulting; if disciplined by a state, province, or other local government and at least one of the grounds for the discipline is the same or substantially equivalent to these principles; if committed an act of misfeasance or malfeasance which is directly related to the practice of the profession as determined by a court of competent jurisdiction, a licensing board, or an agency of a governmental body; or *if violated a Principle set forth in the Code of Ethics for International Board Certified Lactation Consultants which was in force at the time of the violation* [emphasis added]. [and] 22. Accept the obligation to protect society and the profession by upholding the Code of Ethics for International Board Certified Lactation Consultants *and by reporting alleged violations of the Code through the defined review process of the IBLCE* [emphasis added].
Principle 8: Comply with the IBLCE Disciplinary Procedures Every IBCLC shall: 8.2 Agree that a violation of this CPC includes any matter in which:	[The IBCLC must . . .] 21. Submit to disciplinary action under the following circumstance: If convicted of a crime under the laws of the practitioner's country which is a felony or a misdemeanor, *an essential element of which is dishonesty,*

(continued)

Table 3-2   Comparison of 2011 IBLCE Code of Professional Conduct and 2003 IBLCE Code of Ethics (continued)

2011 IBLCE Code of Professional Conduct (CPC) (effective Nov 1, 2011)	2003 IBLCE Code of Ethics (COE) (superseded by IBLCE CPC 2011 on Nov 1, 2011)
8.2.1 the IBCLC is convicted of a crime under applicable law, where dishonesty, gross neglect or wrongful conduct in relation to the practice of lactation consulting is a core issue;	*and which is related to the practice of lactation consulting*; if disciplined by a state, province, or other local government and at least one of the grounds for the discipline is the same or substantially equivalent to these principles; if committed an act of misfeasance or malfeasance which is directly related to the practice of the profession as determined by a court of competent jurisdiction, a licensing board, or an agency of a governmental body; or if violated a Principle set forth in the Code of Ethics for International Board Certified Lactation Consultants which was in force at the time of the violation [emphasis added].
Principle 8: Comply with the IBLCE Disciplinary Procedures Every IBCLC shall: 8.2 Agree that a violation of this Code includes any matter in which: 8.2.2 the IBCLC is disciplined by a state, province or other level of government and at least one of the grounds for discipline is the same as, or substantially equivalent to, this CPC's principle;	[The IBCLC must . . .] 21. Submit to disciplinary action under the following circumstance: If convicted of a crime under the laws of the practitioner's country which is a felony or a misdemeanor, an essential element of which is dishonesty, and which is related to the practice of lactation consulting; *if disciplined by a state, province, or other local government and at least one of the grounds for the discipline is the same or substantially equivalent to these principles*; if committed an act of misfeasance or malfeasance which is directly related to the practice of the profession as determined by a court of competent jurisdiction, a licensing board, or an agency of a governmental body; or if violated a Principle set forth in the Code of Ethics for International Board Certified Lactation Consultants which was in force at the time of the violation [emphasis added].
Principle 8: Comply with the IBLCE Disciplinary Procedures Every IBCLC shall: 8.2 Agree that a violation of this Code includes any matter in which: 8.2.3 a competent court, licensing board, certifying board or governmental authority determines that the IBCLC has committed an act of misfeasance or malfeasance directly related to the practice of lactation consulting.	[The IBCLC must . . .] 21. Submit to disciplinary action under the following circumstance: If convicted of a crime under the laws of the practitioner's country which is a felony or a misdemeanor, an essential element of which is dishonesty, and which is related to the practice of lactation consulting; if disciplined by a state, province, or other local government and at least one of the grounds for the discipline is the same or substantially equivalent to these principles; if *committed an act of misfeasance or malfeasance which is directly related to the practice of the profession* as determined by a court of competent jurisdiction, a licensing board, or an agency of a governmental body; or if violated a Principle set forth in the Code of Ethics for International Board Certified Lactation Consultants which was in force at the time of the violation [emphasis added].

It goes without saying that the IBLCE CPC expects all IBCLCs to practice ethically and professionally, and never find themselves the subject of a complaint. Yet, complaints that are unfounded and even spurious can still be filed. The accused IBCLC will find that his or her due process rights are dramatically truncated under the streamlined procedures in the IBLCE Discipline Committee.

Today, the process is initiated by a written, signed complaint; the respondent (the accused IBCLC) has minimal due process rights to review the full record of evidence, and to present evidence of her own. If misconduct is found, a variety of public or private sanctions can be meted out, with limited right to appeal to the IBLCE Board of Directors.

For such a weighty and formal process, it is maddeningly difficult to determine just how many complaints have ever been filed, what types of ethics violations were alleged, and how the cases were resolved. Because the investigation, hearing phase, and deliberations are all conducted in strict confidence, there is no publicly available record of the number of complaints filed, nor their resolution (IBLCE, 2011c). A few complaints have resulted in public censure, and those persons stripped of their IBCLC credential may be found on the IBLCE website (IBLCE, 2010a). Incidental reference may be found to the work of the IBLCE Ethics and Discipline Committee in the executive summaries of the IBLCE board meetings, posted on the IBLCE website. (In its entirety, the September 2009 executive summary indicates "Ethics and Discipline. Four cases were reviewed." [IBLCE, 2009, p. 1].) Public comment has been made by IBLCE administrators about the discipline process, but only in the most general manner. We know that as of 2005, 20 years after the profession was born and 8 years after implementation of the IBLCE COE, during which time approximately 16,000 certified IBCLCs were practicing all over the world, a total of only 30 complaints had been filed with IBLCE. Of those, 8 were pending in 2005; 11 were dismissed as unsubstantiated; 1 was dismissed for allegations during the accused's pre-IBCLC period; 7 resulted in private reprimands; 1 in public reprimand, 2 in revocation of the credential (Scott, 2005, slides 74–75). As of September 2006 (later in time), a summary is given for 28 complaints (curiously, fewer than in 2005): 2 resulting in revocation of certification; 1 in public reprimand; 5 in private reprimand; 20 in dismissal (Scott & Calandro, 2008, p. 18). By 2010, two IBCLCs had had their certification permanently revoked, and two had been publicly reprimanded (IBLCE, 2010a), but at the time of this writing, no public summary of all IBLCE disciplinary actions has been published for data beyond 2006.

It is readily apparent that this disciplinary and public safety–protecting process is barely used. While one could conclude that is it because the professional conduct of the 22,000+ currently certified IBCLCs worldwide (IBLCE, 2011a) is beyond reproach, it is far more likely that members of the public simply are not filing complaints if they have a quarrel with their IBCLC's professional behaviors.

The IBLCE CPC can be found online at http://www.iblce.org/upload/downloads /CodeOf ProfessionalConduct.pdf. Following is an explanation, bit by bit, of this preeminent practice-guiding document for all IBCLCs, everywhere.

Introduction

> The International Board of Lactation Consultant Examiners® (IBLCE®) is the global authority that certifies practitioners in lactation and breastfeeding care.
>
> IBLCE was founded to protect the health, welfare and safety of the public by providing the internationally recognized measure of knowledge in lactation and breastfeeding care through the IBLCE exam. Successful candidates become International Board Certified Lactation Consultants (IBCLCs).
>
> A crucial part of an IBCLC's duty to protect mothers and children is adherence to the principles and aim of the *International Code of Marketing of Breast-milk Substitutes* and subsequent relevant World Health Assembly's resolutions. (IBLCE, 2011e, CPC p. 1)

The first two introductory paragraphs to the IBLCE CPC tell the reader what the document is, and why it is important to IBCLCs. The information is straightforward: IBCLCs must pass the international certification exam in breastfeeding and human lactation, which is administered by one entity, the International Board of Lactation Consultant Examiners (IBLCE). IBLCE was founded precisely to administer the examination that awards the IBCLC credential. The examination is designed to protect the public health, safety, and welfare by measuring the skill of IBCLCs, who will provide clinical care and education in breastfeeding and human lactation to members of the public at large. Less straightforward is the third introductory paragraph to the IBLCE CPC, regarding IBCLC requirements in support of the *International Code of Marketing of Breast-milk Substitutes* (the International Code, sometimes also called the WHO Code).

It is important to understand the rudiments of the International Code, which predates the profession of lactation consultation, and was "perhaps the most significant international consumer protection standard of modern time" when passed in 1981 (Baumslaug & Michels, 1995, p. 164). It is a minimum model public health policy that seeks to support and promote breastfeeding. It asks governments to pass legislation to support the aims of the International Code and to provide sanctions against inappropriate and unethical marketing of the products covered under its scope (breastmilk substitutes including infant formula, bottles, teats/bottle nipples, and other foods marketed to replace breastmilk for children) (International Code Documentation Centre, 2006).

Anyone may choose to support International Code objectives, regardless of legislative status. If there are to be enforcement or sanctions elements, however, governments first must pass appropriate laws or regulations within their countries. IBCLCs are "health workers" under the International Code. Health workers and healthcare institutions are to have limited interactions with the marketers of the International

Code-covered products, to reduce inappropriate commercial influence on the provision of healthcare to breastfeeding families. Note that the International Code allows the covered products to be sold and purchased; it is meant only to discourage unethical marketing. Also, any IBCLC (or other health worker) is allowed to discuss any product with any mother, in a clinical or educational setting. The International Code is designed to prohibit inappropriate *marketing* of the products within its scope. Clinical discussions about, and sales of, the products are permitted.

The IBLCE CPC contains a shift in IBLCE policy regarding enforceability against IBCLCs of the health worker–related sections of the International Code. Tenet 24 of the old IBLCE COE was clear: it *required* IBCLCs to *adhere* to the principles of the International Code, at risk of having a complaint filed with the IBLCE Discipline Committee (IBLCE, 2003b, COE Tenet 24; see Table 3-2). The language of the IBLCE CPC introduction's third paragraph would appear to retain this requirement ("[a]n IBCLC's **duty** to protect mothers and children is **adherence** to the [International Code]" [IBLCE, 2011e, CPC p. 1] [emphasis added]). However, the Frequently Asked Questions (FAQs) that were published alongside the IBLCE CPC contain examples that retreat from mandatory support for the International Code. For example, the FAQs state that providing free samples of infant formula to families (an overt violation of Article 7.4 of the International Code) "does not constitute an ethical violation by an IBCLC of the IBLCE Code of Professional Conduct" (IBLCE, 2011d, p. 2).

IBLCE has indicated support in spirit for the International Code, stating that it considers the International Code to be a practice-guiding document and encourages all IBCLCs to follow and uphold it, regardless of whether it is legally enforceable in their jurisdiction (Brooks, Stehel, & Mannel, 2013, p. 8). Any IBCLC who endeavors to practice ethically (and avoid the risk of a discipline complaint for failing to meet IBLCE CPC Principles) may simply continue to follow the guidelines suggested for health workers in Article 7 of the International Code. Practice as though IBLCE *does* require IBCLC adherence to the International Code. This was the standard expected under the IBLCE COE; any IBCLC certified before November 2011 assumed the responsibility of embracing best ethical practices that require adherence to health worker provisions of the International Code. Any IBCLC certified after November 2011 may also choose to follow the higher standard earlier required.

Preamble

IBLCE endorses the broad human rights principles articulated in numerous international documents affirming that every human being has the right to the highest attainable standard of health. Moreover, IBLCE considers that every mother and every child has the right to breastfeed. Thus, IBLCE encourages IBCLCs to uphold the highest standards of ethical conduct as outlined in:

- United Nations Convention on the Rights of the Child
- United Nations Convention on the Elimination of All Forms of Discrimination Against Women (Article 12)
- Council of Medical Specialty Societies *Code for Interactions with Companies*

To guide their professional practice, it is in the best interest of all IBCLCs and the public they serve that there is a Code of Professional Conduct which:

- Informs both IBCLCs and the public of the **minimum** standards of acceptable conduct;
- Exemplifies the commitment expected of all holders of the IBCLC credential;
- Provides IBCLCs with a framework for carrying out their essential duties;
- Serves as a basis for decisions regarding alleged misconduct. (IBLCE, 2011e, CPC p. 1 [emphasis in original])

The first paragraph of the Preamble to the IBLCE CPC departs from the IBLCE COE by alluding to and embracing several documents. Two are United Nations Conventions (position statements) about human rights standards. They provide authority for protecting a child's right to good health, and a woman's right to appropriate health care and nutrition during pregnancy and lactation (UNICEF, n.d.b; United Nations General Assembly, 1979). Promoting and protecting breastfeeding are seen as integral to optimal infant and young child feeding (the child's human right) provided by the mother (her human right) (World Health Organization, 2006; United Nations General Assembly, 1979). The third document from the Council of Medical Specialty Societies (CMSS) is a model, voluntary code, to be used by professional associations/societies of U.S. physicians with specialty practices, to avoid commercial influences from pharmaceutical and medical device manufacturers when obtaining continuing education or conducting research (Council of Medical Specialty Societies, 2011).

No explanation is offered by IBLCE for including the statement of support for these documents in the Preamble to the IBLCE CPC. The two United Nations Conventions are germane, topically, to allied healthcare providers working in maternal and child health. However, they provide no specific guidance on professional conduct for IBCLCs, which is the subject matter of the IBLCE CPC. Similarly, the CMSS document describes optimal practices by U.S.-based physician-only professional associations that accept commercial funds for education and research activities. However, IBCLCs are allied healthcare providers (not physicians, who are primary healthcare providers), and IBLCE has international authority (extending beyond the borders of the United States, which is the geographic limit for CMSS). Nonetheless, eschewing undue commercial influence in obtaining health-related education is a concept the ethically practicing IBCLC can certainly embrace.

The second paragraph of the Preamble sets up the basic framework: the IBLCE CPC is the authoritative document describing **minimum** standards of professional conduct (emphasis in the original); the expectation is that IBCLCs will follow this professional guidance in the conduct of their duties, including its process for hearing complaints of misconduct. The IBLCE CPC serves to inform all IBCLCs, and the families they work with, of the *minimum* standards that IBCLCs must meet in their professional practice. Any IBCLC is thus free to practice in a manner that sets a higher bar of ethical conduct (such as continuing to adhere to health worker elements of the International Code). The IBLCE CPC requires that IBCLCs consent to adjudication of any complaints against them under the disciplinary procedures established and enforced by IBLCE. The corollary is that any complaints filed against an IBCLC must contain allegation(s) that an element of the IBLCE CPC has been violated.

Definitions and Interpretations

This section is new to the IBLCE CPC, although elements of the terms described were contained in the earlier IBLCE COE as tenets unto themselves (see Table 3-2). Each will be examined in turn.

> 1. For the purposes of this document, the Code of Professional Conduct for IBCLCs will be referred to as the "CPC." (IBLCE, 2011e, CPC p. 1)

This definition is self-explanatory. IBLCE no doubt sought to reduce confusion with shorthand references elsewhere to the superseded IBLCE Code of Ethics, or the International Code/WHO Code.

> 2. IBCLCs will comply fully with the *IBLCE Disciplinary Procedures*. (IBLCE, 2011e, CPC p. 1)

This definition is clear and succinct: IBCLCs will comply with the IBLCE discipline process. This means an IBCLC agrees to be subject to the authority and jurisdiction of the IBLCE Discipline Committee, should a complaint be filed alleging failure to adhere to a principle of the IBLCE CPC. While this concept was also contained within the former IBLCE COE, Table 3-2 shows that it was buried in rather obtuse language in three separate tenets.

> 3. For the purposes of the CPC, "due diligence" refers to the obligation imposed on IBCLCs to adhere to a standard of reasonable care while performing any acts that could foreseeably harm others. (IBLCE, 2011e, CPC p. 2)
>
> and
>
> 6. "Misfeasance" describes an act that is legal but performed improperly, while "malfeasance" describes a wrongful act. (IBLCE, 2011e, CPC p. 2)

The terms "due diligence," "misfeasance," and "malfeasance" are best discussed together, because they all spring from concepts in tort law. "Due diligence" describes the broad, overarching principle that a healthcare provider (like an IBCLC) who has a specialized skill (to consult on breastfeeding and human lactation) must take reasonable care not to harm someone (a patient/client, or the public at large). Failure to act with due diligence is a tort, under the law. Generally, a tort involves (a) a noncontractual duty from one party to another, (b) a breach of that duty, and (c) injury or damage as a proximate result (Tort, 1979, p. 1335). For example, a medical malpractice lawsuit might allege that a healthcare provider (HCP), with a duty of care to the patient/client, made an error that resulted in injury. Torts are divided into negligent or intentional acts. Misfeasance and malfeasance are subsets of intentional torts: the actor is alleged to have intentionally performed an action, but did so improperly, or wrongfully.

A hypothetical example can explain the concepts. A mother hires an IBCLC to consult with her on suspected oversupply of milk. This is her second baby, now 7 days of age. Mother had recurrent bouts of plugged ducts and mastitis with her first baby, and is alarmed at how much milk she has. The IBCLC will provide a thorough lactation assessment of this mother and baby. She will devise a care plan that takes into account the baby's age and feeding pattern, the mother's lactation history, and the mother's current stage of lactogenesis and estimated breast storage capacity. She will also be available for follow-up care to adjust the care plan as mother's supply calibrates to baby's needs. Failing to use "due diligence" in competently providing all elements of the lactation consultant (assessment, care plan, and follow-up) could result in the harm of plugged ducts, mastitis, and even abscess or premature weaning. The IBCLC might be accused of misfeasance if she gave improper oral instructions on techniques or frequency of milk removal to address plugged ducts (she intended to give instructions to the client, but did so improperly). The IBCLC might be accused of malfeasance if she grabbed and bruised the mother's breast while trying to demonstrate hand-expression (she intended to touch the mother's breast, but did so in a wrongful and injurious manner).

> 4. The term "intellectual property" (Principle 2.5) refers to copyrights (which apply to printed or electronic documents, manuscripts, photographs, slides and illustrations), trademarks, service and certification marks, and patents. (IBLCE, 2011e, CPC p. 2)

This definition makes clear that *all* areas of intellectual property law are to be included in the IBCLC's requirement (which will be reviewed in greater detail below at Principle 2.5) to respect such laws. This obligation has been carried over from Tenet 25 of the old IBLCE COE. Intellectual property rights are a broad area of the law involving rights and protections for authors, artists and inventors.

> 5. The exception to the statement 'refrain from revealing any information' (Principle 3.1) means that, to the extent required, IBCLCs may disclose such information to:
>   a. comply with a law, court or administrative order, or this CPC;
>   b. protect the client, in consultation with appropriate individuals or entities in a position to take suitable action, when the IBCLC reasonably believes that a client is unable to act adequately in her own and her child's best interest and there is thus risk of harm;

    c. establish a claim or defense on behalf of the IBCLC and the client, or a defense against a criminal charge or civil claim against the IBCLC based upon conduct in which the client was involved; or

    d. respond to allegations in any proceeding concerning the services the IBCLC has provided to the client. (IBLCE, 2011e, CPC p. 2)

IBCLCs have an obligation to maintain confidentiality of their clients/patients. The notion of protecting privacy is long established in health care. It springs from the premise that HCPs can more effectively advise and treat those in their care if they have accurate information about the patient. The patient is more likely to reveal information about himself if he is assured the details will not be freely shared with others. While this Definition and Interpretation is the longest in the IBLCE CPC, it is not as complicated as it first appears. It simply spells out those circumstances when it *is* appropriate for the IBCLC to reveal otherwise-confidential information. Sharing otherwise-private information is allowed in situations that make common sense: under court or administrative order; if the client and/or her child are under risk of harm; or if it provides a defense to a complaint or inquiry about the IBCLC's conduct.

Code of Professional Conduct Principles

The CPC consists of eight principles, which require every IBCLC to:

1. Provide services that protect, promote, and support breastfeeding
2. Act with due diligence
3. Preserve the confidentiality of clients
4. Report accurately and completely to other members of the healthcare team
5. Exercise independent judgment and avoid conflicts of interest
6. Maintain personal integrity
7. Uphold the professional standards expected of an IBCLC
8. Comply with the IBLCE Disciplinary Procedures

IBCLCs are personally accountable for acting consistently with the CPC to safeguard the interests of clients and justify public trust. (IBLCE, 2011e, CPC p. 2)

This portion of the IBLCE CPC is akin to a "table of contents," following as it does the introduction, preamble and definitions and interpretations sections. Each of the eight principles is expanded upon in the "chapters" that follow (and will be discussed in turn below). **The noteworthy element here is the admonition that every IBCLC is *required* to practice in accordance with these principles (making the IBLCE CPC a *mandatory* practice-guiding document).** This is designed to safeguard clients/patients, and justifies public trust in the legitimacy of lactation consultation. Similar core concepts underlying lactation consultation were contained in the old IBLCE COE, at the introduction to the tenets (see Table 3-2).

Principle 1

Principle 1: Provide services that protect, promote and support breastfeeding. Every IBCLC shall: (IBLCE, 2011e, CPC p. 2)

The IBLCE CPC opens with this principle, expanded further into five required professional practice elements that are designed to ensure lactation consultant services protect, promote and support breastfeeding. The word "shall" reminds the IBCLC that these are mandatory obligations of competent, ethical practice.

1.1 Fulfill professional commitments by working with mothers to meet their breastfeeding goals. (IBLCE, 2011e, CPC p. 2)

Principle 1.1 recognizes a simple but obvious truth: IBCLCs work with mothers, and mothers have different lactation goals. Clients/patients may seek a lactation consultation with an IBCLC, the internationally certified allied healthcare provider expert in breastfeeding and human lactation, for many reasons. Mother's surgical, medical or personal history may present concerns about establishing appropriate and sustainable volumes of milk. The baby may have a physical condition making feeding-at-breast problematic (e.g., ankyloglossia, or low muscle tone in the mouth and jaw, or a cleft in the lip or palate). Mother may need to be separated from baby (infants with long stays in the neonatal intensive care unit; or, a mother returning to work outside the home within weeks or months of the birth of her breastfeeding child). The baby's physician may order use of formula for medically indicated reasons. Many mothers simply elect to offer nonbreastmilk supplements to their children, early on, in addition to breastfeeding. "Breastfeeding" isn't the measure of whether the IBCLC is acting professionally; "working with mothers" is. The mother decides what her breastfeeding and lactation goals are, and how to meet them, after receiving information and support from the IBCLC.

1.2 Provide care to meet clients' individual needs that is culturally appropriate and informed by the best available evidence. (IBLCE, 2011e, CPC p. 2)

IBCLCs work with mothers all over the world. Mothers come to breastfeeding and parenting with a blend of social, cultural, religious, political, familial and personal beliefs. The IBCLC should provide information and support in a manner that is respectful of the personal beliefs of the mother. The IBCLC will rely upon her own education and specialized training to guide how she will inform and support the mother. An IBCLC, during her consultation, can simply ask the mother if she has any particular customs or beliefs associated with birth and breastfeeding. This is an open-ended inquiry, and provides an opportunity for the IBCLC to explore matters of importance to each individual mother. The IBCLC should involve the mother in the decision-making process. The IBCLC does not impose his or her own interpretation of an appropriate care plan on the mother; the IBCLC talks to the mother to learn her objectives and goals, and then helps to fashion a manageable care plan.

Principle 1.2 also embraces the concept of "evidence-based practice," where clinical decisions in healthcare are "based on the best research evidence available, clinical knowledge and expertise of the practitioner, and in consultation with the individual receiving care" (Riordan & Wambach, 2010, p. 767). Providing "evidence-based" care does *not* require that a valid double-blind research study must first have been conducted on some aspect of breastfeeding and human lactation before an IBCLC may discuss it with a mother. Principle 1.2 recognizes that part of an IBCLC's professional and ethical responsibility (to be "informed by the best available evidence") is to find and evaluate whatever research may have been conducted. It also recognizes inherent limitations of research in the area of human lactation: It would be unethical to randomly assign babies to receive something other than breastmilk, when lifelong morbidities and mortalities could result (ILCA, Spatz, & Lessen, 2011). Thus, many published articles by researchers may be based on case studies, or literature reviews rather than original research, or data evaluations from small self-selecting groups. The IBCLC should take care that her suggestions in the care plan can be substantiated by published, peer-reviewed literature. Where such technical or medical information does not (yet) exist, but the IBCLC has clinical experience relevant to the issue at hand, the mother should be so informed.

> 1.3 Supply sufficient and accurate information to enable clients to make informed decisions. (IBLCE, 2011e, CPC p. 2)

The IBCLC (and the primary healthcare provider) does the informing; the mother does the deciding. This is the essence of "informed decision making." The IBCLC is often working with a mother in a very vulnerable state: perhaps tired or medicated after birth, or suffering emotional highs and lows as her hormones shift after delivery. Mother is likely distressed that breastfeeding is not proceeding as imagined, prompting need for the competent care of an IBCLC. Or, the mother may be problem-free now . . . but using feeding suggestions that could undermine her ultimate goal to exclusively breastfeed. And, there is only so much a mother will be able to remember accurately after a lengthy conversation. It is the obligation of the IBCLC to provide the mother with information relevant to the issues at hand, taking into account all the present circumstances. A distraught or exhausted mother will not be able to absorb huge amounts of information. Does this mother have access to more than one IBCLC visit? If so, the IBCLC should evaluate which matters are critical for immediate discussion, and which can be explained further at the subsequent visit. If the mother may only have one face-to-face consult, the IBCLC should offer suggestions of where the mother can get follow-up support by phone, and give written materials about the care plan that can be reviewed again, later.

1.4 Convey accurate, complete and objective information about commercial products (see Principle 7.1 [sic; probably meant 5.1]). (IBLCE, 2011e, CPC p. 2)

While in a clinical consultation, the IBCLC should be seen as providing good healthcare, not selling any product. The IBCLC may find that a consultation with a mother will involve discussion of the mother's use of a commercial product. It could be a medical device, such as a breast pump, or equipment for supplemental tube feeds at breast. It may be a pharmaceutical product (whether prescribed or over-the-counter). The mother might ask about foods, drinks, herbs and vitamins and their impact on lactation. The mother may want to know about gadgets designed to facilitate breast-feeding (baby-wearing slings, special bras, stools, books, etc.). The IBCLC does not have to avoid discussing these products; indeed, they may be required to implement a lactation care plan. But, to avoid an apparent conflict of interest, the IBCLC should focus on giving, simply, "accurate, complete and objective information" about products.

IBCLC whose practice settings offer retail services along with clinical consultation (e.g., renting breast pumps, or selling bras) must be careful to segregate commercial from clinical recommendations. For example, a mother might be advised to use a rental- or hospital-grade breast pump for the clinical objective of building or preserving milk supply. The IBCLC who offers this product as part of her retail operation should offer the mother several options of where to obtain the equipment, and be careful to explain that the recommendation is being made for clinical reasons, not to secure a sale.

IBCLCs who work in several settings (i.e., at a birthing center, and as a private practitioner) should avoid the appearance of self-referral: offer all mothers a list of all community-based resources for lactation support.

A thorough lactation consultation will involve investigation of all causes and corrections of breastfeeding issues, and use of purchased products should not be promoted over other means to problem-solve. If the mother is seeking to build supply, the baby may do the best job (by more frequent feeds at breast). If the mother and baby must be separated for long stretches of the day, hand-expression may be the most quick and efficient means for the mother to express her breastmilk.

1.5 Present information without personal bias. (IBLCE, 2011e, CPC p. 3)

Breastfeeding, like most aspects of health care and parenting, lends itself to many variations of correct. Recommendations will necessarily vary for different mothers. There will come a time when the IBCLC is suggesting a care plan that differs from what other healthcare providers or family members have told the mother. The IBCLC should supply "sufficient and accurate information" based on the best available evidence base (see Principle 1.3 above). This corollary Principle 1.5 recognizes that IBCLCs must always remove their own personal opinions from the presentation of information.

Offer substantiated, evidence-based information to mothers and colleagues wherever possible. As specialists in the field of human lactation, IBCLCs may learn of research or optimal techniques long before HCPs in related fields. Educate colleagues by presenting to them the same data that shaped the IBCLC's expertise. While differences of opinion about breastfeeding care plans may occur, they are best discussed when the focus is on the evidence, rather than personal viewpoints. Information should be discussed with courtesy and respect for all parties involved.

As a specialist in the field of human lactation, the IBCLC's clinical experience may permit one to "see" patterns that are not obvious to HCPs in other fields. Clinical experience in emerging areas might have valuable bearing on a mother's situation. The IBCLC should present suggestions without personal bias, and be cognizant that as the bearer of new findings or concepts, it may require some diplomacy to encourage acceptance of a novel care plan.

As members of a profession not even 30 years old, IBCLCs are well advised to think about the "public face" they present. Mothers, other HCPs, and public health administrators are often uninformed about the IBCLC's scope of practice and expertise. IBCLCs that practice with courtesy, respect and collegiality will help to promote the profession of lactation consultancy.

Principle 2

Principle 2: Act with due diligence. Every IBCLC shall: (IBLCE, 2011e, CPC p. 3)

The second principle of the IBLCE CPC, expanded further into five required professional practice elements, is designed to define how "due diligence" (see Definition and Interpretation 3) works in day-to-day practice. The word "shall" reminds the IBCLC that these are mandatory obligations of competent, ethical practice.

2.1 Operate within the limits of the scope of practice. (IBLCE, 2011e, CPC p. 3)

The IBLCE Scope of Practice for IBCLCs (IBLCE SOP) (IBLCE, 2008) is a mandatory practice-guiding document describing the "fences" within which the IBCLC may practice. It applies to all IBCLCs around the world, no matter what their geographic or practice setting. It defines the IBCLC's areas of skill and expertise, and the circumstances under which such expertise may be shared with the public (e.g., breastfeeding mothers).

An IBCLC needs only the IBCLC certification in order to practice as an IBCLC; it is a stand-alone credential and profession. Nonetheless, many practitioners come to the field having first earned a degree or credential in another field (i.e., speech pathology, midwifery, doctor of medicine, registered dietitian, registered nurse, etc.). If the IBCLC has such other training, the scope of practice may—as a practical matter—permit for a wider range of clinical competencies. For example, an IBCLC who is also a registered nurse (RN) has a scope of practice including clinical competency to give an injection. An IBCLC does not. Those who wear "many hats" must be clear as to which clinical role they have in relation to the breastfeeding mother. The IBLCE SOP defines those practice areas in which any IBCLC may engage.

The IBCLC profession, being less than 30 years old, means colleagues and administrators may be unfamiliar with the specialized training and expertise of its certificants. The IBLCE SOP clearly defines the IBCLC's authority as a member of the healthcare team if such is challenged. Also helpful in describing the range and boundaries of IBCLC expertise is the *Position Paper on the Role and Impact of the IBCLC* (ILCA & Henderson, 2011), a free download from the website of the International Lactation Consultant Association, www.ilca.org.

> 2.2 Collaborate with other members of the healthcare team to provide unified and comprehensive care. (IBLCE, 2011e, CPC p. 3)

This concept, as basic as it seems in describing an ethical and professional standard of care for a breastfeeding woman, does not have a precise corollary in the old IBLCE COE. However, the IBLCE SOP—issued after the IBLCE COE—does memorialize this mandatory practice-guiding concept: "IBCLCs have the duty to act with reasonable diligence by working collaboratively and interdependently with other members of the health care team" (IBLCE, 2008, SOP p. 4). A duty is a mandatory obligation. Therefore, IBCLCs must keep other members of the mother's healthcare team informed of significant developments in the lactation care plan.

The means to keep other members of the healthcare team apprised of the IBCLC's consultation can vary by work setting and geographical custom. Written charts or reports, if accessible by the other HCPs, serve the purpose. Private practitioners may send, email or fax reports (taking care to protect confidentiality in the mode of communication). The IBCLC should err on the conservative side, and initiate and send a report, if at all unsure that the primary HCPs will be aware of lactation issues. Having a conversation with the HCP works equally well.

The custom has developed in some regions (i.e., Australia and Great Britain, where many IBCLCs came to the field from midwifery) to contact other HCPs only when lactation care goes beyond the routine. Information shared with the HCPs need not be detailed or complex. Include as a minimum the IBCLCs name and contact information, identifying information for the mother, the basic baby data (name, sex, date of birth, and birth weight), date and reasons for the lactation consultation, the IBCLC's assessment, and care plan rudiments. Whenever there is *any* cause for concern for the health of the mother or baby, the IBCLC should initiate a phone or in-person conversation with the mother's or baby's primary HCP.

> 2.3 Be responsible and accountable for personal conduct and practice. (IBLCE, 2011e, CPC p. 3)

IBCLCs work in varied practice settings: hospitals, birth centers, private practice, public health clinics, parenting groups, physician offices, government and public health offices, educational venues and research institutions. Whether employed full-time or part-time as an IBCLC; whether working in clinical contact with mothers or not: The IBCLC should endeavor every day to practice professionally, competently and with demonstrable commitment to purpose.

Network with IBCLC practitioners in the area, formally or informally, to build professional relationships. If the IBCLC is isolated from colleagues, the Internet provides opportunity for online networking, especially through membership in the International Lactation Consultant Association.

Keeping current on research and continuing education on breastfeeding and human lactation is a means by which the IBCLC shows accountability for personal practice. Maintain an easily accessed and updated file proving continuing education activities in human lactation. This will not only be helpful when it comes time to recertify as an IBCLC, but readily demonstrates to employers the individual's efforts to maintain knowledge in one's area of clinical practice.

Being responsible and accountable for personal practice involves understanding and evaluating research. Learn how to identify properly designed studies. Published research involving human lactation is expanding rapidly; the IBCLC may be challenged to explain results that seem contrary to the clinical experience or teaching of other healthcare providers. The competent IBCLC will be able recognize and explain poorly drawn conclusions in research.

Improve clinical and hands-on skills by training with or observing other IBCLCs. The ready availability of teaching videos and webinars on the Internet allow any IBCLC, anywhere, to observe face-to-face care. One must decide (just as with written research) whether such material is valuable and current, but modern technology has widened opportunities for the practitioner to improve skills.

IBCLCs, as allied healthcare providers who assess breastfeeding dyads and draft care plans to address lactation issues, should carry professional liability (malpractice) insurance, no matter what their work setting or geopolitical location. Those who serve in dual professional roles (e.g., labor and delivery nurses who may sometimes work as dedicated IBCLCs at the same institution) should be certain that their professional liability insurance covers all types of clinical work. Those who hold down more than one position (e.g., birthing center IBCLC with a separate job as private practice IBCLC) must be certain that insurance covers activities in each role. Because the IBCLC is not a primary healthcare provider,[1] but operates as a member of the healthcare team, insurance rates are generally affordable all over the world. Insurance should be considered a non-negotiable cost of being a member of the profession, just as taking continuing education classes is a required cost for recertification.

---

[1] There are, of course, primary healthcare providers such as physicians or midwives who also have the IBCLC credential. But it is the "other hat" that makes them primary HCPs, not the "IBCLC hat."

2.4 Obey all applicable laws, including those regulating the activities of lactation consultants. (IBLCE, 2011e, CPC p. 3)

Obviously, everyone should take care to be law abiding citizens, no matter where they live or what profession they practice. This principle reminds the certificant that there are legal obligations that go along with the privilege of being certified as an IBCLC. Plainly put: The IBCLC must obey laws governing practice by IBCLCs or similar allied healthcare providers. The IBCLC must also adhere to the rules and policies in place at the work setting.

As a profession less than 30 years old, there are not many laws or regulations, in the geopolitical jurisdictions of the world, delineating as such an IBCLC's legal responsibilities. This will change; for example, efforts in the United States are underway to enact state-based licensure for IBCLCs. However, as IBCLCs can always be defined as "allied healthcare providers," any statutory or regulatory language defining responsibilities of the allied HCP may guide the IBCLC.

The IBCLC must follow whatever policies and procedures are in place at the work setting: this is a condition of employment. If those recommendations are based on outdated or non-evidence-based assumptions, the IBCLC is encouraged to bring his or her professional expertise to bear to get those policies updated to reflect current acceptable practice.

2.5 Respect intellectual property rights. (IBLCE, 2011e, CPC p. 3)

The IBCLC is required to respect intellectual property rights, a vast area of the law governing copyrights, trademarks and service marks, and patents. Laws to enforce and support the rights of the creators and inventors who have created intellectual property are fairly uniform around the world. IBCLCs will most often find copyright law is the type of intellectual property they will encounter in professional practice.

Materials do *not* have to show a copyright mark (©) to enjoy copyright protection under the law. Mere creation vests in the originator an immediate copyright, including the right to decide who else may reproduce, show or adapt the material. Thus, the IBCLC may *not* use materials created or developed by others (handouts, letters, articles, slides, presentations, photographs or drawings, graphs, etc.) unless there is specific permission granted first. This is true even if the IBCLC has no plans to sell the material, and even if the IBCLC plans to credit the originator (U.S. Copyright Office, 2011).

IBCLCs who are preparing scholarly works (research papers, or articles for publication in a peer-reviewed journal) may cite to sources, without prior permission, under the traditional conventions expected of such academic and professional writing. When offering education presentations that discuss another's work, the original author should be mentioned.

The Internet has greatly increased universal accessibility to material, but it has not diminished the requirement to respect copyright. An IBCLC may share a link to an article or abstract, but should not provide access to a full article unless first given permission by the author and/or publisher.

Seeking permission to use another person's materials does not require a special form or letter: a simple email or letter to the originator will suffice. Describe the material that is sought for re-use, and the conditions under which it will be shown and credited. Retain proof of the permission sought, and granted, to defend any challenge to use.

Principle 3

> Principle 3: Preserve the confidentiality of clients. Every IBCLC shall: (IBLCE, 2011e, CPC p. 3)

The third principle of the IBLCE CPC, expanded further into two required professional practice elements, defines the IBCLC's responsibility to the client/patient to respect her right of privacy. The word "shall" reminds the IBCLC that these are mandatory obligations of competent, ethical practice.

> 3.1 Refrain from revealing any information acquired in the course of the professional relationship, except to another member of a client's healthcare team, or to other persons or entities for which the client has granted express permission, except only as provided in the Definitions and Interpretations to the CPC. (IBLCE, 2011e, CPC p. 3)

This principle was stated in just two words under Tenet 6 of the old IBLCE COE ("Maintain confidentiality" [IBLCE, 2003b, COE p. 1]). The wordier Principle 3.1 pulls in, by reference, No. 5 of the Definitions and Interpretations of the IBLCE CPC, found at the beginning section of the document. When one considers that cumbersome language, the end result is this: the IBCLC will not reveal identifying information about a lactation consultation unless the client/patient permits it, or it is required as part of a court or legal proceeding.

Note that an IBCLC may, pursuant to Principle 2.2 (above), and without separate permission from mother, share information about a lactation consultation with other members of the healthcare team. This is part of the obligation of collaboration, so the family receives "unified and comprehensive care" (IBLCE, 2011e, CPC p. 3). IBLCE CPC Principle 4.1 (below), however, suggests that the mother *does* have to specifically agree to the sharing of her information with other HCPs.

Perhaps the easiest way to reconcile the conflicting language of Principles 2.2, 3.1, and 4.1 is for the IBCLC to take the most conservative route: before commencing any lactation consultation, be certain that the mother agrees (a) to be seen, and (b) to have information about her situation shared, as circumstances warrant, with her own or her baby's HCP.

Consent to be seen, and consent to share clinical information with other members of the healthcare team, are fairly standard forms routinely required of patients/clients.

Those forms also traditionally spell out the caregiver's responsibility to keep the patient/client's information confidential. In a hospital or clinic setting, such paperwork is customarily handled during admission or at the first appointment. The IBCLC who performs the lactation consultation will not need to obtain a second set of permissions, and will follow workplace requirements to record/chart the visit in a manner that prevents others from accidentally learning the details of that consult. However, IBCLCs in private practice or public health, who are the first to see a mother upon referral from another HCP, may need to build a chart from the bottom up (including a record of consents and promise to protect confidentiality).

Some laws will impose further privacy-protecting requirements on the IBCLC who practices within that jurisdiction. For example, "HIPAA" regulations in the United States require that mothers be given a Notice of Privacy Practices by the HCP, describing how her privacy is protected (Health Insurance Portability and Accountability Act of 1996). IBCLCs working in clinical settings should follow their institution's policies on confidentiality (e.g., refrain from using information that can identify the mother if speaking in public areas about a case).

Prior permission is not required, from the mother, for the IBCLC to discuss her case *in anonymous fashion* with colleagues who are not part of the healthcare team. Case studies are a valuable way to share learning with colleagues. The IBCLC must be cognizant to avoid using bits of information that may unwittingly identify the mother. For example, the IBCLC who practices in a small or remote area may find that saying "I worked with a mother of triplets" allows others to quickly detect the patient's identity, whereas the same description would maintain privacy if used at a large hospital, with a fertility clinic, and 5,000 births a year.

Particular care should be taken to avoid use of client/patient identification clues when sharing case studies on websites or conferences. Those settings are in the public domain, and the opportunity for the information to be repeated is increased. Do not share details that have even a remote chance of specifically identifying the mother and baby. The IBCLC may consider adding to any consent forms a section whereby the mother grants permission for anonymous sharing of clinical information with other HCPs, for educational purposes.

> 3.2 Refrain from photographing, recording, or taping (audio or video) a mother or her child for any purpose unless the mother has given advance written consent on her behalf and that of her child. (IBLCE, 2011e, CPC p. 3)

Principle 3.2 is more specific, and restrictive, than its counterpart Tenet 20 in the old IBLCE COE. Whereas the old IBLCE COE merely required "maternal consent" (including verbal assent), the new IBLCE CPC is clear that "advance written consent" must be obtained from a mother before the IBCLC may photograph or record her, or her child. Whereas the former ethics code required consent for use of images for "educational or professional purposes" (e.g., as part of a conference presentation), the advance written permission now required is necessary for "any purpose" (e.g., a photo taken to include only in the clinical record).

The IBCLC may consider adding a section to the consent-to-consult forms signed by the mother, whereby the mother grants permission for recordings of any kind to be used, under such conditions as she requires. The consent form should be signed and dated, and include a description (a handwritten notation being sufficient) of any limitations for recording use.

The IBCLC should also consider whether there are additional requirements or consents, imposed by her employer, for the making and later re-use of recordings. Some institutions will prohibit such images even if the mother fully consents, unless the institution's own permission guidelines are followed.

The ease of taking digital photographs and movies with handheld devices like phones does, however, present an opportunity for the IBCLC. One can document clinical conditions that are fleeting (such as skin color changes associated with vasospasm of the nipple), or record the improvements or healing due to the lactation care plan. The IBCLC should not avoid use of images; rather, simply keep a supply of consent forms available, for the mother to sign in accordance with the guidelines imposed by the IBCLC's workplace and the requirements of IBLCE CPC Principle 3.2.

Principle 4

> Principle 4: Report accurately and completely to other members of the healthcare team. Every IBCLC shall: (IBLCE, 2011e, CPC p. 3)

The fourth principle of the IBLCE CPC, expanded further into two required professional practice elements, describes the IBCLC's responsibility to share information about the lactation consultation other members of the family's healthcare team. The word "shall" reminds the IBCLC that these are mandatory obligations of competent, ethical practice.

> 4.1 Receive a client's consent, before initiating a consultation, to share clinical information with other members of the client's healthcare team. (IBLCE, 2011e, CPC p. 3)

Missing an opportunity to clarify similarly cloudy language at Tenet 23 of the old IBLCE COE, IBLCE's wording in CPC Principle 4.1 seems—at first glance—to require that the IBCLC obtain consent from the mother to have a lactation consultation. But a careful re-reading reveals that the client's consent is (merely) for the sharing of clinical concerns with the rest of the healthcare team. This seems to conflict with the language of IBLCE CPC Principle 2.2, which mandates that the IBCLC collaborate with other members of the healthcare team. The most elemental part of collaboration is sharing of information. It is hard to imagine a situation where a mother would refuse permission for a consult . . . and yet agree to have information about her situation shared with other HCPs. One can safely assume Principle 4.1 is a victim of poor draftsmanship, rather than a mandate to seek only partial consent from a mother.

Perhaps the easiest way to reconcile the conflicting language of Principles 2.2 and 4.1 is for the IBCLC to take the most conservative route: before commencing any lactation consultation, be certain that the mother agrees (a) to be seen, and (b) to have information about her situation shared, as circumstances warrant, with her own or her baby's HCP. While protecting the mother's privacy is not required when sharing information with other HCPs in the healthcare team (after all, they need to know about whom the IBCLC is communicating), the IBCLC should take care that the transmission of such information does not accidently allow outsiders to read the details of the consult or learn the mother's or baby's identification.

In certain rare and unusual circumstances, the mother may have legitimate reasons not to have her identifying information sent to a HCP. For example, if she and her children are at risk and under protection from domestic abuse or threats, the mother will not want a report with her address and phone number included in a report to the pediatrician, if the baby's father can (in his own right) access the pediatric file. The IBCLC should endeavor to speak to the HCP by phone or in person, to verbally describe the lactation assessment and care plan. The IBCLC will also describe in the lactation charting the reasons for offering a verbal rather than written report. The lactation chart is confidential as to both the mother and child.

> 4.2 Inform an appropriate person or authority if it appears that the health or safety of a client or a colleague is at risk, consistent with Principle 3. (IBLCE, 2011e, CPC p. 3)

IBLCE CPC Principle 4.2 corrects and clarifies language omissions in the corollary Tenet 15 of the old IBLCE COE. It is now very clear: when the health and safety of *either* the patient/mother *or* an IBCLC colleague is at risk, one should *inform* "an appropriate person or authority." The earlier ethical code was written such that only the colleague's status was of concern, and further required that a "report" be made. The wording offered by the new IBLCE CPC Principle 4.2 suggests that less formal (and probably earlier) intervention can be made, by informing appropriate superiors. Disclosing the identity of the mother and baby should be avoided, as circumstances warrant, when information is shared with authorities outside the clinical care team.

These admonitions do not have much to do with the overarching concept of Principle 4 (to make accurate and complete reports to the members of the family's healthcare team). Indeed, any reporting here is to administrators or authorities whose responsibility is to oversee the IBCLC, not the breastfeeding family. Nonetheless, while perhaps curiously placed here within the IBLCE CPC, the notions underlying Principle 4.2 are sound.

An IBCLC has a responsibility to look out for mothers and children, and for the profession at large. An IBCLC who is practicing under conditions where health, safety or professional judgment is at risk cannot provide competent, ethical care. One's personal reputation is endangered, as is the reputation of the field of lactation consultancy. When other IBCLCs become aware of, or suspect, such professional liabilities in a colleague, they should share their concerns with the lactation consultant's supervisor or administrator, to trigger appropriate remedial and mitigating measures.

An IBCLC may be unable to professionally and ethically perform his or her duties for any number of reasons: substance abuse, clinical depression or anxiety, personal family crises detracting from concentration, and so on. Sometimes the situation is transitory (e.g., the time period to recover from a mild communicable disease). Regardless, a breastfeeding mother and child are entitled to committed and compassionate attention, and should expect that their IBCLC comes to them able to fulfill all professional responsibilities. Any member of the profession who is aware that a colleague cannot meet those responsibilities should not attempt to "fix it" singlehandedly, but should seek the guidance of appropriate supervisors or authorities.

Principle 5

> Principle 5: Exercise independent judgment and avoid conflicts of interest. Every IBCLC shall: (IBLCE, 2011e, CPC p. 3)

The fifth principle of the IBLCE CPC, expanded further into three required professional practice elements, describes the IBCLC's responsibility to use independent clinical judgment in providing lactation care, and to avoid conflicts of interest that can blur the motives of the IBCLC's clinical assessment. The word "shall" reminds the IBCLC that these are mandatory obligations of competent, ethical practice.

> 5.1 Disclose any actual or apparent conflict of interest, including a financial interest in relevant goods or services, or in organizations which provide relevant goods or services. (IBLCE, 2011e, CPC p. 3)

It is easy to declare that a conflict of interest is something to be avoided; it is harder for the practitioner to know how to spot one. The good news is that full and prior disclosure of the details, and consent from the parties involved, will almost always cure a conflict of interest.

Generally speaking, a conflict of interest arises when the IBCLC is in the position to be perceived as looking out for his or her own interests, rather than those of the patient/client. An example: A mother is being advised to rent a breast pump, to bring in her milk supply for her premature twins. The IBCLC has a pump rental business, in addition to her work as an IBCLC in the neonatal intensive care unit. A conflict of interest arises when the IBCLC steers the mother to her pump rental business, since the IBCLC will make money from the rental. However, to cure the conflict, the mother can be offered a range of pump rental options, including even the IBCLC's pump rental location. In this way, the mother's business is no longer being steered solely to the IBCLC.

An IBCLC who works in a hospital or birth center, and who also has a private practice or retail operation as a second venture, does not—by virtue of this two-job arrangement alone—have a conflict of interest. If the IBCLC had a second job as a car mechanic, few would claim a "conflict of interest." A conflict of interest arises only when the IBCLC in one job is seen to steer work or customers to herself in the second job. To avoid this, referral choices or lists of community resources should include all the available options. It is wise to include websites or toll-free phone numbers for various product manufacturers, as their retail outlets change frequently. The IBCLC can, and should, disclose her own place on the information sheet, taking care not to disparage the other listings or draw undue favorable attention to herself. The decision of where to bring her custom rests with the mother.

An IBCLC should disclose any stipend, honorarium, sponsorship or grant received from any organization or commercial entity in the course of professional work. For example, if the IBCLC speaks at a conference, and her honorarium was paid by the manufacturer of maternity clothing, this fact should be openly disclosed to the conference attendees. Similarly, any research that is funded by a commercial interest should be disclosed when the findings are written and reported.

5.2 Ensure that commercial considerations do not influence professional judgment. (IBLCE, 2011e, CPC p. 3)

Principle 5.2 is similar to 5.1: it requires the IBCLC to use professional behaviors motivated by a desire to provide evidence-based information and support to a breastfeeding family, and not by personal financial gain. Principle 5.1 requires the IBCLC to disclose up front any financial relationship with an organization; Principle 5.2 mandates that the IBCLC also avoid "pushing sales" after the requisite full disclosure.

An IBCLC can, and should, talk about the use of breastfeeding equipment and supplies with a mother. Their brand names, prices, advantages and disadvantages must all be discussed, so the mother can make a fully informed decision about the care plan that will work best for her, given her circumstances. The IBCLC should be certain the mother is aware that this discussion of products is a necessary element in devising her care plan, and not because the IBCLC has a retail interest in the outcome of the consultation. The mother can choose to purchase equipment from the IBCLC; it may well be that convenience or price or availability makes that the best decision, for the mother. She should, however, make that decision from the standpoint of a savvy and well-informed consumer, and not because of pressure from the IBCLC.

5.3 Withdraw voluntarily from professional practice if the IBCLC has a physical or mental disability that could be detrimental to clients. (IBLCE, 2011e, CPC p. 4)

This requirement is similar to Principle 4.2, above, concerning the IBCLC whose behaviors put herself or her clients/patients at risk, and Principle 6.2, below, concerning the IBCLC who is engaged in substance abuse. Principle 5.3 requires that any IBCLC with a disability that will prevent competent and ethical practice, resulting in harm (detriment) to the mother, should withdraw voluntarily from professional practice. The corollary in the old IBLCE COE, Tenet 19, focused more on causality: the IBCLC suffering from untreated substance abuse or mental incompetence who might bring harm to a client/patient. The language of the new IBLCE CPC Principle 5.3 looks less to the cause and more to the undesired result of harm (detriment) to the breastfeeding dyad.

Like Principle 4.2, Principle 5.3 also seems oddly placed. It is part of Principle 5 (about avoidance of conflict of interest and exercise of independent judgment). But like Principle 4.2, the notion underlying Principle 5.3 is certainly sound, despite its curious home in this portion of the IBLCE CPC: Any IBCLC who cannot offer appropriate clinical care should step back from hands-on consultation.

Principle 5.3 appears to address the IBCLC whose condition is incapacitating; as such, withdrawal from "professional practice" is warranted. The IBCLC impaired by substance abuse shall also "withdraw" from professional practice (see Principle 6.2, below). It is not clear if, by "withdraw," IBLCE intends that the IBCLC shall forfeit her credential, or simply temporarily cease clinical interactions. One explanation of old IBLCE COE Tenet 19 suggested that "voluntary surrender of the credential will cause [IBLCE] to look favorably upon resumption of its use once the disability has been ameliorated" (Scott & Calandro, 2008, p. 14). Presumably a similar interpretation would be made under the new IBLCE CPC. Principle 5.3 appears intended to cover all other situations that can give rise to harm or detriment to a mother and baby.

Principle 4.2 (above) encourages the IBCLC to "inform" superiors or authorities if an IBCLC-colleague may be putting herself, her colleagues, or clients/patients, at risk. Guidance and intervention from others is deemed necessary to help remedy the situation. Principles 5.3 and 6.2 place the responsibility on the affected IBCLC to initiate her own "withdrawal" from professional practice.

Principle 6

Principle 6: Maintain personal integrity. Every IBCLC shall: (IBLCE, 2011e, CPC p. 4)

The sixth principle of the IBLCE CPC governs the personal integrity of the certificant, and is expanded further into three required professional practice elements. The word "shall" reminds the IBCLC that these are mandatory obligations of competent, ethical practice.

6.1 Behave honestly and fairly as a health professional. (IBLCE, 2011e, CPC p. 4)

This principle describes the simple notion that IBCLCs must be fair and honest in their professional practice. IBCLCs should abide by their word and use best efforts to serve patients/clients who come under their care. If a mother has been promised follow-up care, make certain it happens, or explain why it cannot. If resources or information have been promised to an HCP, make certain it happens, or explain why it cannot. Provide evidence-based information so the mother can make a fully informed decision about lactation care for herself and her family; equably support her decision even if the IBCLC might have wished for a different course of action. A fair fee should be charged for services rendered, in keeping with community standards and regulations for reimbursement.

Spending focused and caring time with the client/patient in the IBCLC's care may offer the most honest and fair professional service an IBCLC can provide. Resolving lactation issues may require some detective work, and assessment of the mother will be more accurate when she feels trust in her IBCLC. Accurate assessment of a feed necessarily requires the IBCLC to be there at the start, middle and finish of the baby's time at breast. These professional behaviors will offer the client/patient a truly honest, and fair, consultation.

> 6.2 Withdraw voluntarily from professional practice if the IBCLC has engaged in substance abuse that could affect the IBCLC's practice. (IBLCE, 2011e, CPC p. 4)

Principle 6.2 requires the IBCLC who is impaired by addiction or substance abuse to withdraw from professional practice. Principle 5.3 (above) similarly requires the IBCLC to initiate self-withdrawal from professional practice if disability would be detrimental to or harm clients/patients. Compare to Principle 4.2 (above) where an IBCLC is required to seek the guidance and intervention of a supervisor or other authority if an IBCLC colleague could risk the health and safety of self, or others. Colleagues might need to help an IBCLC realize that she is breaching IBLCE CPC Principle 6.2 because of substance abuse that impairs professional capacity. As discussed above at Principle 5.3, it is not clear if, by "withdraw," IBLCE intends that the IBCLC shall forfeit her credential, or simply temporarily cease clinical interactions.

> 6.3 Treat all clients equitably without regard to age, ethnicity, national origin, marital status, religion, or sexual orientation. (IBLCE, 2011e, CPC p. 4)

The IBCLC should treat all families fairly and equally, harboring no ill will or prejudice based on the characteristics or circumstances of the client/patient. The same skilled level of care will be given to all mothers seen by the IBCLC, no matter the personal beliefs or tastes of the IBCLC. The IBCLC may be required to learn about unfamiliar traditions and customs in order to understand the mother's goals and needs.

If the IBCLC realizes that personally held beliefs make it difficult to provide competent, dispassionate care, every effort should be made to refer the mother to another colleague. The personal reasons prompting the referral should not be shared with the mother; she simply may be told, "It is not possible right now for me to provide the lactation consultation services you require, but I will find a colleague who can see you."

Principle 7

Principle 7: Uphold the professional standards expected of an IBCLC. Every IBCLC shall: (IBLCE, 2011e, CPC p. 4)

The seventh principle of the IBLCE CPC describes the professional standards an IBCLC is expected to uphold, and is expanded further into four required practice elements. The word "shall" reminds the IBCLC that these are mandatory obligations of competent, ethical practice. The entire IBLCE CPC purports to mandate ethical and professional behaviors. Principle 7 focuses on how the IBCLC presents herself as a credentialed member of the profession at large; Principles 1–6 look more to individual professional behaviors in the clinical context.

7.1 Operate within the framework defined by the CPC. (IBLCE, 2011e, CPC p. 4)

Principle 7.1 simply means that every IBCLC is expected to use professional behaviors that conform with those described in the IBLCE CPC.

7.2 Provide only accurate information to the public and colleagues concerning lactation consultant services offered. (IBLCE, 2011e, CPC p. 4)

Any advertising or marketing of IBCLC services will accurately and honestly describe what a lactation consultation involves: how fees, payment or reimbursement are handled; the IBCLC's obligation to share clinical concerns with other HCPs; the protection of privacy; the mother's role in devising and implementing a care plan; how follow-up is handled.

It is impossible for the IBCLC to promise a particular breastfeeding outcome. The variables in any lactation situation are simply too many. The mother may find, much to her dismay, that she cannot provide every feed at breast until the child self-weans. The IBCLC can promise to provide evidence-based information and support, so the mother can adjust to the reality of her situation, whatever it might be. The IBCLC can promise to deliver professional services in a responsive, efficient and ethical manner.

It is ethical and desirable for IBCLC services to be marketed. Private practitioners can distribute brochures and business cards. Hospitals can advertise that they have IBCLCs, dedicated to providing care to breastfeeding mothers. Physician offices can let patients know that IBCLCs on staff are available for pre- and postnatal consultations. The breastfeeding advocate's customary concern about "marketing" has only to do with unethical marketing of the product types covered by the International Code. IBCLCs sell health care, not products. It is important that members of the public at large know how and where to access IBCLC services in the community.

7.3 Permit use of the IBCLC's name for the purpose of certifying that lactation consultant services have been rendered only when the IBCLC provided those services. (IBLCE, 2011e, CPC p. 4)

If a mother expects that she will be seen by an IBCLC, then it is an IBCLC who is responsible for the consultation. An IBCLC may work with or supervise other breastfeeding helpers. Indeed, mother-to-mother counselors are the backbone of most community-based breastfeeding support around the world. The patient/client must always have a clear understanding of who is offering support, and the limitations of care a non-IBCLC can provide. Often, it is not necessary for the mother to be seen by an IBCLC, an allied healthcare provider. She may find that a conversation with a compassionate breastfeeding counselor about her baby's common breastfeeding behaviors is just the reassurance she needed. However, the mother should not be led to think a non-credentialed person is an IBCLC. And, in a similar vein, HCPs or third-party reimbursement agencies should be informed that the dyad was seen by an IBCLC only if that was the case.

IBCLCs may be serving as mentors, helping to train and educate those who are in active pursuit of requirements to become an IBCLC. As time progresses, those students will operate with diminishing "over the shoulder" supervision. These clinical training arrangements are a perfectly acceptable and ethical means to educate new entrants into the field. The mother should always be informed that part (or nearly all) of her consult is being spent with a student. Note that the supervising IBCLC will always have to "sign off on" whatever assessments, clinical contacts, and care plans are devised by the student. The mother thus will always have an IBCLC ultimately accountable for the consult.

7.4 Use the acronyms "IBCLC" and "RLC" or the titles "International Board Certified Lactation Consultant" and "Registered Lactation Consultant" only when certification is current and in the manner in which IBLCE authorizes their use. (IBLCE, 2011e, CPC p. 4)

All of the terms inside quotation marks in Principle 7.4 are registered certification marks of IBLCE (IBLCE, 2003c, 1997 [renewed 2007]). IBLCE thus controls the manner in which one may have the privilege of using "IBCLC" or its variants when describing his or her professional qualifications. Note that only actively certified IBCLCs may use such a designation.

Aspiring IBCLCs, or retired IBCLCs, may *not* use the acronym or descriptors "IBCLC," "RLC," "International Board Certified Lactation Consultant," or "Registered Lactation Consultant." Continuing to represent oneself as an IBCLC when such certification has lapsed, or allowing oneself to be so described by others, is a breach not only of the IBLCE CPC but of the trademark protections afforded to IBLCE for the registered acronyms and phrases.

Use of terms such as "IBCLC candidate" or "Student IBCLC" are potentially misleading to the public. As cumbersome as it may be, the student is advised to use a generic descriptor such as "student lactation consultant" or "applicant for the certification exam administered by IBLCE."

Principle 8

> Principle 8: Comply with the IBLCE Disciplinary Procedures. Every IBCLC shall: (IBLCE, 2011e, CPC p. 4)

The eighth and last principle of the IBLCE CPC governs the disciplinary procedures which are intended to enforce the IBLCE CPC, and by extension the health, safety, and welfare of the public at large. It is expanded further into five required professional practice elements. The word "shall" reminds the IBCLC that these are mandatory obligations of competent, ethical practice.

> 8.1 Comply fully with the IBLCE Ethics & Discipline process. (IBLCE, 2011e, CPC p. 4)

The IBCLC must submit to the jurisdiction of IBLCE, and the disciplinary procedures they have established to enforce the IBLCE CPC, as a condition of IBCLC certification (Brooks, Stehel, & Mannel, 2013; IBLCE, 2011c). The IBLCE CPC is enforced through the IBLCE Ethics & Discipline Committee, composed of a subset of members of the Board of Directors for IBLCE.

The IBCLC is advised to become familiar with the procedures set out in the IBLCE Disciplinary Procedures. The entire document underwent substantial and substantive revision, and was made effective November 1, 2011. IBLCE's explanation for the overhaul is simply that "it is a best practice to periodically review policies and procedures. IBLCE reviewed its procedures with respect to ethics complaints and elected to streamline the same" (IBLCE, 2011d, p. 2). Streamlining was indeed accomplished; the earlier disciplinary procedures were described in 52 pages; the new ones are described in 5.

It goes without saying: the IBLCE CPC expects all IBCLCs to practice ethically and professionally, and never find themselves the subject of a complaint. Yet, complaints that are unfounded and even spurious can still be filed. The accused will find that his or her due process rights at IBLCE are dramatically truncated under the streamlined procedures.

The old "IBLCE Disciplinary Procedures" (IBLCE, 2010b) set out at Section XIX a detailed process for how a case would proceed involving an IBCLC against whom a complaint was initially determined to have merit. It described a formal administrative hearing, including the accused's right to counsel, and an opportunity to hear and cross-examine witnesses, even though the formalities of trial evidence were not required. A record was to be kept (presumably in case of an appeal). It was all done under oath. It was a thorough (though by necessity lengthy) description of a hearing, designed to protect the rights of the accused while permitting examination of allegations of misconduct.

The new "Disciplinary Procedures for the Code of Professional Conduct for IBCLCs for the International Board of Lactation Consultant Examiners (IBLCE)" (IBLCE, 2011c) have retreated from this process, significantly. Sections III and V give the Chair of the IBLCE Ethics & Discipline Committee "sole discretion" to determine if a complaint that comes into the IBLCE is frivolous or invalid. Thus, one person is the gatekeeper for all procedures that are to follow. "Sole discretion" is powerful under the law, allowing decisions to be made without explanation or justification to outsiders. If a complaint is deemed to have merit, the accused will be sent a summary of the complaint; there is no guarantee of receiving the original complaint, in full. It is unclear if the accused is informed, initially, who filed the complaint. The accused has thirty days to respond (IBLCE, 2011c).

A three-member Review Subcommittee of the IBLCE Ethics & Discipline Committee is then appointed to "clarify, expand or corroborate the information provided by the submitter" (IBLCE, 2011c, p. 2). It is unclear if the "submitter" is the original complainant who submitted a complaint, or the accused who submitted a response in the 30-day window. "The Review Subcommittee may be assisted in the conduct of its investigation by the IBLCE staff or legal counsel" (IBLCE, 2011c, p. 3). No right to counsel is assured to the accused.

The Review Subcommittee or staff "may at its discretion contact such other individuals who may have knowledge of the facts and circumstances surrounding the complaint" (IBLCE, 2011c, p. 3). Such self-initiated investigation, by the body that is expected to ultimately and fairly adjudicate the matter, is extraordinary. Customarily, the parties to an action (here, the complainant and the accused) are asked to present their own witnesses, evidence, or explanations. The "judges," who are meant to decide the case after weighing the evidence, do not commence investigation on their own. The 2011 IBLCE Disciplinary Procedures invite legitimate inquiry into the objectivity of the adjudicators, and whether rudimentary due process is being afforded to the accused, especially since the right to counsel (permitted under the old [2010] IBLCE Disciplinary Procedures) is nowhere guaranteed in the new [2011] IBLCE Disciplinary Procedures. IBLCE, however, maintains that the [2011] disciplinary procedures comport with due process and conflict of interest considerations, and that the CPC, the [2011] Disciplinary Procedures, and the FAQs [IBLCE, 2011d] have been reviewed and streamlined (IBLCE, 2011d).

The Review Subcommittee makes a finding, and recommendation of sanction, which it presents to a larger IBLCE Ethics & Discipline Panel, again composed of members of the IBLCE Board of Directors. "There is no formal hearing or trial-type proceeding, no hearing or witnesses, and the rules of evidence are not applicable. The Panel may at its discretion permit an informal oral statement to be made by the [accused] by conference call. Legal counsel is not expected to participate in the process, unless requested by the [accused] and approved by the Ethics & Disciplinary

Panel. IBLCE and the Ethics & Disciplinary Panel may consult IBLCE legal counsel" (IBLCE, 2011c, p. 3). Thus, the accused must first seek permission to be represented by counsel, in a disciplinary matter, while the adjudicators have counsel available to them throughout the process. IBLCE does not explain why it feels the Panel requires legal counsel, when the accused is guaranteed no such right, and the document is entirely silent on whether the complainant should be advised by counsel.

All disciplinary investigations and deliberations are conducted in confidence, and the record is sealed. If the Panel finds that there has been a violation of the IBLCE CPC, a range of sanctions may be imposed, from a private reprimand up to and including revocation of certification. Appeal is allowed on only two grounds: material errors of fact, and failure by the IBLCE Ethics & Discipline Panel to follow its procedures (IBLCE, 2011c, pp. 4–5). "The appeal shall not include a hearing or any other similar trial-type proceeding. [L]egal counsel is not expected to participate in the appeal process, unless requested by the appellant and approved by the Appeal Board. IBLCE and the Appeal Board may consult IBLCE legal counsel" (IBLCE, 2011c, p. 5).

To summarize, any disciplinary actions considered by IBLCE after November 1, 2011, to enforce the IBLCE CPC, are conducted as follows: Nothing under oath. No right to face the accuser. No right to see the original complaint. All investigatory proceedings conducted in private, and in confidence, without the accused there. Investigations may be conducted sui generis by those serving in an adjudicatory capacity. Accused must receive permission before being allowed to seek advice from a lawyer, while IBLCE has legal counsel assured throughout and the complainant's use of a lawyer is not mentioned at all. Appeal is allowed only for procedural errors or material errors of fact, yet the record containing the facts alleged and investigated is under seal.

> 8.2 Agree that a violation of this CPC includes any matter in which: (IBLCE, 2011e, CPC p. 4)

Principle 8.2 asserts that an IBCLC agrees that a violation of the IBLCE CPC is automatically triggered if any of the three subsections (8.2.1, 8.2.2, or 8.2.3) apply as to an IBCLC certificant. But that begs the question: if the IBCLC "agrees" that one of the Principle 8.2 subsections applies, which means there has been a violation of the IBLCE CPC, then what shall the IBCLC now do with this information? There is no obligation for the IBCLC to report this to IBLCE.

The IBLCE CPC departs dramatically from the IBLCE COE in that it no longer requires an IBCLC to report violations (by self, or other certificants) of the ethical precepts mandated by the IBLCE CPC. Tenet 22 under the old IBLCE COE required every IBCLC to "report alleged violations of the [COE]" in an effort to "protect society and the profession" by triggering an investigation under the IBLCE disciplinary process (IBLCE, 2003b, COE p. 2). The closest corollary under the new IBLCE CPC is in the Definitions and Interpretation section, and in Principle 8.1, where IBCLCs are told they must "comply fully" with the IBLCE Disciplinary Procedures (see Table

3-2). Missing now is the former and corresponding obligation for IBCLC certificants, perhaps the best equipped persons to recognize lapses in IBCLC professional ethical practice, to initiate a disciplinary action in the very adjudicatory body designated to enforce professional ethical practice.

> 8.2.1 the IBCLC is convicted of a crime under applicable law, where dishonesty, gross neglect or wrongful conduct in relation to the practice of lactation consulting is a core issue; (IBLCE, 2011e, CPC p. 4)

Criminal convictions occur when someone has been arrested for breaking the law, is prosecuted by the government, and found guilty. Civil lawsuits (i.e., in tort, the basis for most lawsuits against HCPs) seek redress for civil (or noncriminal) wrongs. An IBCLC may become involved as a defendant, in a criminal court proceeding (which is, of course, outside of IBLCE jurisdiction), and involving some aspect of his or her work as an IBCLC. If the IBCLC is accused and found guilty of a crime that includes (1) dishonesty (e.g., lying), (2) gross negligence (the IBCLC's conscious and voluntary disregard for reasonable care caused injury), or (3) wrongful conduct (the IBCLC's actions caused injury), then the conviction is prima facie evidence that the IBCLC also violated the IBLCE CPC.

The criminal matter must involve an examination of the IBCLC's work and responsibilities in order to trigger an automatic IBLCE CPC violation. "Crimes" refer only to matters prosecuted by the government, in a criminal trial. The IBCLC would be the defendant in such a case. If a defendant is found guilty, sanctions can include jail, probation, or fines. To compare, a civil lawsuit involves two parties, and may involve all sorts of matters in dispute: contracts, torts, trusts and estates, etc.

> 8.2.2 the IBCLC is disciplined by a state, province or other level of government and at least one of the grounds for discipline is the same as, or substantially equivalent to, this CPC's principle; (IBLCE, 2011e, CPC p. 4)

Principle 8.2.2 seems to be missing something, and defies extrapolation. It starts out on a promising note: it mentions a disciplinary proceeding. Since Principle 8.2.1 describes the limited circumstances in which an IBCLC is the subject of a *criminal* trial involving IBCLC work, it seems logical that Principle 8.2.2 would follow with a discussion of IBCLC liability found under a *civil proceeding*. But the critical language confusingly mentions, instead, "grounds for discipline [the] same as, or substantially equivalent to, this CPC's principle" (IBLCE, 2011e, CPC p. 4). "This CPC" means "this Code of Professional Conduct." Yet the CPC has 8 broad principles, expanded further into 28 articulated subsections. There is no way of knowing which of them is "this CPC's principle." Until there is cause for IBLCE to explain the meaning and intent of Principle 8.2.2, it is any IBCLC's guess as to whether an adjudication, brought by a "state, provincial or other level of government," gives rise to an automatic violation of the IBLCE CPC.

8.2.3 a competent court, licensing board, certifying board or governmental authority determines that the IBCLC has committed an act of misfeasance or malfeasance directly related to the practice of lactation consulting. (IBLCE, 2011e, CPC p. 4)

Principle 8.2.3 describes a noncriminal proceeding where a certificant is examined about his or her professional activities as an IBCLC. If the IBCLC is found, in the course of professional practice, to have committed the intentional torts of misfeasance or malfeasance (see Definitions and Interpretations 6), then a violation of the IBLCE CPC is automatically triggered.

An example of a noncriminal proceeding is a case heard by a licensing agency, in those jurisdictions where an IBCLC is required to have a license to practice as an allied healthcare provider. Or, the IBCLC may work in a special jurisdictional region, subject to the laws and procedures established for those locations (e.g., military bases and facilities, or lands reserved by treaty or law to the control of certain peoples).

The IBLCE Scope of Practice: A "Must"

All IBCLCs everywhere must practice within the confines of the IBLCE Scope of Practice for IBCLCs (IBLCE SOP, 2008). The current version was adopted in March 2008, and defines the fences or boundaries within which an IBCLC may (indeed, has a *duty*) to practice. Like that little word "shall" used in the IBLCE CPC, "duty" carries with it, in traditional legal analysis, a powerful responsibility. It means:

A human action which is exactly conformable to the laws which require us to obey them. Legal or moral obligation. Obligatory conduct or service. Mandatory obligation to perform. (Duty, 1979, p. 453)

Thus, for the first time, IBCLC clinical responsibilities (duties) are described in the IBLCE SOP in proactive terms. Rather than offering an inventory of subject matters the IBCLC is expected to master prior to taking the IBCLC certification exam,[2] the IBLCE SOP now describes what the IBCLC is expected and authorized to do with all that lactation-related knowledge. For the IBCLC whose role and responsibilities are often unclear to her HCP colleagues or administrators, the IBLCE SOP is succinct and powerful proof of the skills and expertise an IBCLC can bring to bear in a clinical setting.

---

[2] In 1999, ILCA published *The International Board Certified Lactation Consultant: Scope of Practice and Education Guidelines*. This lengthy document was developed by the Professional Education Council, a group of lactation educators that at the time took on special projects for ILCA. Much of what appeared in this document was later broken into three stand-alone publications: (1) the *ILCA Standards of Practice*, (2) the *Clinical Competencies for IBCLC Practice*, and (3) the *IBLCE Competency Statements for IBCLC Practice*. Despite the existence of the 1999 ILCA document, the professional conduct of IBCLCs had primarily been guided by the *IBLCE Code of Ethics* and the *ILCA Standards of Practice* (Barger et al., 2007) until the 2008 version of the IBLCE SOP was enacted.

Preamble

International Board Certified Lactation Consultants (IBCLCs) have demonstrated specialized knowledge and clinical expertise in breastfeeding and human lactation and are certified by the International Board of Lactation Consultant Examiners (IBLCE).

This Scope of Practice encompasses the activities for which IBCLCs are educated and in which they are authorized to engage. The aim of the Scope of Practice is to protect the public by ensuring that all IBCLCs provide safe, competent, and evidence-based care. As this is an international credential, the Scope of Practice is applicable in any country or setting where IBCLCs practice. (IBLCE, 2008, SOP paras. 1 & 2)

These two introductory paragraphs actually pack a legal wallop. They identify the IBCLC as having special knowledge in lactation, and explain that this scope of practice defines her boundaries of clinical practice. Like scopes of practice for licensed HCPs, this IBLCE SOP has the overriding goal to protect public health and safety. And, it is international in scope.

That seems fairly boring and straightforward, but recall the discussions in earlier chapters that scopes of practice are customarily tied to licensure, which is customarily issued by authorities with very limited geographical reach. This IBLCE SOP provides validation to any IBCLC who is challenged on her right, as a member of the healthcare team, to assess and care for the breastfeeding dyad. Many IBCLCs in the 21st century still find their independent authority being questioned in the workplace, and these two paragraphs go a long way to stilling those doubting voices.

The IBLCE SOP enumerates six major duties that all IBCLCs, everywhere, must fulfill. We'll explore each in detail.

Duty to Uphold the Standards of the IBCLC Profession

IBCLCs have the duty to uphold the standards of the IBCLC profession by:

- Working within the framework defined by the IBLCE Code of Ethics, the Clinical Competencies for IBCLC Practice, and the International Lactation Consultant Association (ILCA) Standards of Practice for IBCLCs
- Integrating knowledge and evidence when providing care for breastfeeding families from the disciplines defined in the IBLCE Exam Blueprint
- Working within the legal framework of the respective geopolitical regions or settings
- Maintaining knowledge and skills through regular continuing education (IBLCE, 2008, para. 3)

This duty pulls in a description of the various sources of authority governing an IBCLC's practice. It whizzes by so fast, especially coming right after those first two legally powerful paragraphs, that the significance of this duty can be underappreciated. So let us savor what is being described: the IBCLC upholds the high standards of the only allied healthcare profession specializing in breastfeeding and human lactation because her practice is guided by:

- The mandatory IBLCE Code of Ethics, superseded by the mandatory IBLCE Code of Professional Conduct. Note that the IBLCE SOP was issued in 2008; the IBLCE CPC was issued in 2011. Thus, the IBLCE SOP refers to the predecessor document on ethical practice, the IBLCE COE. As explained above, the IBLCE CPC, like the IBLCE COE, is administered by IBLCE to "protect the health, welfare and safety of the public by providing the internationally recognized measure of knowledge in lactation and breastfeeding care through the IBLCE exam" (IBLCE, 2011e, CPC p. 1). And, the IBLCE CPC offers an enforcement mechanism via the IBLCE Ethics & Discipline Committee.
- The IBLCE Exam Blueprint, an "indication of the breadth of information" one must master for the certification exam (IBLCE, 2011b, para. 1), covering 13 disciplines and 12 chronological parameters.
- The voluntary ILCA Standards of Practice, "stated measures or levels of quality that are models for the conduct and evaluation of practice" (ILCA, 2006, para. 3).
- The Clinical Competencies for IBCLC Practice, described originally as a "checklist [of] the clinical/practice skills that an entry level IBCLC needs in order to be satisfactorily proficient to provide safe and effective care for breastfeeding mothers and babies" (IBLCE, 2003a, p. 1). In 2010 the document was revised by IBLCE, and slightly re-named as *Clinical Competencies for the Practice of IBCLCs* (IBLCE CC). It now describes actions that "encompass the responsibilities/activities that are part of the IBCLC's practice [and] to inform the public of the field in which IBCLCs can provide safe, competent and evidence-based care" (IBLCE, 2010c, p. 1).[3]

---

[3] The 2010 IBLCE CC document was reconfigured to replace the 2003 look, which read like a syllabus for an entry-level didactic and clinical course on breastfeeding and human lactation. The 2010 IBLCE CC reads more like an expanded (to 76 points) scope of practice, using "duty" language that echoes that of IBLCE SOP.

This is confusing, to be sure. Which is the "real" IBLCE SOP, the 2008 one that is titled as such, or this 2010 document that has all the same language of the original, plus a whole lot more? Adding to the confusion is language in the 2010 IBLCE CC that asks IBCLCs to "report immediately to IBLCE any IBCLC who is functioning outside" the IBLCE SOP, the IBLCE COE, and the IBLCE CC (IBLCE, 2010c, p. 4). The cavalier use of that legally laden term "duty," and allusions to the IBLCE discipline process, appear here in the 2010 IBLCE CC for the first time, with no explanation from IBLCE as to why.

Thus, we are left to wonder what prompted these linguistic changes. While the 2010 IBLCE CC is not a stellar example of draftsmanship, it is probably safe to assume that the intent of IBLCE was not to replace the IBLCE SOP, but rather simply to make the IBLCE CC language simpatico with it. That makes a certain amount of stylistic sense. IBCLCs should hope that is the case: the legal and ethical ramifications of having an IBLCE-drafted document, in which a 76-point set of required "duties" is now thrust upon all IBCLCs, everywhere, presents enforcement problems of staggering proportion.

- Retaining and improving her knowledge through regular continuing education.
- The "legal framework" of her location, a catchall encompassing laws, regulations, and institutional policies in the IBCLC's work setting. It simply means: IBCLCs have to follow the rules of the place where they work. Despite international certification demonstrating IBCLCs are all educated and trained in the same lactation-related subjects, we work in vastly different settings. Policies and procedures for IBCLCs can differ in hospitals that are across the street from one another. An example is IBCLCs who are being thwarted in their ability, at the birthing hospitals where they work, to discuss ankyloglossia or hormonal contraception with breastfeeding mothers (Noel-Weiss & Walters, 2006). This duty in the IBLCE SOP is a simple reminder that "it is what it is" for the practitioner in her workplace, and she must operate within the parameters that are her conditions of employment. Of course, this does not prevent the IBCLC from seeking to change policies by educating her peers and superiors. But until that can be accomplished, the IBCLC is obliged to work "within the legal framework of the respective geopolitical regions or settings."

Duty to Protect, Promote, and Support Breastfeeding

IBCLCs have the duty to protect, promote and support breastfeeding by:

- Educating women, families, health professionals, and the community about breastfeeding and human lactation
- Facilitating the development of policies which protect, promote, and support breastfeeding
- Acting as an advocate for breastfeeding as the child-feeding norm
- Providing holistic, evidence-based breastfeeding support and care, from preconception to weaning, for women and their families
- Using principles of adult education when teaching clients, health care providers, and others in the community
- Complying with the International Code of Marketing of Breast-milk Substitutes and subsequent relevant World Health Assembly resolutions (IBLCE, 2008, SOP para. 4)

The obligations described in this paragraph summarize the responsibilities defined for the IBCLC. Breastfeeding advocacy is given a wide-ranging definition: from preconception to weaning; for everyone from mothers on up to the community at large. Bullet points one and two provide authority for the IBCLC, working in a facility that needs improvements in its breastfeeding support, to educate her colleagues and to seek substantive policy changes. Of course, diplomacy, hard work, and a lot of research-based suggestions will be required of the IBCLC seeking to suggest institutional change, but if she runs into procedural flak, she can suggest that "my scope of practice imposes a duty that I take very seriously to educate my health professional colleagues about breastfeeding and human lactation, since it affects practice areas outside my own."

Bullet point three is salient to the IBCLC who may live in a culture or setting that assumes bottle feeding as the norm. Many seemingly innocuous messages that undermine breastfeeding lurk in our workplace or community: An oversized baby bottle used as a coin bank, to collect donations for a baby-benefitting charity; an ad for a daddy playgroup in the community newsletter, showing father lovingly giving a baby a bottle. Some grandparents or even healthcare co-workers show contempt for the evidence against use of pacifiers or bottles and teats during the early days, as a risk for early weaning (ILCA, Overfield, Ryan, Spangler, & Tully, 2005), saying that "one bottle won't hurt." If eye rolling ensues when the IBCLC begins her teaching, citing this portion of this duty may diffuse those who mistake the IBCLC message as a personal agenda, rather than a professional public health directive.

Bullet point four reminds us that breastfeeding is not something that exists, prim and contained, within the halls of a postpartum floor. The IBCLC who offers "holistic care" is concerned about the whole person, including medical, biologic, and social factors, not just treatment of symptoms. Breastfeeding mothers and their children live, work, shop, worship, and play in the community. Lactation occurs over months and years, and as the infant grows into a toddler and child, the needs of the breastfeeding dyad will change. Thus, this portion of this duty signifies that the IBCLC has expertise she can bring to bear on a huge range of situations. Needless to say, evidence-based practice will guide how the IBCLC provides her expertise.

Bullet point five is another clarion call to the IBCLC to provide education to families, HCPs, and the community at large. "Principles of adult education" is a reference to a fairly new field of study, which examines the learning styles used by adults, which differ from those of children. Four learning theories for adults are action learning, experiential learning, project-based learning, and self-directed learning (Conlan, Grabowski, & Smith, 2003). Given the context provided elsewhere in the IBLCE CPC and IBLCE SOP, it is safe to assume this means: teach so they can learn. Materials and teaching tactics (i.e., small group projects vs. a lecture format) will have to be adapted to suit your audience.

The sixth and final bullet point in this portion of the IBLCE SOP is the *duty* to protect, promote, and support breastfeeding by compliance with the WHO Code. While the IBLCE CPC in its Introduction retains similarly strong "duty language" regarding WHO Code compliance, the requirement is not embodied in the actual principles of the IBLCE CPC. Thus, it is incumbent upon each individual IBCLC to self-impose compulsory support of the WHO Code.

Duty to Provide Competent Services

IBCLCs have the duty to provide competent services for mothers and families by:

- Performing comprehensive maternal, child, and feeding assessments related to lactation
- Developing and implementing an individualized feeding plan in consultation with the mother
- Providing evidence-based information regarding a mother's use, during lactation, of medications (over-the-counter and prescription), alcohol, tobacco and street drugs, and their potential impact on milk production and child safety
- Providing evidence-based information regarding complementary therapies during lactation and their impact on a mother's milk production and the effect on her child
- Integrating cultural, psychosocial, and nutritional aspects of breastfeeding
- Providing support and encouragement to enable mothers to successfully meet their breastfeeding goals
- Using effective counseling skills when interacting with clients and other health-care providers
- Using the principles of family-centred care while maintaining a collaborative, supportive relationship with clients (IBLCE, 2008, SOP para. 5)

This duty spells out how the competent IBCLC practices. It is the section of the IBLCE SOP that defines our narrow but deep focus on lactation. Each bullet point will be explored in turn, as this is the duty that represents the "fence" within which our clinical authority rests.

Bullet point one states the obvious: a comprehensive assessment of the mother and child, with regard to lactation, and an assessment of an honest-to-goodness breast-feeding at breast, will be needed if the IBCLC is to be able to spot issues that may require a care plan. IBCLCs see mothers and babies very early in the game. If there are feeding difficulties, they show up early and often, since the infant's primary biologic job is to breastfeed effectively. More often than not, a mother who requires an IBCLC's care will find her breastfeeding issue readily identified and addressed. But not every *feeding* difficulty is a *lactation* difficulty. It may be that the baby has a heretofore undiag-nosed condition that makes breastfeeding difficult (although, often, bottle feeding may be similarly problematic). Example: the baby who cannot maintain latch and transfer milk because of torticollis. This baby will need the care of a physical or craniosacral therapist; mother may need to start expressing her milk to protect her supply, and to offer supplements of expressed breastmilk to the baby (Genna, 2013). Or, the baby may be fatiguing at breast due to a congenital heart disease, again requiring a specialist for the baby and a care plan to protect breastfeeding (Genna, 2013). Note that it is *not* the IBCLC's duty within this scope of practice to make these diagnoses. Rather, her thorough lactation assessment may bring the IBCLC to the conclusion that "something else" is going on; she will refer elsewhere for appropriate diagnosis and treatment (IBLCE, 2011e, CPC Principles 2.1, 2.2; IBLCE, 2008, SOP para. 8), but she will maintain contact with the mother to provide lactation support.

Bullet point two is noteworthy in that it imposes a *duty* on the IBCLC to develop a lactation care plan *in consultation with the mother*. The competent IBCLC does not whip out her one-size-fits-all care plan, plop it into mother's hands, and consider the job done. Each care plan should be individually crafted to the mother. Certainly IBCLCs offer the same *kinds* of advice, over and over, to the patients in their care. They can use convenient handouts, perhaps with check boxes, but the best ones will have blank lines for writing down individualized care. Each mother should feel that her care plan is designed to address her particular needs. She should be consulted when it is devised. Ask her: What are your breastfeeding goals? What help do you have when you get home? Can you handle this time-intensive care plan? Do you know whom to call if you have questions or concerns?

Bullet point three is a clear pronouncement: mothers are entitled to evidence-based information about the impact, on lactation, of their use or ingestion of drugs, alcohol, and tobacco. Information never hurt any mother. The lactation consultant, who is the only allied healthcare provider specializing in breastfeeding, is the obvious HCP to whom the mother can turn for accurate information. The IBCLC is *not* authorized, under this portion of this duty, to instruct a mother on what medications she can or should take, but the IBCLC *can* tell the mother how breastfeeding will be affected (if at all) should various substances be ingested.

This is a topic that arises frequently for the IBCLC. Mothers universally want to know what foods, beverages, or medicines they should take, or avoid, while breastfeeding. Often the mother simply needs reassurance that her baby will be just fine, even if the mother's HCP prescribed a medicine or vitamin. But, frustratingly, many mothers are erroneously told—by friends, neighbors, relatives, and by pharmacists, doctors, dentists—that they must wean, or discard their breastmilk ("pump and dump"), when they take various medications or have certain foods and drinks. And it is no surprise that this is the common recommendation to mothers: pharmaceutical package inserts for every drug, whether prescription or over-the-counter, contain customary warnings to "Avoid taking if pregnant or breastfeeding," or perhaps, "If pregnant or breastfeeding, ask a health professional before use," regardless of the actual lactation or pediatric risks involved with the use of the medication (*Physician's Desk Reference*, 2009). This phrasing is unlikely to engender feelings of safety, and most mothers will interpret it as a big red stop sign. The annual *Physician's Desk Reference* is a widely available resource in pharmacies and doctors' offices, and it is the drug information resource to which many HCPs turn. It is merely a compendium of all pharmaceutical package inserts, with generic warnings, whereas the competent IBCLC keeps evidence-based information about specific medications and their actual effect on mothers' milk at her fingertips.

The fourth bullet covers another area about which IBCLCs receive frequent questions: the impact of complementary therapies on lactation. *Complementary therapy* is an umbrella term to cover a broad range of products and services that a mother may inquire about: acupressure, acupuncture, aromatherapy, chiropractic, craniosacral therapy, herb use, homeopathy, or massage therapy, to name a few. If the IBCLC is not well versed in these treatment options, the IBLCE CPC and IBLCE SOP ask her to "know what she does not know" and refer to someone who is knowledgeable (IBLCE, 2011e, CPC Principles 2.1, 2.2; IBLCE, 2008, SOP para. 8). And as we've learned, an IBCLC can never go wrong, legally or ethically, merely in providing information and support to a mother. This portion of this duty makes it clear: the IBCLC is to provide evidence-based information about all kinds of care, including complementary therapy options, as the mother's interest or situation warrants.

Bullet point five describes the competent IBCLC as integrating "cultural, psycho-social, and nutritional aspects" into breastfeeding care. That's another sentence that packs a wallop: it is a reminder that nothing is "off limits" when discussing lactation with a mother, because breastfeeding "goes everywhere," just as the mother does. Her family situation (living alone? supportive family nearby?), her own history (depression? sexual abuse? infertility?), her postpartum plans (immediate return to work or school? extra home-based support because baby was born prematurely?), and her own general health (history of allergy? how about the father?) all play a role in how the IBCLC may help her to protect breastfeeding.

Bullet point six should be reread, once more, slowly. Helping mothers "to successfully meet their breastfeeding goals" is an entirely different venture than simply helping mothers "to breastfeed." Surely, a mother who wants to breastfeed at breast will have *that* as her goal, and the IBCLC is the go-to specialist for assistance. Happily, most mothers who have the goal "to breastfeed," and have a healthy baby and milk supply, will just march straight to the goal line without ever having to call the IBCLC for help. But IBCLCs, by the very nature of their work, will tend to see the mothers with difficult and complex lactation issues. Maybe supply will never be enough to meet the baby's need because of mother's breast surgery or insufficient glandular development history. Maybe mom has to return to work outside the home within weeks of delivery. Maybe the mother has a severe medical condition whose treatment options truly are incompatible with breastfeeding (think chemotherapy for cancer). Maybe the baby has congenital anomalies making it difficult or impossible to latch and suckle. Maybe the baby was born weeks or months early, and is in the intensive care unit struggling merely to breathe, much less feed. All of these women, in compassionate consultation with a competent IBCLC, can "successfully meet their breastfeeding goals" as interpreted for their situation. The breast surgery mom may use a supplementer tube at breast; the working mom can be supported to express her milk when away from baby; the cancer patient can be validated for offering short-term breastfeeding before her own treatment starts; the mother whose baby cannot feed at breast can be reminded of the tremendous value that only her expressed milk provides. And all of these mothers may benefit from knowing that human milk banks are an option (Human Milk Banking Association of North America, n.d.).

Bullet point seven is blissfully straightforward: when you are communicating with patients/clients or other HCPs, use your best counseling skills, so your message sticks.

The last portion of this duty, bullet point eight, suggests offering lactation support using principles of "family-centred care." This approach to care "recognizes that the perspectives and information provided by families, children and young adults are essential components of high-quality decision-making, and that patients and family are integral partners with the health care team" (American Academy of Pediatrics [AAP], 2012a, p. 1). In short, the baby comes with a family, and families inherently promote the health and well-being of their children. Consultation of the lactating mother should take into account her family circumstances and be built upon the supports her family situation permit.

Duty to Report Truthfully and Fully

> IBCLCs have the duty to report truthfully and fully to the mother and/or infant's primary healthcare provider and to the healthcare system by:
>
> • Recording all relevant information concerning care provided and, where appropriate, retaining records for the time specified by the local jurisdiction (IBLCE, 2008, SOP para. 6)

This duty seems to be aligned, at least in spirit, with IBLCE CPC Principle 4.1, which requires the IBCLC (after consent) to share *clinical information* with HCPs. However, this language in the IBLCE SOP seems to impose proactive obligations on the IBCLC, to (a) chart accurately, and (b) go forth and report (presumably by sending a copy of the chart or a summary of the visit to the mother's and baby's HCPs). A reading of this language, on its face, does not make it very clear. No test cases have been brought to IBLCE, which is the self-appointed enforcement authority for the IBLCE SOP, seeking clarification. Which presents an obvious legal and ethical dilemma for the IBCLC: does she, or does she not, have to send reports of all her consultations to the maternal and child HCPs? And just when would it ever be *inappropriate* to retain records for the time period prescribed by the law?

It is probably safe to assume that this *duty* is meant to be compatible with the IBLCE CPC, and while Principle 4.1 of the IBLCE CPC is itself ambiguous, it is a safe and plausible construction of IBLCE SOP paragraph 6 to conclude that, in the interests of being able to accurately report clinical concerns and information to the other HCPs, the IBCLC should keep good detailed records as per IBLCE SOP paragraph 6.

Duty to Preserve Client Confidence

IBCLCs have the duty to preserve client confidence by:

- Respecting the privacy, dignity, and confidentiality of mothers and families (IBLCE, 2008, SOP para. 7)

This is old news to IBCLCs and is clear and direct. It is the *duty* of all IBCLCs, everywhere, to preserve the privacy of the patient/client. Use the patient's name only when in discussion with her other HCPs; discuss her case anonymously with others who may offer clinical insight but are not in the mother's actual circle of care. And don't discuss the case with anyone else. Period.

Duty to Act with Reasonable Diligence

IBCLCs have the duty to act with reasonable diligence by:

- Assisting families with decisions regarding the feeding of children by providing information that is evidence-based and free of conflict of interest
- Providing follow-up services as required
- Making necessary referrals to other health care providers and community support resources when necessary
- Functioning and contributing as a member of the health care team to deliver coordinated services to women and families
- Working collaboratively and interdependently with other members of the health-care team
- Reporting to IBLCE if they have been found guilty of any offence under the criminal code of their country or jurisdiction in which they work or is [sic] sanctioned by another profession
- Reporting to IBLCE any other IBCLC who is functioning outside this Scope of Practice (IBLCE, 2008, SOP para. 8)

Reasonable diligence is another one of those phrases that, in the eyes of the law, carries significant meaning:

A fair, proper, and due degree of care and activity, measured with reference to the particular circumstances; such diligence, care, or attention as might be expected from a man of ordinary prudence and activity. (Diligence—reasonable, 1979, p. 412)

This last duty in the IBLCE SOP has several bullet points that seem something of a shotgun scatter. A few ethics, communication, and referral matters, already addressed elsewhere in the IBLCE SOP and even IBLCE CPC, are highlighted here. One would think the IBCLC should use reasonable diligence in the exercise of *any* activity under the IBLCE SOP: the duty to uphold the standards of the profession; the duty to promote, protect, and support breastfeeding; the duty to provide competent services; the duty to report truthfully and fully; and the duty to preserve client confidence. Don't all these duties deserve "a fair, proper, and due degree of care?" Reasonable diligence really addresses *how* one performs a duty.

Thus, bullet point one should sound familiar (asking us to provide evidence-based and conflict-free information to families), as should bullet point two (provide needed follow-up), bullet point three (refer as necessary), bullet points four and five (work collaboratively as a member of the healthcare *team*), and bullet points six and seven (report yourself or others to IBLCE if you have broken rules or laws). Rather than repeat the rationale for such professional behaviors here, perhaps it is easiest simply to conclude that the IBLCE SOP, by singling out these responsibilities, is drawing attention to their significance for the well-practicing IBCLC.

The ILCA Standards of Practice: A "Should"

Promulgated by the International Lactation Consultant Association (ILCA), the Standards of Practice for International Board Certified Lactation Consultants (ILCA Standards) is a model document, meaning it is a compendium of best professional practices in which the IBCLC *should* engage. Failure to do so, however, brings no sanctions (except, perhaps, gossip among your colleagues if they find your professionalism subpar).

How is ILCA different from IBLCE? ILCA is:

> The professional association for International Board Certified Lactation Consultants (IBCLCs) and other health care professionals who care for breastfeeding families. Our vision is a worldwide network of lactation professionals. Our mission is to advance the profession of lactation consulting worldwide through leadership, advocacy, professional development, and research. (ILCA, 2012b, para. 1)

ILCA provides a myriad of educational and professional development opportunities for its members, promotes IBCLCs and the profession to the public at large, engages in international policy making as a nongovernmental organization (NGO) with recognized status at the World Health Organization (WHO), and publishes the highly regarded *Journal of Human Lactation* (ILCA, 2005).

Membership in ILCA is voluntary. Whereas every IBCLC in the world had to successfully pass the certification exam administered by the IBLCE, membership in ILCA is entirely up to the IBCLC (or other HCP or volunteer caring for breastfeeding families). In January 2011, there were 22,736 IBCLCs worldwide, with 56% residing in all the Americas or Israel, 21% in Australia, Asia Pacific or Africa , and 22% in Europe, North Africa and the Middle East (IBLCE, 2011a). ILCA membership in December 2011 hovered at just over 6,000, from 84 countries (approximately 80% residing in the

Americas or Israel, 11% in Australia, Asia Pacific or Africa, and 6% in Europe, North Africa and the Middle East) (ILCA, 2012a). Thus, about one quarter of those who hold the international certification are members of the international professional association.

Perhaps the easiest way to remember the distinctions: The IBCLC *must* pass the certification exam administered by IBLCE; therefore, she *must* follow the IBLCE CPC and IBLCE SOP administered by the IBLCE. As an IBCLC, she *should* join her professional association ILCA, and she *should* follow the ILCA Standards promulgated by that organization.

Now, a closer look at the ILCA Standards. In 1991, ILCA published *Recommendations and Competencies*, the precursor to the ILCA Standards of Practice. The *ILCA Standards of Practice for IBCLC Lactation Consultants* were first issued in 1995, about one year before the first IBLCE COE. The ILCA Standards underwent a revision in 1999, and the third edition was issued in 2005 (ILCA, 2005).

Preface

> This is the third edition of *Standards of Practice for International Board Certified Lactation Consultants (IBCLCs)* published by the International Lactation Consultant Association (ILCA).
>
> All individuals practicing as a currently certified IBCLC should adhere to ILCA's *Standards of Practice* and the International Board of Lactation Consultant Examiners (IBLCE) *Code of Ethics for International Board Certified Lactation Consultants* in all interactions with clients, families, and other health care professionals. ILCA recognizes the certification conferred by the IBLCE as the worldwide professional credential for lactation consultants.
>
> Quality practice and service are the core responsibilities of a profession to the public. Standards of practice are stated measures or levels of quality that are models for the conduct and evaluation of practice. Standards of practice:
> * Promote consistency by encouraging a common systematic approach
> * Are sufficiently specific in content to guide daily practice
> * Provide a recommended framework for the development of policies and protocols, educational programs, and quality improvement efforts
> * Are intended for use in diverse practice settings and cultural contexts (ILCA, 2006, paras. 1–3)

The preface, again, lays out what this document is and why it matters. It establishes that IBCLCs are the premiere healthcare providers for lactation. Critically, the "IBCLC *should* adhere to" the ILCA Standards and IBLCE Code of Ethics (this document, published before the creation of the IBLCE Code of Professional Conduct, necessarily referring to the predecessor document the IBLCE Code of Ethics). We know from the earlier discussion that the IBCLC already *must* follow the IBLCE CPC, but it certainly does no harm to "pull" the mandatory professional practice-guiding document from IBLCE into the ILCA Standards, and suggest the practitioner "should" be doing what she already "must" be doing. The current ILCA Standards were issued in 2005, three years prior to the mandatory IBLCE SOP, so no mention is made of that practice-guiding document in this preface.

We also learn a little bit about the concept of professional standards of practice. They are models of conduct. They describe the manner in which an IBCLC *should* practice if she takes pride in her work, her level of professionalism, and in offering quality care. Because the bullet points go to a description of what a standard of practice—in any profession—serves to accomplish, they are not as important as the rest of the ILCA Standards, which describe with specificity the IBCLC's model conduct.

Standard 1. Professional Responsibilities

The IBCLC has a responsibility to maintain professional conduct and to practice in an ethical manner, accountable for professional actions and legal responsibilities.

1.1. Adhere to these ILCA *Standards of Practice* and the IBLCE Code of Ethics [now the Code of Professional Conduct]
1.2. Practice within the scope of the *International Code of Marketing of Breast-milk Substitutes* and all subsequent World Health Assembly resolutions
1.3. Maintain an awareness of conflict of interest in all aspects of work, especially when profiting from the rental or sale of breastfeeding equipment and services
1.4. Act as an advocate for breastfeeding women, infants, and children
1.5. Assist the mother in maintaining a breastfeeding relationship with her child
1.6. Maintain and expand knowledge and skills for lactation consultant practice by participating in continuing education
1.7. Undertake periodic and systematic evaluation of one's clinical practice
1.8. Support and promote well-designed research in human lactation and breast-feeding, and base clinical practice, whenever possible, on such research

If things are starting to look familiar, that is rather sensible. Many of the model behaviors described as an IBCLC professional responsibility echo those we have examined in detail under the IBLCE CPC and IBLCE SOP. And that is as it should be: it would be rather odd to have the best practices (which a model standards of practice represents) be entirely different from mandatory behaviors. Shouldn't we be requiring the best, as well as asking for it? And, that is as the ILCA Standards are constructed. With all we have learned, this will be a brief review.

The ILCA Standards do set some things out with a bit more clarity than the sister documents. Standards 1.1 and 1.2 mention some familiar IBCLC-related documents: the IBLCE COE (now replaced by the IBLCE CPC) and the WHO Code. At 1.3 we revisit conflicts of interest (COIs), but here the reference is specifically made to the tensions between selling or renting equipment, and using it in a clinical context.

That is an easy COI to identify and avoid. Standards 1.4 and 1.5 clearly state that our advocacy goes to mother, child *and* the breastfeeding relationship.

Standard 1.6 reminds us to stay on top of our game through continuing education, while Standard 1.7 is a model of professionalism that asks us to regularly step back and assess whether we, in fact, *are* on the top of our game. IBLCE recertification requires 75 continuing education hours every 5 years and a retaking of the test every 10 years (IBLCE, 2012), so any IBCLC who plans to retain her certification will be able to meet the educational component promoted at Standard 1.6. Standard 1.7's "periodic and systematic evaluation of one's clinical practice" may be difficult for some IBCLCs. Those working in a hospital or birthing center, with many other IBCLCs, probably have a performance review as part of their regular job benefits, but the private prac- titioner working alone, or as the sole IBCLC in the public health clinic, or the lone IBCLC who staffs a pediatric or obstetric practice, may find it difficult to gauge her professional progress with no peers at work. It is important to reach out in this situa- tion: Join (or start) the local chapter of ILCA, or sign up for one of the many email lists or Web forums that serve lactation consultant interests. One such award-winning list is Lactnet, a major email list service for professional and lay breastfeeding supporters, where messages come to one's email inbox, rather than requiring a visit to an on-line message board. It has over 3000 members worldwide (Bruce, Myr, Koch, Gribble, & Pohl, 2010).

Standard 1.8 is a reminder of the importance of high-quality research in the field of human lactation: use evidence-based practice, and promote well-designed studies to build our body of knowledge.

Standard 2. Legal Considerations

The IBCLC is obligated to practice within the laws of the geopolitical region and set- ting in which she/he works. The IBCLC must practice with consideration for rights of privacy and with respect for matters of a confidential nature.

2.1. Work within the policies and procedures of the institution where employed, or if self-employed, have identifiable policies and procedures to follow

2.2. Clearly state applicable fees prior to providing care

2.3. Obtain informed consent from all clients prior to:
- Assessing or intervening
- Reporting relevant information to other health care professional(s)
- Taking photographs for any purpose
- Seeking publication of information associated with the consultation

2.4. Protect client confidentiality at all times

2.5. Maintain records according to legal and ethical practices within the work setting

Standard 2 describes in clear, unambiguous terms some important legal considerations of practice, and in a book about legal and ethical issues for the IBCLC, it seems only fitting that we examine these elements in detail.

The introduction sets out an important parameter that may ease the confusion or fears of practicing IBCLCs: if you follow the laws of your land and the rules of your place of work, you will be operating to the highest professional standard. To repeat earlier analysis: workplace setting rules and procedures may vary, even wildly, within the same region. An IBCLC may be worried that she is practicing at risk of liability, if her clinical approach (dictated by her facility's policies and procedures) differs from her colleagues across town. Not so. The ambitious IBCLC may always seek to change policies within her facility, if she feels newer research (perhaps which she learned from her colleague across town) suggests a revision in policy. But she doesn't have to. And she will be using IBCLC best practices if she operates within the predefined parameters of her employer. The need to respect privacy and confidentiality is mentioned here, as well, as an umbrella concept governing all legal considerations of IBCLC practice.

Standard 2.1 seems to be a mere repeat of what was discussed in the introductory paragraph to Standard 2, and in a way, it is. Practicing "within the laws of the . . . setting in which she/he works" is pretty much the same as working "within the policies and procedures of the institution where employed." But Standard 2.1 makes it plain. Administrative policies and procedures are like laws, in that they are established after a thorough examination of their need; they are published; practitioners are expected to follow them; sanctions will result for those who do not. Standard 2.1 also specifically calls upon the self-employed private practice lactation consultant (PPLC) to prepare a policy and procedure manual (PPM), just like any large hospital, clinic, or medical practice, spelling out the professional and conscientious manner in which the business is to be conducted. There are a whole host of legitimate legal reasons why a small business owner (like an IBCLC in private practice) would want a PPM (and her accountant and lawyer can easily describe them). But it should also be emphasized that an excellent means of achieving a high personal standard of professionalism is to sit down and write the template for just how it is that the PPLC will engage in any clinical consultation. IBCLCs that are self-employed, but not in a private clinical practice as such (think childbirth preparation instructor, or lactation educators), reap equal professional development benefits from this exercise.

Standards 2.2 and 2.3 remove some of the fog that descended when we analyzed the IBLCE CPC Principle 4.1. Here we see, plainly, that the IBCLC operating under best practices, as she *should*, will tell the mother up front what costs are involved to provide services. The IBCLC will also obtain "informed consent" from the mother *before* any of several activities occurs: (1) the consult itself (since by its very nature a consultation involves "assessing or intervening"), (2) reporting "relevant information" to the HCP, (3) taking any photograph, and (4) "publication" of any information associated with the consult.

If we have to ask a mother permission to share relevant information with HCPs, it helps to know what is considered relevant. Here, the practices within your region may guide you: some IBCLCs send reports of any and all consults; some IBCLCs will send reports only in situations where red flags raise concerns and the need for follow-up care from other HCPs. When in doubt, send the report or make the phone call. Invariably, the primary HCP will appreciate that clinical concerns prompted the outreach. As to "publication of information" concerning the consult, most of us think of publication as something that newspapers, magazines, and scholarly journals do. But in the eyes of the law, "publication" occurs when information under your control becomes easily accessible to others; when you "exhibit, display, disclose, or reveal" it (Publication, 1979, p. 1105). If you stand in a crowded elevator and say, in an audible voice, "Mrs. Jones in Room 423 has a raging case of herpes simplex, and we are concerned about protecting the baby" (Riordan & Wambach, 2010) you are publishing this information associated with the consultation every bit as much as if it appeared on the front page of the local newspaper. Which is a lovely segue to Standard 2.4: if you protect client confidentiality at all times, you will not have to worry about whether or not you inadvertently published information without consent from the mother.

Standard 2.5 addresses the time period an IBCLC should keep charts and other records of practice. How long the PPLC or hospital must store clinical records (securely and privately) is a function of the laws of each state or country, but is rarely clear at that. A large medical practice or hospital will have long-standing policies governing this; the staff in the medical records department can probably rattle off from memory the necessary time frames for keeping all sorts of different records. For the PPLC, an oft-mentioned rule of thumb is 21 years after the baby is born, on the premise that your files will back you up if you are sued for malpractice by the "baby" who is now aged 20 years 11 months. In the United Kingdom, the recommendation is to keep records until the "child" is 25 or 26 years of age (NHS Choice, 2011).

An IBCLC should endeavor to keep records so that, many months or years later, she can successfully recreate the consultation in her mind. While record retention is usually discussed in the context of litigation (to prove we did nothing wrong), there may be plenty of other reasons to keep client records for 10 or 20 years. You would find it helpful to have good background information and clinical history if a mother visits you with the birth of every child. All those back files will be useful for lactation research. Such records will also enable you to monitor trends in the practice to adjust marketing or services; 10 years ago everyone bought books, but today everyone wants online information—maybe it is time to investigate social marketing to capture all the Millennial Moms.

If you are an IBCLC with control over your own records, the important step is to create a procedure regarding document retention and destruction, put it into your PPM (remember Standard 2.1), and then simply follow it. If you want to be absolutely certain and safe, have your policy require file retention for 21 years. If you feel 18 years (the age of majority in most jurisdictions) is long enough, list that. However you decide to store and periodically destroy your files, the key is to do so methodically. There are myriad options, and in the 21st century immense amounts of data can be stored in small bits of digital space, unlike generations past that had to find facilities to store hundreds of cartons of paper in an environment that was protected from destructive elements and prying eyes. Commercial enterprises will, for fairly reasonable rates, convert your paper files into computer files, under pledges of confidentiality, and provide secure storage, offsite, even shredding the paper versions once the digital record has been created. If you do not convert your files to digital form, your PPM can describe how you shred the contents of files every few years, keeping a record (by name or file number) of files so destroyed. Then, if that 20-year-old does come back to sue you on the eve of his 21st birthday, and files of your consult with his mother were destroyed or shredded according to the document retention plan described in your PPM, you will be able to defend any allegation of spoliation (an elegant word that means "destruction of evidence [which] constitutes an obstruction of justice") (Spoliation, 1979, p. 1257).

Standard 3. Clinical Practice

The clinical practice of the IBCLC focuses on providing clinical lactation care and management. This is best accomplished by promoting optimal health, through collaboration and problem-solving with the client and other members of the health care team. The role of the IBCLC includes:

- Assessment, planning, intervention, and evaluation of care in a variety of situations
- Anticipatory guidance and prevention of problems
- Complete, accurate, and timely documentation of care
- Communication and collaboration with other health care professionals

3.1. Assessment
    3.1.1. Obtain and document an appropriate history of the breastfeeding mother and child
    3.1.2 Systematically collect objective and subjective information
    3.1.3 Discuss with the mother and document as appropriate all assessment information

3.2. Plan
    3.2.1 Analyze assessment information to identify issues and/or problems
    3.2.2 Develop a plan of care based on identified issues
    3.2.3 Arrange for follow-up evaluation where indicated

3.3. Implementation
    3.3.1 Implement the plan of care in a manner appropriate to the situation and acceptable to the mother
    3.3.2 Utilize translators as needed
    3.3.3 Exercise principles of optimal health, safety, and universal precautions

3.3.4 Provide appropriate oral and written instructions and/or demonstration of interventions, procedures, and techniques

3.3.5 Facilitate referral to other health care professionals, community services, and support groups as needed

3.3.6 Use equipment appropriately:
- Refrain from unnecessary or excessive use
- Assure cleanliness and good operating condition
- Discuss the risks and benefits of recommended equipment including financial considerations
- Demonstrate the correct use and care of equipment
- Evaluate safety and effectiveness of use

3.3.7 Document and communicate to health care providers as appropriate:
- Assessment information
- Suggested interventions
- Instructions provided
- Evaluations of outcomes
- Modifications of the plan of care
- Follow-up strategies

3.4. Evaluation

3.4.1 Evaluate outcomes of planned interventions

3.4.2 Modify the care plan based on the evaluation of outcomes

This standard, covering the best clinical practices an IBCLC *should* use, is lengthy, but its specificity makes it pretty clear, and many of the concepts should be familiar after the discussion of the IBLCE CPC and IBLCE SOP earlier in the chapter.

Again, the introductory paragraph is a clue about what is to follow. We learn that excellent clinical practice, for an IBCLC, is accomplished when the mother and the entire healthcare team are "in on the plan." As a practical matter, the IBCLC will, in the moment, construct the care plan with the mother's assistance, and then share this plan (if the situation warrants) with the primary HCPs for the mother or baby to keep them apprised of the IBCLC's interventions.

Bullet point one describes a comprehensive IBCLC role: "assessment, planning, intervention, and evaluation of care" covers a broad range of skills, considering a broad range of possibilities. Anticipatory guidance, mentioned in bullet point two, means "fair warning" to the mother of what issues may come down the road, and how she can prevent other problems. For example, the mother with low milk supply will be encouraged to increase the amount of breastfeeding and/or expression that is occurring every day; anticipatory guidance is the part where the IBCLC tells the mom it make take 48–72 hours for her to see or feel any difference, so she knows to hang in there with those first 10 or 20 feeding or pumping sessions to achieve the eventual result (West & Marasco, 2009).

Bullet point three is another obvious one: Record it when it happens. Whether you chart by hand on paper, or electronically, it is important that you make (or enter) notes of the consult and follow-up phone calls, emails, or visits. Most of us are pretty good about this at the actual consult: we have our charts and forms and handouts all lined up ready to go, and it is easy to jot down findings as the session progresses. Where we get sloppy is in follow-up care, especially since our cell phones have made us so mobile. Imagine you are at the grocery store on Saturday morning, and the mother you saw on Thursday calls you to ask some follow-up questions and to give you a progress report. Fantastic! How do you plan to make notes of this 10-minute call? Will you even remember to do so upon your return to your office? Or, what about that Millennial Mom who sends an email with questions at 2 a.m.? (At least she didn't call in the dead of night with her nonemergency question.) Are those emails being printed out and added to the paper file, or linked to the electronic chart for the mother?

Bullet point four in the ILCA Standards introduction is a general reminder that the IBCLC does not operate in a vacuum. There are other HCPs in the picture; indeed, the baby and mother both probably have someone else as the *primary* HCP. Information and communication never harmed any mother and child, and it doesn't harm HCPs: when in doubt, share your report and concerns with others in the family's circle of care.

Assessment is the first clinical practice area that is described under ILCA Standard 3, and the IBCLC *should* use several best practices to make a competent assessment. Standard 3.1.1 suggests obtaining a pertinent history of both mother and child, geared toward matters that may affect breastfeeding and lactation. To meet Standard 3.1.2, as you build your history and start to take notes in the consult, separate your objective notes (what you can physically and dispassionately see, hear, feel, and measure during the consult) from your subjective notes (information supplied by the mother or family members to describe the problem) (Altman, 2008). Subjective charting might indicate: "Mother says 'Baby eating all the time; my nipples are sore.' Father supplies log kept since birth: shows Baby fed 6 times on Day 1, 12 times on Day 2, 8 times on Day 3 but 'we stopped marking in the middle of that night.'" Your objective notes might include: "Baby is 4 days old; born at 6 lbs. 8 oz. Weighed 6 lbs. 6 oz. at start of consult. Suckled for 12 minutes on right; self-detached; mother has lateral crease on nipple face. No broken skin on nipple. Cheeks "dimpled" during feed; audible swallows heard. Baby cued 10 minutes later by placing hands to mouth; latched onto left and actively suckled for less than two minutes before falling asleep at breast. Mother detached baby; observed lateral creasing across nipple face but no broken skin. Baby transferred 1.75 oz., total, from both breasts." Following Standard 3.1.3 is easy and sensible: you simply share with the mother what you learn ("Oh, it looks like your baby is getting plenty of milk for a four-dayer!").

Crafting a care plan for the mother is probably the most important part of the consult. Standard 3.2 describes the steps an IBCLC *should* take: Standard 3.2.1 is the instruction to step back from all that assessing you just did, to figure out what is going on. What are true issues (sore nipples, in our example)? What may be addressed with simple information and reassurance? That baby who is "nursing all the time" is feeding well within the range of normal, but does mother know what "normal" is? Standard 3.2.2 suggests development of a plan to address the real issues (do not neglect to include the mother, in a meaningful way, to develop a manageable care plan [IBLCE, 2008, SOP para. 5]). Standard 3.2.3 reminds us to "arrange for follow-up evaluation" (akin to IBLCE CPC Principles 2.1 and 2.1 and IBLCE SOP para. 8). In our example, let us assume that the IBCLC suspects the baby's shallow latch, causing nipple creasing and subsequent pain, is due to baby's clenched jaw. Mother thinks infant massage or infant craniosacral therapy will help resolve the baby's hypertonia. The IBCLC may, but does not have to, take on the secretarial role of actually making an appointment for the mother with a therapist specializing in these treatments. To "arrange for follow-up evaluation" can mean simply to instruct the mother to make an appointment with one of the specialists you have listed on a handout of local resources (as you tuck it with the rest of her paperwork from the consultation), perhaps suggesting that she check with her insurance company first to see what they will cover.

Implementation of the care plan is covered generally under Standard 3.3, and Standard 3.3.1 states that the implementation of the care plan must happen "in a manner appropriate to the situation and acceptable to the mother." This may require some clever thinking on the part of the IBCLC and mother. Imagine we have a mother returning to work, who wants to preserve her supply and feed the baby at breast when she is home. "No sweat!" the IBCLC thinks. "Just express milk at work!" Now imagine the mother works as an emergency room doctor, who may at any given moment be involved in complex life-saving procedures from which she cannot simply duck out for 15 or 20 minutes to express her breastmilk. Imagine, further, she does not want her employer to know she is expressing breastmilk while at work. The competent and conscientious IBCLC does not prejudge any mother (IBLCE, 2011e, CPC Principles 1.1, 1.5, & 6.3), even though it is agonizing to the IBCLC that this doctor, who can be a positive role model to so many colleagues and patients, doesn't even want the world to know she is expressing milk. But a care plan that is "acceptable to the mother" has to be one that she accepts. Telling her to find two to three breaks while on shift won't cut it. You may have to explore options like "reverse cycling," where the majority of feeds occur in the evening and night, rather than the daylight hours, so that the need to express milk is reduced during the hours that mother is away from her baby (Berggren, 2005).

Use translators if mother's language differs from the IBCLC (Standard 3.3.2). That makes sense. Think about health, safety, and universal precautions (Standard 3.3.3): That makes sense, too, but note that this is more than a reminder that mother should wash her hands after changing the baby's diaper and before breastfeeding. Health and safety may mean the IBCLC should find out: Does mother work around dangerous products or chemicals, and do they have any impact on her breastmilk? Does someone in the family smoke cigarettes? drink alcohol—perhaps to excess? Do the parents know how to create a safe sleep environment that allows baby to be at arms' reach (American Academy of Pediatrics, 2011; McKenna & McDade, 2005)? If powdered formula supplementation is in the care plan, does mother know how to safely measure and prepare it (WHO, 2007)? If liquid formula is part of the care plan, has it been subject to recall (U.S. Food & Drug Administration, 2012)?

Under Standard 3.3.4, the IBCLC should give meaningful instructions. Leave a written care plan that repeats what was discussed with the mother. If she is going to use and clean equipment, show her how to do it, and watch her while she does so to make certain she does it properly. Describe hand-expression; model it using your hands on your own clothed breast, and ask mother to do the same thing, using her own hands, on her own unclothed breast. If she wants more assistance, ask her if you may touch her (the permission being a requisite element of good manners, and not a legal requirement), and show her how it is done. First place your hands over hers, so she can sense the movements that are suggested. As a last resort, the IBCLC can palpate the mother's breast to demonstrate hand-expression. These teaching techniques are time consuming, but they are effective, which is why they are best practices.

Standard 3.3.5 is a close cousin to 3.2.3; the wording here reminds us that mother may need referral to someone other than a healthcare provider. Often, referral to a nursing mothers' group (like La Leche League) is the best and only connection this mother will require, to give her the support and confidence she needs to continue breastfeeding her child. Social service agencies may offer food and medical assistance the mother may not have known was available to her, her baby, or her other family members. We see mothers with lactation issues, but they are mothers living their modern-day lives, being pulled in many directions. Any element of a mother's life that becomes overwhelming or chaotic poses a threat to the breastfeeding part of her life. Imagine the mother who has had the role of transporting her ailing grandfather to and from dialysis treatment. Now she has an infant, and there are no comfortable accommodations for the breastfeeding dyad at the facility, where the grandfather's treatment may take several hours. If transportation can be arranged for the grandfather, then the mother will be better able to stay with and meet her infant's needs. No, IBCLCs are not social workers, but when we consult mothers, we built rapport. That makes our advice to seek help from other resources (some of whom we might even specifically name) trustworthy.

Standard 3.3.6 describes crisply and clearly how the use of breastfeeding products and supplies should be addressed in a clinical situation. A healthy dose of skepticism is a good start for any IBCLC. She should ask herself, "Do I really need to introduce something that has been invented and manufactured to improve a basic biological function?" The answer may well be yes; if so, the bullet-point suggestions are a good roadmap to show the mother how to use it, clean it, and get it at a reasonable cost. IBCLCs will also remain cognizant of avoiding, or curing, any conflicts of interest (recall IBLCE CPC Principles 1.4, 5.1, and 5.2; IBLCE SOP, para. 8; and ILCA Standard 1.3).

Some clarity is offered, in Standard 3.3.7, of the IBCLC responsibilities with regard to sharing of clinical information with HCPs. We are told to "document and communicate" to HCPs "as appropriate" the elements of our consults (assessment, plan, instructions, follow-up, etc.). This means document as you should in your own charts or files, then contact the HCP with your concerns, and if you do, share enough information to put that HCP on the same informational footing as you.

Standard 3.4 asks that we check in with the mother to see whether the care plan we devised is working or needs to be modified. Lactation problems can change wildly from one day to the next. Best practices include the IBCLC seeking follow-up information to adapt—and one day discard, when goals are met—the care plan.

Standard 4. Breastfeeding Education and Counseling

Breastfeeding education and counseling are integral parts of the care provided by the IBCLC.

4.1.   Educate parents and families to encourage informed decision-making about infant and child feeding

4.2.   Utilize a pragmatic problem-solving approach, sensitive to the learner's culture, questions and concerns

4.3.   Provide anticipatory guidance (teaching) to:
  • Promote optimal breastfeeding practices
  • Minimize the potential for breastfeeding problems or complications

4.4.   Provide positive feedback and emotional support for continued breastfeeding, especially in difficult or complicated circumstances

4.5.   Share current evidence-based information and clinical skills in collaboration with other health care providers

As we wind up examination of the ILCA Standards of Practice, we again see familiar suggestions: education of families and HCPs is a big part of our role. Effective teaching allows for informed decision making. Involving family members in discussing care that accounts for their personal needs and special considerations will make it feasible for them to follow the care plan.

Perhaps special attention should be drawn to Standard 4.4. Women who are having breastfeeding difficulties are *not* having fun. Care plans are often laborious and stressful. Mothers in the postpartum period (and beyond) are tired. Pain and feelings of disappointment or failure are happening every day, at a time when joy and exhilaration were dreamt of. These mothers *need* "positive feedback and emotional support for continued breastfeeding, especially in difficult or complicated circumstances." This is not a laborious task for the IBCLC: teaching proper equipment use and cleaning will take far longer than simply connecting eye to eye, and telling the patient/client, "You are doing an incredible job in a really tough situation. It hurts to have nipple pain! I can see real improvement in healing in just the last 24 hours. Keep it up. Your baby knows you are doing this all for him, because your baby knows you love him."

The International Code of Marketing of Breast-milk Substitutes: A "Should" Unless It Is a "Must"

The fourth and final practice-guiding document is something of a hybrid for IBCLCs. The International Code of Marketing of Breast-milk[4] Substitutes (referred to, in shorthand, as either "the WHO Code" or "the International Code") was adopted by the member countries of the World Health Organization in 1981 as a call to action: by governments of nations around the world, to enact legislative to enforce it; and to companies, to stop predatory marketing practices on the vulnerable population of families with young children.[5] We will explore the WHO Code in greater detail in a later chapter. For our purposes here, we will give just a snapshot.

Manufacturers of four product types (bottles, teats, infant formula, and other foods pushed on babies as full or partial replacement of breastfeeding) are not supposed to market them directly to the public, nor is the healthcare system (and its HCPs) to be used to market the products. It is a powerful policy-promoting document that recognizes public health interests do not mix well with commercial interests. It is a *model* document, meaning that in and of itself it is not a law or regulation.

> It is an international standard, not an international law. [T]he Code is really a simple document that recommends that member governments restrict advertising and sales promotions of breastmilk substitutes. Each nation is free to adapt the Code within the national and legal frameworks of its own society. (Baumslag & Michels, 1995, p. 164)

---

[4] The original document uses the spelling *breast-milk* throughout, common nomenclature for the day. In the 21st century, *breastmilk* (all one word) is frequently used in professional journals for maternal and child health, though *breast-milk* or *breast milk* still appear in mainstream media. A society moves from hyphenated words to nonhyphenated words (*to-morrow* and *to-day* were once the accepted spellings) as a fluid process of use and convention. Some scholarly journals or societies will establish rules for nomenclature and spelling in their materials (Thorley, 2010).

[5] Approximately every 2 years, the member countries of the World Health Assembly (WHA) meet. WHA is empowered through passage of resolutions to provide clarification to sections of World Health Organization documents like the International Code. Thus, the International Code today is composed of the original language as passed in 1981, along with several subsequently adopted resolutions that have offered interpretation of or expanded explanation of sections of the International Code. Resolutions may *not* be used to substantively change the original International Code; for example, breast pumps (not originally defined as a product covered by the International Code) cannot be brought under the WHO Code through the back door by passage of a resolution. Proper reference to the Code is this mouthful: "International Code of Marketing of Breast-milk Substitutes and all subsequent relevant World Health Assembly resolutions."

When a country enacts WHO Code language into law, an enforcement mechanism is created for that country, which carries more punch than in countries where no legislative action has been taken. Where countries have chosen to legislate all or part of the WHO Code, they have turned the model document (a "should") into law (a "must"). Note that *any* company or HCP is free to choose to follow and support the aims of the International Code; companies and HCPs need not "wait" for regulations or laws to be enacted to elect to support the broad public health imperatives endorsed by the WHO Code. Another example of when the WHO Code "should" is transformed into a "must" is when a birthing facility has elected to seek "Baby-Friendly" designation; they will be required to purchase formula (rather than receive free samples from the manufacturer, prohibited under the WHO Code) (UNICEF, n.d.a; Baby-Friendly USA, 2010).

This model document of *shoulds* had earlier been turned into a *must* for IBCLCs, under Tenet 24 of the old IBLCE COE. It remains a mandate under the IBLCE SOP (in paragraph 3). And the ILCA Standards of Practice (at Standard 1) asks similar allegiance to the International Code. As described earlier in this chapter, the IBLCE CPC has apparently withdrawn the mandatory element of WHO Code compliance from the ethical guidelines in the IBCLC's penultimate practice-guiding document, by placing within the nonbinding introduction to the IBLCE CPC mandatory-sounding language about the IBCLC's "duty" to "adhere" to the WHO Code.

Let us assume that all IBCLCS, everywhere, choose to support the WHO Code. What does that require? The language of the entire WHO Code and subsequent relevant WHA resolutions is most easily accessed at the website for the International Baby Food Action Network (International Baby Food Action Network [IBFAN], n.d.a), an organization that "consists of public interest groups working around the world to reduce infant and young child morbidity and mortality" (IBFAN, n.d.b). The portions of the WHO Code that cover health workers can be found at Article 6 (healthcare systems) and Article 7 (health workers). What it asks is really pretty simple, especially if the IBCLC is already following the IBLCE CPC, IBLCE SOP, and ILCA Standards of Practice cautioning against conflicts of interest when using or discussing *any* commercial products:

1. Promote and protect breastfeeding (WHO, 1981, Article 7.1).
2. Do not accept any "material or financial inducements" (gifts or money) from those who market the products falling under the WHO Code (WHO, 1981, Article 7.3).
3. Do not accept free samples of WHO-Code-covered products, unless you are doing legitimate scientific research (WHO, 1981, Article 7.4).
4. Do not give free samples of WHO-Code-covered products to families, period (WHO, 1981, Article 7.4).
5. If you do accept any money or gifts from a WHO-Code-covered marketer, disclose it (WHO, 1981, Article 7.5).

The IBCLC should find it easy to keep her nose squeaky clean, for purposes of all four of her practice-guiding documents (not just the WHO Code), by following these fairly easy-to-understand explanations. Yet, IBCLCs universally agonize over their legal and ethical duties under the International Code (Noel-Weiss, 2009), as we will explore in a later chapter.

For All IBCLCs, in Some Places

All IBCLCs live some place, and as residents of that geopolitical jurisdiction, they will be expected to follow the laws of the land. This is what we expect of citizens, generally, and what IBCLCs are admonished to do under all four practice-guiding documents. Each country (state, province, county, city, municipality, etc.) passes laws that are enforced within its borders. As the IBCLC moves from one place to another, or perhaps commutes to work in a place that is different from where she lives, she and her IBCLC colleagues are bound by the laws where they practice. This places the IBCLC in a legal or ethical quandary if she finds that her customary practices either are not permitted under the law in her new place of work or residence, or must be revised to comport with the new regulatory scheme.

Privacy laws are a good example. In the European Union (EU), the laws governing how and when the private information about an individual may be shared with others is severely restricted. The EU Directive on Data Protection of 1995 required each nation to pass a national privacy law, and mechanisms to protect citizens' privacy. In the United States, an IBCLC is able to forward to the local nursing mothers' support group the mother's name, address, phone number, baby's name, and their dates of birth, if general authority granting such permission is in her lactation consultation (or hospital admission) consent form. This would not be allowed in EU countries. There, the mother must give her *express* permission for personal information to be forwarded, she must know it is going to the mothers' group, and double-check that what is to be sent is correct (Europe Summaries of EU Legislation, 2011). Put another way: the United States would allow the information to be sent under authority of "umbrella consents" (probably quickly signed, unread during admission while in active labor) unless the mother specifically describes who may *not* get her information. In the EU, the reverse is true: the information may be sent only if the mother specifically *agrees* to each singular instance of sharing.

Similarly, laws or regulations to register and operate a small business (like a breast-feeding clinic) will vary from place to place. Whether and how the allied healthcare provider is permitted to advertise may be subject to local regulation. The rules the government health ministry has established for education and outreach to breastfeeding mothers, and compiling statistics of these contacts with mothers, will depend on the country involved. This book cannot synopsize all laws in all places, but the prudent IBCLC will know that a move to a new location may require learning new ways to practice her profession, just as she must learn how to get her driver's license, or how taxes are structured, in her new locale.

The good news is the IBCLC profession is global. Using either the IBLCE or ILCA websites, any IBCLC can find practitioners in her new location. A bit of proactive networking may be an excellent way to get settled and established, and to ask new colleagues if there are any local laws about which the IBCLC should be aware.

For Some IBCLCs, in Some Places

Some IBCLCs will have to follow rules of the road that apply only to a small set of colleagues. The IBCLCs working in one government agency, or in one hospital, or in one outpatient clinic, will have policies and procedures unique to that place of work. The IBCLCs working there will be required to follow those rules. An example: Facility No. 1 has a "warm line" where discharged mothers may call the hospital with routine questions or concerns about breastfeeding. A simple phone log is kept to track these calls. Facility No. 2 has a policy forbidding IBCLCs from offering clinical advice to discharged patients over the phone; the mothers are to be referred to the primary HCP. Both models for follow-up care are perfectly legitimate models. The IBCLC working in Facility No. 2 will follow the rules of her institution should a mother call on the phone; otherwise, she risks a reprimand or other disciplinary action.

Ironically, it is these job-place-related rules, more so than her four practice-guiding documents, that can make an IBCLC fretful about legal or ethical consequences of her actions. Having to adjust her style of practice may seem like a compromise; that she is providing less than professional care for the dyads she sees. But lactation consultation, as with any healthcare profession, is not an exacting science, like mathematics, with one equation to find one answer. It is a mish-mash of human beings, their needs and concerns, realities of everyday life, and, if we're lucky, excellent research to give us some comfort in what options we can discuss in a care plan. But the list of variables to consider is endless. Having to follow rules or policies at your workplace, whether liberating or constricting to your practice style, is just another variable to consider. An IBCLC can take it upon herself to commence the steps to achieve change within her institution. Sometimes change comes quickly, sometimes slowly, and sometimes not at all. It will require some perseverance, but the process itself can be professionally empowering as the IBCLC masters the research in the practice area affected by the policies in place, fashions an argument demonstrating that clinical outcomes may improve by changing the policies, and then convinces her colleagues and superiors to give the change a try.

Let's explore a few examples where different workplace policies can affect lactation practice for some IBCLCs.

Charting, Files, and Paperwork

Learning (or deciding) how to memorialize contacts with breastfeeding mothers will consume an enormous amount of time, and yet this is the practice area that varies with every single facility or practice, and between every single IBCLC. Some facilities use electronic charting; others rely on paper charts. The lactation consultant may put her notes on the mother's chart, or on the baby's chart, or on her own chart, accessible by HCPs for the dyad. Some institutions will have very rigid rules of proper charting, down to a prescribed list of acceptable abbreviations. Some private practitioners may use very loose charting on the (flimsy) theory that they have only themselves to answer to.

The need to keep accurate records is clear (IBLCE, 2011e, CPC Principles 3.2 & 4.1; IBLCE, 2008, SOP para. 6; ILCA, 2006, Standard 3). If the IBCLC is employed by an institution, she will have to follow whatever guidelines are in place for charting, note-taking, and document retention. That is simply a condition of employment, akin to work hours and break times, the salary and benefits, whom to call when a schedule change is needed, and so on. If the IBCLC is self-employed, or works in a setting where clinical consults are a rarity (a public health office, for example, which uses education and classes to accomplish its mission), she may need to invent a system of her own. Even if there is never a situation of clinical contact, it may still behoove the IBCLC to keep some sort of informal statistics. If she is running a drop-in breastfeeding class every week, it may be wise to track how many parents show up, and perhaps their questions or areas of concerns. Is the class growing in size over time? Are the mothers asking how to get support upon their return to school or work? Is there more interest in how breastfeeding affects the mother's body or the baby? Tracking trends over time may be a good way to (a) establish that the classes are valuable; (b) demonstrate the importance of an IBCLC to provide evidence-based information, and (c) notice patterns in concerns raised, so as to adapt classes to better meet community needs.

Noncompete Clauses, or Conflict of Interest Clauses, in Employment Contracts

Imagine the IBCLC who works very hard, 40 hours a week, in a postpartum unit seeing mothers and babies. She loves her work; many IBCLCs are passionate about lactation. So she has opened her own private practice, and on the weekends or her days off, she sees mothers in her home office. She also rents and sells breastfeeding products, especially hard-to-find items (like varied pump flange sizes, or tubes for offering supplements at breast or by finger), filling a niche market in her community. Many an IBCLC, who has a day job in the local hospital or clinic, has been told that it is "against facility policy" to inform postpartum mothers of this after-hours business; if it happens, the IBCLC may lose her hospital job. Reasons given: "It is a conflict of interest to list you on the local community resource sheet;" or, "You can't open a private practice. You have a noncompete clause in your employment contract."

As we said above, the IBCLC is bound under the rules and policies of the place where she works. Some of these rules may induce eye rolling, but they are the policies in place, nonetheless. One's choices are to change the policy, or change the place of work. But if the IBCLC is to be dissuaded from operating and marketing her own private practice, it ought at least to be for a valid reason, and often the phrases "conflict of interest" and "noncompete clause" are thrown about without an actual analysis of whether, in fact, a true conflict of interest exists.

Let's start with the definition offered earlier: "A conflict of interest is a set of circumstances that creates a risk that professional judgment or actions regarding a primary interest will be unduly influenced by a secondary interest" (Lo & Field, 2009, p. 46). When working in the hospital, our IBCLC sees dyads on the postpartum floor after delivery of the baby and *before* discharge. That is her primary interest. When our IBCLC works as a private practitioner, she sees mothers *after* discharge, either in the home, or in the IBCLC's office. That is her secondary interest. The only way to make this "conflict of interest" real is to turn our IBCLC into an unethical practitioner, where she uses her time on the postpartum floor to somehow inappropriately steer business to her shop. Is that likely? No more likely than the pediatrician who makes hospital rounds on families with no designated HCP, leaving behind office information should the families wish to continue seeing that practitioner upon discharge.

Is it a violation of a "noncompete" clause for our hospital-based IBCLC to open her own private practice? Hardly. Contract law will allow for "noncompete" clauses, but the courts look upon them with a very critical eye, as the notions of free commerce and competition are undercut by such clauses. They are customarily used in agreements involving high-level executives, to prevent them from taking client lists or trade secrets if they leave a firm and work for a direct competitor (think high-level investment advisors or software designers, or inventors of secret recipes for one-of-a-kind foods or perfumes and such) (Sfikas, 2005). Hanging out a shingle as a solo private practice lactation consultant can hardly be said to "compete" with a delivery hospital that employs hundreds of doctors, nurses, administrators, custodians, and lactation consultants.

Effecting Change Is an Option

If the policies of your place of work are consistently presenting roadblocks to excellent practice, an IBCLC can effect change. Think of the roadblock as an opportunity for a "teachable moment." Perhaps the pediatric staff is prickly about ankyloglossia because they are unaware of recent research demonstrating that breastfeeding, which they are to support and promote under the AAP Policy on Breastfeeding and Use of Human Milk (AAP, 2012b) and the U.S. Surgeon General's *Call to Action to Support Breast-feeding* (U.S. Dept. of Health and Human Services, 2011), can be adversely affected when the baby with the short frenulum injures mother's nipples and fails to transfer enough milk to gain appropriately (Knox, 2010). Ask to have 10 minutes at the next pediatric staff meeting to share some of these new articles. Ask to do an in-service on the topic with nurses. Doing the preparatory research will enhance your knowledge, and you can build your curriculum vitae with these professional education sessions. If issues involving unethical marketing (like distribution of free formula samples) are of concern, consult with the risk management and quality improvement departments at the hospital, to find out how other clinical departments handle these issues (and to give you some ammunition to effect change in the maternity unit). Lobbying for change can be a long process and may need to be preceded by building trust and rapport with the staff. As members of a fairly new profession, IBCLCs will have to become change agents to effect change.

When the Law or Policy Conflicts with the Practice-Guiding Document

If all IBCLCs everywhere must follow the four practice-guiding documents, if all IBCLCs in some places have laws that apply only in their geopolitical setting, if some IBCLCs in some places have special rules that apply only in their workplace, what happens if these laws and rules seems to be in conflict?

Generally speaking, for the IBCLC, laws will trump policies will trump practice-guiding documents. Put another way, the practice-guiding documents must yield to a work-place policy that is in conflict, and the work-place policy must yield to laws or regulation of the land.

As an example, let us consider the fairly controversial topic of mother-to-child transmission of HIV-1 via breastfeeding. Imagine an IBCLC in the United States sees a pregnant mother, who has tested positive for HIV. As an IBCLC, her practice-guiding documents will encourage her to provide evidence-based information and support to the mother regarding possible transfer of HIV through breastmilk to her baby (mother-to-child-transmission, or MTCT). The IBCLC is aware of recent studies in Africa that show prophylactic antiretroviral treatment of mothers and infants, along with *exclusive* breastfeeding in the early months, resulted in lowered transmission rates of HIV (Horvath, Madi, Iuppa, Kennedy, Rutherford, & Read, 2009; Kilewo et al., 2009). However, the current recommendation of the American Academy of Pediatrics is that breastfeeding is contraindicated for HIV-positive mothers in the United States, while recognizing that "in the developing world, where mortality is increased in non-breastfeeding infants from a combination of malnutrition and infectious diseases, breastfeeding may outweigh the risk of the acquiring HIV infection from human milk" (AAP, 2012b, e832–e833). At our IBCLC's hospital, the pediatric department's policies and procedures are aligned with the AAP statement: HIV-positive mothers are advised that breastfeeding is contraindicated, and the mother will be told by her pediatrician that she should not breastfeed her child.

The IBCLC has practice-guiding documents that require her to provide relevant evidence-based information to the mother, and that evidence suggests means by which the HIV-positive mother can breastfeed. But the IBCLC's work setting has a policy of giving the AAP-guideline recommendations to the HIV-positive mother. The IBCLC is a member of the healthcare team; it is the baby's primary HCP who will have the final word in treatment options ordered for a baby. The practice-guiding documents yield to the policies in the workplace; in this case, the clinical recommendation of "no breastfeeding."

Bear in mind, this example is being used merely to demonstrate how the IBCLC's practice-guiding documents, while describing proactive duties and strong responsibilities, do not always carry the weight of being the definitive source of authority for providing health care. Of course, individual cases can always be discussed individually and health care fashioned to meet the patient's needs. Let's play with the facts a bit: imagine our IBCLC was counseling an HIV-positive mother who had delivered her baby quite by surprise during a vacation trip to the United States. She is about to return to her homeland of Kenya. She was receiving antiretroviral drug therapy in pregnancy. She wants to continue her drug therapy, exclusively breastfeeding her child, and give the baby antiretroviral drugs as well. The U.S.-based doctor may certainly take this mother's particular situation into consideration, and realize that the AAP guideline (which is, after all, a guideline, and not a hard-and-fast requirement) is not suitable for this family. The IBCLC can go a long way toward helping this family to come to this result, by education, advocacy, and collaboration with the pediatrician and obstetrician.

What good, you may wonder, are the practice-guiding documents, if they can be trumped by hospital policy that may not be based on the latest evidence? Their value is that they can be offered as a powerful and persuasive reason to effect change. A classic example is the formula discharge bags (or packs), handed out on some postpartum floors. These free gifts from the formula manufacturers (containing samples and coupons) are intended to be handed out at discharge by the nurse or other HCP, a classic violation of the *International Code of Marketing of Breast-milk Substitutes*. They imply to the mother that these products are endorsed by the medical institution, and necessary for the baby; their mere distribution has a negative impact on breastfeeding exclusivity and duration (Ban the Bags, n.d.a). Some hospitals require their HCPs (including IBCLCs) to dispense them. By showing to their superiors their practice-guiding documents requiring support for the WHO Code, IBCLCs have been able to effectively argue that the ethics of their profession require that they not be associated with such shallow marketing tactics. Advocacy efforts at the hospital level, and with state and federal government agencies, has created a successful

"Ban the Bags" movement that has curtailed this practice in many places (Ban the Bags, n.d.b).

Summary

All IBCLCs, everywhere, have rules of the road to guide their practice: (1) the mandatory IBLCE Code of Professional Conducts, (2) the mandatory IBLCE Scope of Practice, (3) the model ILCA Standards of Practice, and (4) the model-unless-it-is-mandatory *International Code of Marketing of Breast-milk Substitutes*. Table 3-1 offers a comparison of the requirements of each of the four current practice-guiding documents. Table 3-2 compares the 2011 IBLCE Code of Professional Conduct with its predecessor the IBLCE Code of Ethics. All IBCLCs in the same geopolitical region will have to follow the laws of that land (for example, countries that have legislated the WHO Code). Some IBCLCs in some places will be required to follow the policies of those workplaces, and it is these day-to-day restrictions on practice that can be the source of considerable tension, confusion, or frustration. However, they are the one area where the diligent and diplomatic IBCLC may be able to effect some change.

REFERENCES

Altman, D. (2008). *History and assessment: It's all in the details* (Monograph No. 3). Amarillo, TX: Hale Publishing.

American Academy of Pediatrics. (2011, November). American Academy of Pediatrics policy statement on SIDS and other sleep-related infant deaths: Expansion of recommendations for a safe infant sleeping environment. *Pediatrics, 128*(5), 1030–1039. Retrieved from http://pediatrics.aappublications.org/content/early/2011/10/12/peds.2011-2284.full.pdf+html

American Academy of Pediatrics. (2012a, February). American Academy of Pediatrics policy on patient- and family-centered care and the pediatrician's role. *Pediatrics, 129*(2), 394–403. Retrieved from http://pediatrics.aappublications.org/content/129/2/394.full.pdf+html

American Academy of Pediatrics. (2012b, March 1). American Academy of Pediatrics policy on breastfeeding and use of human milk. *Pediatrics, 129*(3), e827–e841. Retrieved from http://pediatrics.aappublications.org/content/early/2012/02/22/peds.2011-3552.full.pdf

Baby Friendly USA. (2010). *Does the BFHI enhance breastfeeding?* [Frequently Asked Questions]. Retrieved from http://www.babyfriendlyusa.org/eng/06.html

Ban the Bags. (n.d.a). *About banthebags.org*. Retrieved from http://banthebags.org/about

Ban the Bags. (n.d.b). *Bag-free hospitals and nursing centers*. Retrieved from http://banthebags.org/bag-free-hospitals

Barger, J., Burger, S., Lauwers, J., Leeper, K., Myr, R., Sandink, A., . . . Thorley, V. (2007, September). *Report of the ILCA Scope of Practice Task Force* (Monograph). Raleigh, NC: International Lactation Consultant Association.

Baumslag, N., & Michels, D. (1995). *Milk, money and madness: The culture and politics of breastfeeding*. Westport, CT: Bergin & Garvey.

Berggren, K. (2005). *Reverse cycling*. Retrieved from http://www.workandpump.com/reversecycling.htm

Brooks, E., Stehel, E., & Mannel, R. (2013). The IBLCE code of professional conduct for IBCLCs. In International Lactation Consultant Association, *Core curriculum for lactation consultant practice* (R. Mannel, P. Martens, & M. Walker, Eds., 3rd ed., pp. 5–37). Burlington, MA: Jones & Bartlett Learning.

Bruce, K., Myr, R., Koch, K., Gribble, K., & Pohl, L. (2010, October 31). *To manage your subscription* [Online forum message]. Retrieved from http://community.lsoft.com/archives/lactnet.html

Conlan, J., Grabowski, S., & Smith, K. (2003). Adult learning. In M. Orey (Ed.), *Emerging perspectives on learning, teaching and technology*. Retrieved from http://projects.coe.uga.edu/epltt/index.php ?title=Adult_Learning

Council of Medical Specialty Societies. (2011, March). *Code for interactions with companies* (Model policy). Retrieved from http://www.cmss.org/uploadedFiles/Site/CMSS_Policies/CMSS%20Code%20for %20Interactions%20with%20Companies%20Approved%20Revised%20Version%203-19-11CLEAN.pdf

Diligence—reasonable. (1979/1891). In H. Black (Ed.), *Black's law dictionary* (5th ed., p. 412). St. Paul, MN: West.

Duty. (1979/1891). In H. Black (Ed.), *Black's law dictionary* (5th ed., p. 453). St. Paul, MN: West.

Europe Summaries of EU Legislation. (2011, February 1). *Protection of personal data*. Retrieved from http:// europa.eu/legislation_summaries/information_society/l14012_en.htm

Genna, C. W. (2013). *Supporting sucking skills in breastfeeding infants* (2nd ed.). Burlington, MA: Jones & Bartlett Learning.

Health Insurance Portability and Accountability Act of 1996, Pub. L. No. 104-191, 45 C.F.R. § 160 & 164 (2002).

Horvath, T., Madi, B. C., Iuppa, I. M., Kennedy, G. E., Rutherford, G. W., & Read, J. S. (2009). *Interventions for preventing late postnatal mother-to-child transmission of HIV (review)*. Retrieved from http:// onlinelibrary.wiley.com/doi/10.1002/14651858.CD006734.pub2/pdf/standard

Human Milk Banking Association of North America (HMBANA). (n.d.). *Mission/description*. Retrieved from http://www.hmbana.org/index/missiondescription

International Baby Food Action Network (IBFAN). (n.d.a). *The full code and subsequent WHA resolutions*. Retrieved from http://www.ibfan.org/issue-international_code-full.html

International Baby Food Action Network (IBFAN). (n.d.b). *IBFAN home page*. Retrieved from http://www .ibfan.org/index.html

International Board of Lactation Consultant Examiners. (1997, March 11; renewed 2007). *U.S. Certification Mark 2042667 [IBCLC]*. Washington, DC: U.S. Patent and Trademark Office.

International Board of Lactation Consultant Examiners. (1999, April 22). *Code of ethics* [Archival document]. Retrieved from http://web.archive.org/web/*/http://iblce.org

International Board of Lactation Consultant Examiners. (2003a). *Clinical competencies for IBCLC practice*. Retrieved from http://replay.waybackmachine.org/20090202031539/http://iblce.org/clinicalcompetencies.php

International Board of Lactation Consultant Examiners. (2003b). *Code of ethics for international board certified lactation consultants*. Retrieved from http://www.iblce.org/upload/downloads/CodeOfEthics.pdf

International Board of Lactation Consultant Examiners. (2003c, August 5). *U.S. Certification Mark 2749041 [Registered Lactation Consultant]*. Washington, DC: U.S. Patent and Trademark Office.

International Board of Lactation Consultant Examiners. (2008, March 8). *Scope of practice for international board certified lactation consultants*. Retrieved from http://www.iblce.org/upload/downloads/Scope Of Practice.pdf

International Board of Lactation Consultant Examiners. (2009, September 8). *IBLCE executive summary of board of directors meeting (Sept. 2009)*. Retrieved from http://www.iblce.edu.au/documents/iblcesummary BODSept09.pdf

International Board of Lactation Consultant Examiners. (2010a, April 22). *Sanctions imposed against IBCLCs.* Retrieved from http://iblce.org/upload/downloads/SanctionsList.pdf

International Board of Lactation Consultant Examiners. (2010b, September 26). *IBLCE disciplinary procedures.* Retrieved from http://www.iblce.org/upload/downloads/IBLCEDisciplinaryProcedures.pdf

International Board of Lactation Consultant Examiners. (2010c, December 6). *Clinical competencies for the practice of IBCLCs.* Retrieved from http://www.iblce.org/upload/downloads/ClinicalCompetencies.pdf

International Board of Lactation Consultant Examiners. (2011a, January). *Number of IBCLCs in the world.* Retrieved from http://www.iblce.org/upload/downloads/NumberIBCLCsWorld.pdf

International Board of Lactation Consultant Examiners. (2011b, July 5). *IBLCE exam blueprint* [Fact sheet]. Retrieved from http://www.iblce.org/upload/downloads/IBLCEExamBlueprint.pdf

International Board of Lactation Consultant Examiners. (2011c, September 24). *Disciplinary procedures for the code of professional conduct for IBCLCs for the international board of lactation consultant examiners (IBLCE).* Retrieved from http://www.iblce.org/upload/downloads/IBLCEDisciplinaryProcedures.pdf

International Board of Lactation Consultant Examiners. (2011d, October 31). *Frequently asked questions (FAQs) regarding the code of professional conduct for IBCLC.* Retrieved from http://iblce.org/upload/downloads /CodeOfConductFAQs.pdf

International Board of Lactation Consultant Examiners. (2011e, November 1). *Code of professional conduct for IBCLCs.* Retrieved from http://iblce.org/upload/downloads/CodeOfProfessionalConduct.pdf

International Board of Lactation Consultant Examiners. (2012). *Recertification requirements.* Retrieved from http://americas.iblce.org/recertification-requirements

International Code Documentation Centre (ICDC). (2006). *International code of marketing of breastmilk substitutes and relevant WHA resolutions.* Penang, Malaysia: IBFAN Penang.

International Lactation Consultant Association. (2005). *Lactation consulting: The first twenty years—A history* (J. Lauwers, Ed.) [Pamphlet]. Raleigh, NC: International Lactation Consultant Association.

International Lactation Consultant Association. (2006). *Standards of practice for international board certified lactation consultants.* Retrieved from http://www.ilca.org/files/resources/Standards-of-Practice-web.pdf

International Lactation Consultant Association. (2012a, January 22). *ILCA board of directors' meeting Dec 1–4, 2011 executive summary.* Retrieved http://www.ilca.org/files/members_only/ExecSummary_Dec%20 2011.pdf

International Lactation Consultant Association. (2012b). *Welcome to ILCA* [Home page]. Retrieved from http://www.ilca.org/i4a/pages/index.cfm?pageid=1

International Lactation Consultant Association, & Henderson, S. (2011, June). *Position paper on the role and impact of the IBCLC* (Monograph). Retrieved from http://www.ilca.org/files/resources/ilca_publications /Role%20%20Impact%20of%20the%20IBCLC-webFINAL_08-15-11.pdf

International Lactation Consultant Association, Overfield, M., Ryan, C., Spangler, A., & Tully, M. R. (2005). *Clinical guidelines for the establishment of exclusive breastfeeding* (Monograph). Raleigh, NC: International Lactation Consultant Association.

International Lactation Consultant Association, Spatz, D., & Lessen, R. (2011). *Risks of not breastfeeding* (Monograph). Morrisville, NC: International Lactation Consultant Association.

Kilewo, C., Karlsson, K., Massawe, A., Lyamuya, E., Swai, A., Mhalu, F., & Ngarina, M. (2009, November 1). Prevention of mother-to-child transmission of HIV-1 through breast-feeding by treating mothers with triple antiretroviral in Dar es Salaam, Tanzania: The Mitra Plus study [Abstract]. *Journal of Acquired Immune Deficiency Syndromes, 52*(3), 406–416. Retrieved from http://www.ncbi.nlm.nih.gov /pubmed/19730269

Knox, I. (2010, September). Tongue tie and frenotomy in the breastfeeding newborn. *NeoReviews, 11*(9), e513–e519. Retrieved from http://www.lunalactation.com/KnoxTT.pdf

Lo, B., & Field, M. (Eds.). (2009). *Conflict of interest in medical research, education, and practice.* Retrieved from http://www.ncbi.nlm.nih.gov/books/NBK22942

McKenna, J., & McDade, T. (2005, June). Why babies should never sleep alone: A review of the co-sleeping controversy in relation to SIDS, bedsharing and breast feeding [Abstract]. *Paediatric Respiratory Review, 6*(2), 134–152. Retrieved from http://img2.timg.co.il/forums/1_147673444.pdf

NHS Choice (National Health Service, United Kingdom). (2011, December 9). *How long should health records (medical records) be kept for?* Retrieved from http://www.nhs.uk/chq/Pages/1889.aspx?Category ID=68&SubCategoryID=160

Noel-Weiss, J. (2009, July 24). *Ethics and lactation consultants: A needs assessment.* Lecture presented at ILCA Annual Conference, Orlando, FL.

Noel-Weiss, J., & Walters, G. (2006). Ethics and lactation consultants: Developing knowledge, skills, and tools. *Journal of Human Lactation, 22*(2), 203–212. doi:10.1177/0890334406286955

Physician's desk reference (64th ed.). (2009). Montvale, NJ: PDR Network.

Publication. (1979/1891). In H. Black (Ed.), *Black's law dictionary* (5th ed., p. 1105). St. Paul, MN: West.

Riordan, J., & Wambach, K. (2010). *Breastfeeding and human lactation* (4th ed.). Sudbury, MA: Jones & Bartlett.

Scott, J., & Calandro, A. (2008). The code of ethics for international board certified lactation consultants: Ethical practice. In International Lactation Consultant Association (ILCA), R. Mannel, P. J. Martens, & M. Walker (Eds.), *Core curriculum for lactation consultant practice* (2nd ed., pp. 5–18). Sudbury, MA: Jones & Bartlett.

Scott, J. W. (1996, December). Code of ethics for international board certified lactation consultants. *Journal of Human Lactation, 12*(4), 344–347. doi:10.1177/089033449601200449

Scott, J. W. (Speaker). (2005, July 5). *From code to consultation: Applying IBCLC ethics to practice* [MP3]. ProLibraries.com, for La Leche League International. Retrieved from http://www.prolibraries.com

Sfikas, P. (2005). Are covenants not to compete becoming unenforceable? A growing trend explored. *Journal of the American Dental Association, 136*, 1309–1311. Retrieved from http://jada.ada.org/cgi/reprint /136/9/1309

Spoliation. (1979/1891). In H. Black (Ed.), *Black's law dictionary* (5th ed., p. 1257). St. Paul, MN: West.

Thorley, V. (2010, November 3). Why do we say breastmilk? [Electronic mailing list message]. Retrieved from http:// community.lsoft.com/SCRIPTS/WA-LSOFTDONATIONS.EXE?A2=ind1011A&L=LACTNET &P=R1191&1=LACTNET&9=A&I=-3&J=on&d=No+Match%3BMatch%3BMatches&z=4

Tort. (1979/1891). In H. Black (Ed.), *Black's law dictionary* (5th ed., p. 1335). St. Paul, MN: West.

UNICEF. (n.d.a). *The baby-friendly hospital initiative.* Retrieved from http://www.unicef.org/programme /breastfeeding/baby.htm

UNICEF. (n.d.b). *Fact sheet: A summary of the rights under the convention on the rights of the child.* Retrieved from http://www.unicef.org/crc/files/Rights_overview.pdf

United Nations General Assembly. (1979, December 18). *Convention on the elimination of all forms of discrimination against women.* Retrieved from http://www.hrweb.org/legal/cdw.html

U.S. Copyright Office. (2011, August). *Circular 1: Copyright basics.* Retrieved from http://www.copyright.gov /circs/circ01.pdf

U.S. Dept. of Health and Human Services. (2011, January). *Surgeon general's call to action to support breastfeeding.* Retrieved from http://www.surgeongeneral.gov/topics/breastfeeding/calltoactiontosupportbreastfeeding.pdf

U.S. Food & Drug Administration (FDA). (2012, March 5). *Recalls, market withdrawals, & safety alerts.* Retrieved from http://www.fda.gov/Safety/Recalls/default.htm

West, D., & Marasco, L. (2009). *The breastfeeding mother's guide to making more milk.* New York, NY: McGraw Hill.

World Health Organization. (1981). *International code of marketing of breast-milk substitutes.* Retrieved from http://www.who.int/nutrition/publications/code_english.pdf

World Health Organization. (2006). *The international code of marketing of breast-milk substitutes: Frequently asked questions* [Brochure]. Retrieved from http://whqlibdoc.who.int/publications/2008/9789241594295 _eng.pdf

World Health Organization (Ed.). (2007). *Safe preparation storage and handling of powdered infant formula: Guidelines.* Retrieved from http://www.who.int/foodsafety/publications/micro/pif_guidelines.pdf

Chapter 4

I Think This Is Trouble.
What Do I Do Now?

Congratulations! You are an International Board Certified Lactation Consultant (IBCLC), you have found a wonderful position where you help breastfeeding families every day, your colleagues welcome your expertise, and you get great personal satisfaction from your nurturing profession and the opportunity to hone clinical skills.

Then, one day, those little hairs go up on the back of your neck. Something just happened and your inner voice said, "Wait. That isn't right."

Perhaps you witness an IBCLC colleague, or another healthcare provider (HCP), in a stomach-sinking interaction with one of your breastfeeding mothers. The pediatrician offered outdated or unfounded clinical advice (suggesting "timed feedings" as the way to prevent sore nipples, a technique questioned by research back in the 1980s [de Carvalho, Robertson, & Klaus, 1984]). The 45 minutes you just spent boosting the confidence of the first-time mother with a well-suckling infant was instantly undermined when the bedside nurse casually remarked, "Oh, heavens, don't let that baby use you as a pacifier!" An IBCLC colleague gives some formula samples to a mother of a 36-hour-old infant, who "wants Dad to bond with the baby by feeding," and you know she regularly attends lunches paid for by formula manufacturers and medical device manufacturers.

Our inner radar is quite accurate when it comes to legal and ethical issues. We all know that sensation of witnessing something off-kilter, even if we can't precisely cite which International Board of Lactation Consultant Examiners Code of Professional Conduct (IBLCE CPC, 2011c) or International Board of Lactation Consultant Examiners Scope of Practice (IBLCE SOP, 2008) or International Lactation Consultant Association Standards of Practice (ILCA Standards, 2006) section has been violated. It doesn't take long in the practice of any healthcare profession to find that what was learned in the classroom does not always take place in the real-world clinical setting. There will also be times we come up against something more grave than a mere difference in personality or technique. IBCLCs agonize over what to do with this information. We are far more distressed about what to do about perceived ethics violations of our co-workers than we are about our own ethical inequities (Noel-Weiss, 2009). Let's explore how an IBCLC might deal with an unsettling scenario.

Define the Problem and Consider Your Options

As simple as this seems, it is an excellent first step: stop a minute, step back, and try to isolate the ethical problem. It will clarify what you can, or should, do next. You aren't trying to fix it now, just define it. You may be pleasantly surprised to realize there is no issue at all. A colleague's rushed and rude bedside manner is irksome, but it does not rise to the level of unethical behavior. Sometimes the problem isn't related to lactation at all. Perhaps this is a workplace squabble: if you witnessed an unprofessional shouting match between colleagues, the practice-guiding documents of your profession do not require any action on your part. The dilemma may seem more manageable if it can be put into some sort of context, only parts of which may be within your control.

Figure 4-1 represents a flow chart of yes/no options for the IBCLC deciding whether she should "do something" when those little hairs stand up on the back of her neck. Don't be put off by the size of the chart. It is meant to synthesize the variables that come into play: we want to chip away at them bit by bit, to feel less overwhelmed by an unethical situation. And, to be clear: it is the rare IBCLC, in a real-life scenario, who will plod these steps, chutes-and-ladders style, to arrive at a conclusion. However, in the safe context of reading a book, this table allows for reflection about what should be spinning through your mind when confronted by an ethical or legal dilemma in your practice. The various steps will be discussed in the following sections.

Ack! Ethical or Legal Dilemma! Should I Take Action? Part One

No
Let's take the easiest route first: that of no action. And, yes, this is a perfectly viable option to explore. Some of us are movers and shakers; some of us are not. You are entitled to the personality and professional style you have; indeed, your quiet, competent style may be the attribute that allows you to build trust and rapport with your patients/clients. Taking no action is an option that can be exercised most of the time. It doesn't hurt, however, to double-check the rules of the road.

When the law or your healthcare responsibilities give you a "duty of care," your failure to do so is an "omission" or "breach" that may give rise to culpability for failure to act (Duty of care, n.d.; Omission, 2012). However, if you are witnessing the unethical or illegal behavior *of someone else,* your role is simply that of a witness. You are not required to do anything when you are merely a bystander to the action. So that begs the ultimate question: do you, as the IBCLC, have "a duty of care" requiring you to take action, even if you don't want to?

Review the Four Practice-Guiding Documents for the IBCLC Profession
The first level of analysis involves your four practice-guiding documents. The IBLCE CPC and IBLCE SOP are mandatory practice-guiding documents the IBCLC *must* follow. Reporting requirements (in the form of a written complaint to the IBLCE

Discipline Committee) *are* an element of IBLCE CPC Principles 8.1 and 8.2; reports to non-IBLCE authorities are suggested by IBLCE CPC Principles 2.4, 4.2, 5.3, and 6.2. Reporting is required by IBLCE SOP paragraphs 3 and 8. If the IBCLC finds that these principles and duties have come into play, especially with regard to her own [mis]conduct, she may not have the option of "no action." She may have to gird herself, and file a complaint or report with IBLCE.

The ILCA Standards of Practice are a model of professional practices that the IBCLC *should* follow, but failure to do so carries no sanction nor reporting requirement. The IBCLC who wants to take "no action" will find comfort in knowing that nothing in the ILCA Standards compels otherwise.

For the IBCLC, the *International Code of Marketing of Breast-milk Substitutes* (WHO Code, sometimes called International Code) is a model document (a "should") that IBCLCs *should* support, unless they *must*. How does that work? The IBLCE CPC in its Introduction discusses "an IBCLC's duty to protect mothers and children [by] adherence to the principles and aim of the *International Code of Marketing of Breast-milk Substitutes*" (IBLCE, 2011c, CPC p. 1)—such "duty language" ordinarily imposing an obligation of mandatory professional behaviors. Yet, the accompanying Frequently Asked Questions document to the IBLCE CPC steps back from requiring IBCLC adherence to the International Code (IBLCE, 2011b), something that had been required under Tenet 24 of the predecessor document, the IBLCE Code of Ethics (IBLCE COE) (IBLCE, 2003). To further complicate matters, the International Code *will* be deemed a mandatory practice-guiding document for the IBCLC if she works in a country that has legislated the International Code, or she works in an institution that has been designated with, or is working toward, Baby-Friendly status (Baby-Friendly USA, 2010; UNICEF, n.d.).

To briefly review: The WHO Code contains a handful of obligations on the part of health workers (who include IBCLCs). They have a proactive obligation to disclose whatever money or gifts are received from marketers of products within the scope of the International Code (World Health Organization [WHO], 1981, Article 7.5). There are several prohibited behaviors for health workers, such as do not accept "material or financial inducements" from marketers (WHO, 1981 Article 7.3) and do not distribute free samples (WHO, 1981, Article 7.4) nor accept free samples unless it is for legitimate research (WHO, 1981 Article 7.4). If there has been legislation enacted in her country to enact and enforce the WHO Code, the IBCLC may be obligated under provisions of those laws or regulations. But the WHO Code itself does not contain any sorts of "reporting" requirements (in the form of a written complaint to the IBLCE Discipline Committee), and so the IBCLC who wishes to take "no action" will not be required to do so under the policy-promoting principles outlined in the *International Code of Marketing of Breast-milk Substitutes*. Note that this is different from reporting marketing violations of the WHO Code, which anyone is encouraged to do, to the monitoring groups designed to track such events (International Baby Food Action

Figure 4-1   Decision Steps for the IBCLC Facing an Ethical or Legal Dilemma

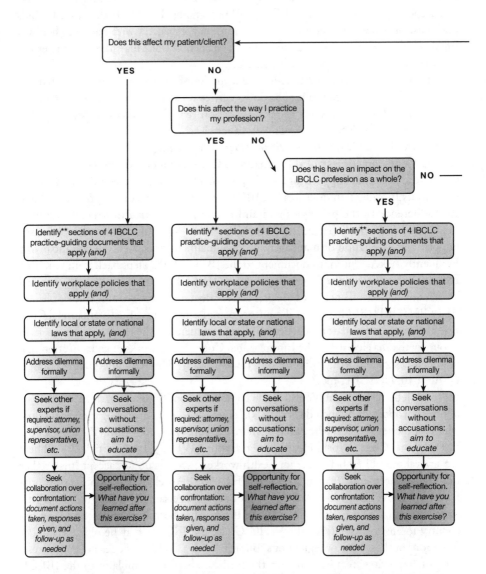

* Reporting requirements: The IBLCE Code of Professional Conduct (IBLCE CPC) and IBLCE Scope of Practice for IBCLCs (IBLCE SOP) are mandatory practice-guiding documents the IBCLC must follow. Reporting requirements (in the form of a written complaint to the IBLCE Discipline Committee) are an element of IBLCE CPC principle 8; reports to non-IBLCE authorities are suggested by IBLCE CPC principles 2.4, 4.2, 5.3, and 6.2, and IBLCE SOP paras. 3 and 8. The ILCA Standards of Practice (ILCA Standards) are a model of professional practices that the IBCLC should follow, but failure to do so does not carry any sanction and there is no reporting requirement. For the IBCLC, the *International Code of Marketing of Breast-milk Substitutes* (WHO Code) is a model document that IBCLCs *should* support, unless they *must* support it because they live in a country where it has been legislated, or work in an institution designated or working toward Baby-Friendly status. Reports of marketing violations can be sent to WHO Code monitoring organizations; if the WHO Code is enacted into law in an IBCLC's country, she will follow reporting requirements set forth in the specific laws/regulations in her country.

Figure 4-1   Decision Steps for the IBCLC Facing an Ethical or Legal Dilemma (continued)

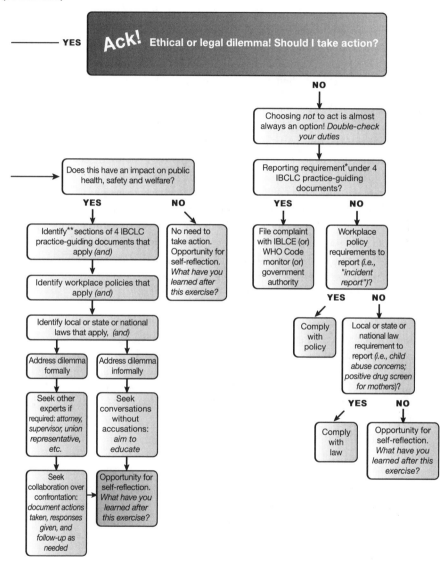

Identify relevant sections: Table 3-1 may assist in making this analysis by the IBCLC manageable. **The IBLCE Code of Professional Conduct (IBLCE CPC) and IBLCE Scope of Practice for IBCLCs (IBLCE SOP) are mandatory practice-guiding documents the IBCLC *must* follow. The ILCA Standards of Practice (ILCA Standards) are a model of professional practices that the IBCLC *should* follow, but failure to do so carries no sanction. For the IBCLC, the *International Code of Marketing of Breast-milk Substitutes* (WHO Code) is a model document that IBCLCs *should* support, unless they *must* support it because they live in a country where it has been legislated, or work in an institution designated or working toward Baby-Friendly status. If the WHO Code has been enacted into law in the IBCLC's country she will follow those geopolitical laws/regulations. Not all elements of these practice-guiding documents will apply.

Network [IBFAN], n.d.). Such reporting is not the same as filing a complaint report with IBLCE about IBCLC behaviors. And note, too, that countries that have legislated the International Code may have sections in their law that *do* allow or require health workers to report marketing violations to the health minister. Again, that is a different scenario than the one we are exploring here: the IBCLC in her clinical practice, exploring her options for appropriate action and possible requirement to file a complaint, now that those hairs have gone up on the back of her neck.

Review Workplace Policy Requirements for the IBCLC

We have learned that some IBCLCs, in some places, have their own set of rules of the road. The larger the institution (hospital, governmental agency, teaching university) the more formalized the policies are likely to be. As a matter of common sense and professionalism, the IBCLC will acquaint herself with these policies, as they represent a condition of her employment. If the IBCLC has witnessed what she suspects to be unethical or illegal behaviors, her desire to take "no action" may not be an option. For example, many institutions require that "incident reports" be filed whenever something has gone awry. It can be something as simple as an accident ("revolving door pinched incoming visitor's fingers"), or it can be something as grave as a malpractice allegation. The reasoning behind such reporting requirements is to protect public health and safety, and to improve risk management and quality within the facility (Taylor et al., 2004).

Review Statutory or Regulatory Requirements for the IBCLC

We have also learned that all IBCLCs, in some places, have legal obligations affecting practice. Local laws of the land may not allow the IBCLC to take "no action." For example, an IBCLC is a "mandatory reporter" of suspected child abuse in the laws of many countries of the world (Higgins, Bromfield, Richardson, Holzer, & Berlyn, 2010 [Australia]; U.S. Dept. of Health and Human Services Administration for Children & Families, 2010 [United States]; Social, Health & Family Affairs Committee, & Rupprecht, 2010 [Council of Europe]). Concerns about potential child neglect has prompted some jurisdictions to pass regulations that require reports to the child protective services agency if the birth mother has tested positive for various controlled substances (U.S. Dept. of Health and Human Services Administration for Children & Families, 2009; Kandall, 1993). Often the policy of the workplace (see the paragraph above) will indicate that the worker must abide by whatever reporting requirements are mandated by law.

Use This Opportunity for Self-Reflection

Regardless of where the IBCLC ends up: reporting, or not reporting, despite her initial desire to take no action, she will have gone through a mental exercise to reach her decision. We can all benefit from a bit of introspective reflection after the fact. What did the IBCLC learn? What can she do in the future to avoid being put into this uncomfortable circumstance? Can she adjust her own professional practice to prevent mistakes or clarify expectations?

Ack! Ethical or Legal Dilemma! Should I Take Action? Part Two

Yes

Let's assume the IBCLC has come up against a situation that is causing consternation, and she is inclined to do something about it. Yet, she is likely to feel overwhelmed about where to begin, and even to have a sensation that she'll get "in trouble" if she doesn't choose the right path. Let's try to break it down. Remember that Figure 4-1 puts this into a flow chart to navigate the various steps requiring a decision. The pathway is much the same as for our "no action" IBCLC; the only difference is in how we interpret the rules to serve our goals.

What or Whom Does the Dilemma Affect?

Recall that the IBCLC's core responsibilities, as a part of the healthcare team, is to provide information and support to the dyad, so the mother can make an informed decision. Recall also that the rules of the road for the IBCLC are found in the four practice-guiding documents, and the policies and laws specific to the IBCLC's workplace and residence. Keeping these obligations in her "rear brain," the IBCLC should ask in her "front brain," "Who is affected by this ethical dilemma I have come up against?"

If the patient/client will somehow feel the pinch in this quandary, the IBCLC's obligations are more obvious, and usually will require quicker action. If a mother has been (erroneously) told by her obstetrician that breastfeeding is contraindicated because of maternal medications, the mother can't wait 2 or 3 weeks for the IBCLC to call a staff meeting to discuss protocols for reviewing medications and mothers' milk. The IBCLC will need to intervene right away to preserve the breastfeeding relationship and milk production.

The next rung of analysis: Does this dilemma affect the way the IBCLC practices? If the answer is a generic yes, the time pressures are reduced for the IBCLC who chooses to slay whatever dragons are preventing her from providing best practices as an IBCLC. In our example involving maternal medications, the IBCLC runs immediate interference on a case-by-case basis for mothers given erroneous information, but the IBCLC can take more time to approach her supervisors about reviewing this topic for a possible change in policy or consultation protocols.

The IBCLC next should ask: Will this dilemma somehow affect my profession as a whole? This seems a presumptuous analysis: While some workdays make us feel like Atlas bearing the weight of the world, it is not required that we spend *all* our waking hours "promoting the profession." However, imagine the IBCLC who has just learned the hospital may cut costs by laying off all the IBCLCs, replacing them with breastfeeding counselors (with no certification or licensure). This *is* happening, in today's tight economy (Barney, 2008; Bartick, 2011). The IBCLC certainly has a personal stake in this drama, but the threat to her job is because of her job *title*, and not her personal skills. In this dilemma, where the short-term savings to the hospital do not account for the long-term patient satisfaction and overall reduction in healthcare costs (United States Lactation Consultant Association [USLCA], Gutowski, Walker & Chetwynd, 2010; USLCA, Clegg, Francis, & Walker, 2010), the IBCLC who seeks to preserve her job is underscoring the important role her entire profession contributes in providing quality health care at the institution.

The last question the IBCLC will ask is: does this dilemma have an impact on the public health, safety, and welfare? Again, this may seem awfully far-reaching; the IBCLC is just one cog in the very big wheel of life. Imagine, however, the IBCLC working as a prenatal educator in a public health agency that serves a low-income and under-educated population, primarily of women of child-bearing age. The IBCLC learns the department head has changed; the new boss's priority is obesity reduction, and he plans to phase out the prenatal educators and hire a registered dietitian to formulate programs to tackle the obesity epidemic. Certainly the IBCLC, who seeks to preserve her job *and* educate her new boss that breastfeeding is actually an excellent means to prevent childhood obesity (Metzger & McDade, 2010), has an impact on the public health, safety, and welfare of an entire generation.

Review the Four Practice-Guiding Documents for the IBCLC Profession

It does not matter at which point the IBCLC answered "yes" in her analysis of whether the dilemma affected a patient/client, the practice of the profession, the profession as a whole, or the public health, safety, and welfare. The next step is the same, regardless, and echoes what our "no action" IBCLC had to do: review the four practice-guiding documents for the IBCLC. The IBLCE CPC and IBLCE SOP are mandatory practice-guiding documents the IBCLC *must* follow. The ILCA Standards are a model of professional practices that the IBCLC *should* follow, but failure to do so does not carry any sanction. For the IBCLC, the *International Code of Marketing of Breast-milk Substitutes* is a model document (a "should") that IBCLCs *should* support, unless she *must* (i.e., the WHO Code has been legislated in her country, or her institution is seeking, or has, designated status as Baby-Friendly). Not all elements of these practice-guiding documents will apply; Table 3-1 from the previous chapter may assist in making this analysis by the IBCLC manageable.

When she skims these documents, the IBCLC is looking for pertinent sections. Using the example of the mother who was told to stop breastfeeding due to maternal medications, it is easy to "weed out" sections of the four practice-guiding documents that do not pertain. Reviewing the IBLCE CPC as one example, the irrelevant principles seem to be 2.3, 2.4, 2.5, 3.1, 3.2, 4.2, 5.1, 5.2, 5.3, 6.2, 6.3, 7.1, 7.2, 7.3, 7.4, 8.1, and 8.2. That leaves Principle 1.1 (work with mothers to meet their breastfeeding goals), Principle 1.2 (meet clients' needs informed by best available evidence), Principle 1.3 (supply information to support informed decision-making), Principle 1.4 (convey accurate, objective information about products), Principle 1.5 (present information without personal bias), Principle 2.1 (operate within scope of practice), Principle 2.2 (collaborate with healthcare team), Principle 4.1 (consent to share healthcare concerns with healthcare team), and Principle 6.1 (behave honestly and fairly). Thus, by looking over the IBLCE CPC, that "What do I do?" moment has now taken on some manageable parameters. The IBCLC can form an action plan based on 9 principles, rather than all 26. The IBCLC can approach the mother's HCP and use good manners and an open mind to offer and discuss evidence-based information about the medication involved, because the mother wishes to breastfeed, and the IBCLC's role is to be her advocate.

Review Workplace Policy Requirements for the IBCLC

After the IBCLC has reviewed her practice-guiding documents, which ought to help shore up any lingering doubts she may have had about the professional rights and duties she brings to bear in advocating for the mother, baby, and breastfeeding, the next step is to look at the workplace policies that apply to the IBCLC. For a private practitioner, or a lone IBCLC working in a midwifery or pediatric office, the policies and procedures may be simple and easy to review. Those working in larger institutions probably will have more to consider.

Recall that workplace policies (on their face) will trump the four practice-guiding documents. Why? The employer uses its policies to manage its workplace, and the IBCLC hired to work there must, as a condition of employment, follow them. The policies are designed to meet various internal and external quality control and risk management objectives. The objectives can be those set by the facility; they may be a requirement from an outside entity (e.g., the Joint Commission, which accredits hospitals in the United States in part by looking at their policies) (Joint Commission Resources, 2012). While the four practice-guiding documents establish rights and authority for the IBCLC, she is but one practitioner. The institution's policies affect all practitioners; hence, they will trump the practice-guiding documents in the first analysis. The IBCLC may well decide that it is time to effect change in the policies of her workplace, so that at some future point they better align with the processes envisioned by the IBLCE CPC, IBLCE SOP, ILCA Standards, or WHO Code. But until there is that paradigm shift, the IBCLC will have to resolve her immediate dilemma by recognizing that her workplace policies may require her to take some form of action or follow a set procedure.

Let's go back to our mother on medications, and assume she is on fluoxetine for depression, something she took throughout pregnancy. The mother has told the IBCLC that fluoxetine has worked well for her, and she has her heart set on nursing her baby. However, the pediatrician has told the mother that her baby should discontinue breastfeeding because the doctor is concerned that the newborn will continue to absorb fluoxetine. The IBCLC is aware, however, of research that indicates that use of antidepressants or other treatments *can* be compatible with breastfeeding (Weissman et al., 2004). "The risk of medication use must [be] weighed against the risk of ongoing, untreated depression for both mother and child, and the risks associated with not breastfeeding" (Kendall-Tackett, 2009, para. 2). The IBCLC notes that by all outward measures the baby is doing just fine: waking to feed, nursing well, self-detaching contentedly.

Let us further assume the obstetrician, who is not treating the mother for depression, defers to the pediatrician's recommendation that fluoxetine is not compatible with breastfeeding. Assume further that the standard policy and procedure at the hospital requires that the primary healthcare provider (here, the pediatrician) must agree to and sign off on any changes in orders. Imagine now that the pediatrician cannot be reached; her partner is in surgery and unavailable, and the resident covering the nursery does not want to go against the lead doctor's orders in a non-life-threatening situation.

So what is the IBCLC to do? Waiting may be the only viable option right now. The IBCLC should enlist the support of the nurses who have the mother and baby in their care, as the IBCLC is a member of the healthcare team serving the dyad. For now, the written policy is clear: the primary HCP (pediatrician) must agree to and sign off on changes in orders (current instruction to provide formula). Even with the additional support of the nurses, all of these allied care givers must wait for the "green light" from the primary care giver. The IBCLC (perhaps now with the nurses to back her up) can initiate a conversation with the pediatrician upon her return, as the IBCLC practice-guiding documents allow and encourage the IBCLC to do, but until the doctor changes the formula-only order, the IBCLC is stuck.

Nonetheless, the IBCLC has power and resources to give the mother immediate support, acting in her IBCLC role as part of the healthcare team. The IBCLC can share with the mother research-based information about the use of antidepressants, and encourage her discuss this with her psychologist (who prescribed the fluoxetine in the first place), who is her primary healthcare provider for depression. The IBCLC can encourage the mother to have the psychologist contact the pediatrician so the two of them can discuss the best options, in light of the IBCLC's assessment, the mother's desires, and the health history of both mother and baby. The IBCLC can send an email or phone message with her assessment and recommendations with both the psychologist and pediatrician; the doctors may check emails or messages long before returning to the postpartum floor. The mother can be shown how to hand- or pump-express her breastmilk, carefully saving and labeling it, to preserve milk production while the no-breastfeeding care plan is being reviewed. All of these options are well within the IBCLC's Scope of Practice (IBLCE, 2008, SOP paras. 3, 4, 5, 6, & 8).

Review Statutory or Regulatory Requirements for the IBCLC

The IBCLC facing that uncomfortable ethical or legal dilemma has one more level of analysis to consider: are there any regulations or laws that apply, from the local, state, or national level? That may well determine the course of action the IBCLC will have to take. As with our example of the "no action" IBCLC, there may be requirements to call social services/child protective services, if certain conditions have occurred prior to/at delivery. Did the mother come to the emergency room in labor, with no history of prenatal care? In many jurisdictions, a mandatory blood test to screen for narcotics or various diseases will occur; the positive results may be considered evidence of child abuse and neglect permitting the infant to be removed from the mother's care until an investigation can be made of the suitability of the home environment (Dailard & Nash, 2000). Customarily it is the mother's or baby's HCP who will initiate the contact with social services, not the IBCLC. But the IBCLC will have a role to play as she consults about lactation matters for the mother, who is breastfeeding a newborn, and who may very well find her baby taken away in a matter of days by child protective services.

Decide Whether to Address the Dilemma Informally, or Formally

By now, the IBCLC has a pretty sound footing on what issues are at play, and what authority or persuasion she can exert as an allied healthcare provider. The next decision may be, tactically, the most difficult one. Up until now, in our model, the IBCLC has been doing a lot of head-scratching, personal research, and policy review—all by herself. To be honest, most IBCLCs in a real-life situation who feel those hairs going up on the backs of their necks will immediately turn to a trusted peer and discuss the situation with whispers and side-long glances. Even if this "informal consultation" has occurred, the next step for the IBCLC is to decide whether she wants to address the dilemma using informal or formal means.

Informal. IBCLCs may dread informally "confronting" a colleague with whom they have a professional difference of opinion, but it is probably the most common means used to address conflicts. One need only look at how many written complaints have been filed with the IBLCE Ethics & Discipline Committee in 25 years to realize the formal process is rarely initiated. How and when you raise the sensitive topic with your HCP colleague depends on a host of intangible variables: your mood; the pace of the workplace; your colleague's mood and power position in relation to you (did your boss make the mistake, or a student you are training?). The goal should be to seek a conversation, without accusation. Aim to educate. You may have to win the war and not the battle.

Indeed, despite the presence of IBLCE CPC Principles 8.1 and 8.2 and IBLCE SOP paragraph 8 (regarding the discipline process at IBLCE), IBLCE has itself suggested that when an IBCLC becomes aware of ethical discrepancies by another IBCLC, the best and first approach is to discuss the situation informally (Scott, 2005). Self-policing professions like lactation consultation are more interested in attaining compliance with their codes of conduct than in punishment of offenders (Miller, 2006). And that is as it should be.

Formal. If the situation calls for a formal approach, it might be worth it to touch base with whatever "experts" are called for by the process. If the workplace requires the filing of an incident report, the IBCLC's supervisor, or the manager in the risk management or quality assurance department will be able to advise on the correct procedures. If there are issues involving child abuse or neglect allegations, the institution probably has a very structured process to establish that the mother's rights were preserved, and that laws were obeyed. The IBCLC's contribution to the report will no doubt be reviewed and triple-checked by those with primary healthcare or social services responsibility.

There is no question that using formality in addressing an ethical dilemma sets up defensive responses. If an IBCLC files a complaint with IBLCE against a colleague, the IBLCE Disciplinary Procedures (IBLCE, 2011a) describe the quasi-trial-like process that ensues. When the complainant (our IBCLC) initiates the process, her name will be made known to the respondent (the IBCLC against whom the allegations are made). Investigation and review are then undertaken by the IBLCE Discipline Committee, and the complainant may have very little (if any) direct contact with the respondent or the investigators. But her complaint will be scrutinized and her name will be attached to it. It behooves the IBCLC getting ready to file to have the materials reviewed beforehand, perhaps by a friendly colleague unconnected to the case at hand. It requires enough bravery to "go public" on a complaint; being secure that every *t* was crossed and *i* dotted will shore up the strength of one's convictions should there be any repercussions from the filing.

As lofty as this seems, the goal in filing a formal report or complaint should be to seek collaboration rather than confrontation. The more formal the process, the more carefully the IBCLC will want to document her own actions, document responses given, and follow up as needed. As an example, let's assume the IBCLC is alarmed by the number of nipple shields that are being distributed by the night-shift nursing staff, without consideration for whether they are clinically indicated, without proper instruction about their use, and without referral to the IBCLC for follow-up, all of which can disrupt breastfeeding (Genna, 2009). The IBCLC tried informal conversations with the nursing staff to no avail. She raised it in passing with the nurse manager; there was no change in practice. It now appears that a more formal approach will be required. The IBCLC can request time at the next staff meeting to do an in-service about appropriate nipple shield use; she should track the email request she makes, perhaps in follow-up to a verbal request for time on the agenda. She can prepare an evidence-based presentation, discussing recent research and clinical outcomes involving nipple shields with copies for attendees. If the staff or manager concur that new procedures should be implemented regarding nipple shield distribution or teaching, the IBCLC should send a note to the supervisor or meeting leader confirming the discussion, and asking how she can help in drafting the new procedures. And so on and so on. Yes, more work. But through this process the IBCLC can demonstrate all of the steps she took to implement clinical changes to improve patient safety and satisfaction. It is an approach that is much more likely to receive buy-in (and implementation) by the rest of the staff seeing breastfeeding dyads.

Use This Opportunity for Self-Reflection

Last but not least, when all the dust has settled, take some time to reflect on what happened. What personal professional development occurred? Was this the first time the

IBCLC had to publicly disagree with another HCP whose practices are notoriously breastfeeding-unfriendly? How might this have been handled differently, viewed now with the clarity of hindsight? What aspects of the dilemma, causing sleepless nights, turned out to be groundless? Every situation presents an opportunity for self-reflection and self-growth. Don't let this one get away.

Seeking Guidance for Dilemmas in Places You Hadn't Considered

It ought to surprise no IBCLC that the place to look for authority and guidance, when dealing with a legal or ethical dilemma, are the practitioner's rules of road: the four practice-guiding documents and whatever laws or workplace rules apply to the IBCLC. Experience as a practitioner will provide plenty of perspective in avoiding, or dealing with, an IBCLC legal or ethical dilemma. But your own personal excellence—taking it upon yourself to be the best practitioner you can be—will go a long way to preventing uncomfortable scenarios. No, you can't prevent all problems, but being comfortably astute about your zone of authority, and the subject matter of your expertise, will provide confidence in problem solving. Let's review some options for being that excellent practitioner.

Stay on Top of Research

We know that we have to pay attention to evidence-based practice (IBLCE, 2011c, CPC Principle 1.2; IBLCE, 2008, SOP paras. 3, 4, 5, 6, & 8; ILCA, 2006, Standard 1.8). We know evidence-based practice is the gold standard of care for HCPs (Riordan & Wambach, 2010). Whole publications have been devoted to the use of evidence in clinical management of breastfeeding (ILCA, Spatz, & Lessen, 2011; Walker, 2011; Wight, Morton, & Kim, 2008). How is the IBCLC supposed to learn everything that is out there? That is impossible. But there are some tried-and-true options within the reach of any IBCLC to keep her on top of her game, as is her professional expectation (IBLCE, 2011c, CPC Principles 1.2, 1.3, 1.5; IBLCE, 2008, SOP paras. 3, 4, 5, 6 & 8; ILCA, 2006, Standards 1.8 & 4.5).

Join Your Professional Association: Local, National, or International Level
When you spend time with people in your line of work, who have demonstrated they strive to achieve excellence by investing membership money in their own professional development, some of that is bound to rub off. Most organizations have periodic gatherings; continuing education recognition points (CERPs), or their equivalent from another organization awarding education credits, may even be offered for a brief substantive presentation. Networking with colleagues is an opportunity to learn—even to complain—in a safe environment when you will have wise and sympathetic ears. The group may host a lactation conference, and may have books and resources to share. It

probably has a website, email list, or social media presence. Even IBCLCs in remote parts of the world can connect with colleagues in the Internet age, and it is foolhardy not to. Rubbing elbows with other IBCLCs, even in an informal way, will clue you in to the topics that are hot, novel care plan options, fascinating or horrid research articles, and political issues in your neck of the woods.

The International Lactation Consultant Association (ILCA, www.ilca.org) is an organization dedicated to meeting the educational and professional development needs of IBCLCs and others who care for breastfeeding families. It is "a worldwide network of lactation professionals [whose] mission is to advance the profession of lactation consulting worldwide through leadership, advocacy, professional development, and research" (ILCA, 2012b, para. 1). There are other professional associations of IBCLCs, based in smaller geopolitical regions. Some are affiliates of ILCA (such as the Association of Lactation Consultants in Ireland [ALCI] [ILCA, 2012a]) and some are independent of ILCA altogether (European Lactation Consultants Alliance, n.d.). If you truly have no idea who else is an IBCLC in your area, join ILCA, troll its membership directory for nearby practitioners, and call and invite a colleague to lunch.

Read Journals in Breastfeeding and Human Lactation

What ILCA has that the other associations do not is the *Journal of Human Lactation* (JHL), the premiere peer-reviewed quarterly journal. "Lactation research has blossomed into the realms of public health, epidemiology, neonatology, nutrition, microbiology, genetics, pharmacology, anatomy, obstetrics, psychology, nursing, [and] pediatrics. [O]ne of the greatest challenges for involved professionals is to extract research information from journals in all this fields. *JHL*'s strength is its ability to channel all these disciplines . . ." (Merewood, 2012). One of the great advantages of ILCA membership is that printed paper copies of JHL are delivered directly to members, who are also entitled to full online access to every JHL issue ever published. Many academic and institutional libraries subscribe to JHL, so nonmembers of ILCA with appropriate library privileges can access issues. Nonmember individuals can also subscribe to the journal (although the subscription price per person in the United States is more [$190 in 2012] than to join the organization [$181 in 2012], where the JHL is one of several member benefits included in the fee).

Academic journals are rated and ranked in an annual analysis conducted by Thomson Scientific, and released as the Journal Citation Reports (JCR) Data. Journal rankings are important for several reasons: faculty seeking tenure are expected to publish in ranked journals; some non-U.S.-based universities grant funding if faculty has published in ranked journals; librarians make subscription decisions based on rankings. This process is quite competitive and only about the top 10% of the journals in any particular discipline are reviewed for the JCR. They devise an "impact factor," a number that reflects how often a JHL article has been cited by authors publishing in *other* academic journals. In other words, it is a measure of a journal's esteem if researchers are using (and citing to) articles in JHL to support their work (Brooks, 2007).

An *impact factor* is a means of measuring how often a journal's articles are being cited in other publications in a given time period. *Rankings* describe how often the journal is cited, compared to other journals in that field. "All things being equal, the larger the number of previously published articles, the more often a journal will be cited" (Garfield, 2012, para. 4). Since lactation crosses disciplines, it is ranked in three categories: pediatrics, nursing, and obstetrics/gynecology. In 2010, JHL had an impact factor of 1.329, and rankings as follows: 54/109 in pediatrics; 50/77 in obstetrics and gynecology; and 21/89 in nursing (Sage Publications, 2012).

It is doubtful that any IBCLC reads every issue of any journal cover to cover, but a scan at least of the abstracts will tuck more into your brain than you realize. If an issue arises in your practice (about nipple shields, public health initiatives to promote breastfeeding, or rates of breastfeeding in your country; whatever is the subject matter of interest), you may recall that you saw something about that in JHL. And off you will go, with your research mission focused on a topic.

In November 2010, the United States Lactation Consultant Association (USLCA) launched the first issue of *Clinical Lactation*, meeting an oft-mentioned need by IBCLCs for evidence-based lactation articles focusing on clinical practice. It is available in paper and online versions (the latter allowing for links to video clips demonstrating various aspects of the companion article). While the journal is too new to have an impact factor or ranking, its focus on evaluation and treatment of clinical lactation issues provides a unique opportunity for the IBCLC seeking to encourage new thinking or even policy change in her institution. ILCA members who live in the United States automatically are members of USLCA, and receive this new journal as a member benefit. Individual subscriptions (for non-USLCA members) to this publication are reasonable, with options for paper and/or online versions.

There are a few other journals dedicated to the topics of breastfeeding and human lactation; it behooves the IBCLC to be aware of them. Journals dedicated to this topic may be paper and/or online publications. Knowing what is out there, even if you are not a subscriber, can allow you to focus research on a topic should the need arise. *Breastfeeding Medicine* is published by the Academy of Breastfeeding Medicine, "a worldwide organization of physicians dedicated to the promotion, protection, and support of breastfeeding and human lactation. Our mission is to unite members of the various medical specialties with this common purpose" (Academy of Breastfeeding Medicine [ABM], 2008, para. 2). Individual subscriptions to the journal may be made; the online only version was $278 annually in 2012. *International Breastfeeding Journal* is a free "open access, peer-reviewed online journal that will encompass all aspects of breastfeeding" (BioMed Central Ltd., 2012, para. 1). Research involving breastfeeding and human lactation is burgeoning; other journals from various fields may include articles about breastfeeding and human lactation, though they are not dedicated to this topic exclusively (e.g., *Journal of Epidemiology*, *Journal of Allergy and Clinical Immunology*, or *BJOG: An International Journal in Obstetrics and Gynaecology*).

Gain Access to Free Full-Text Resources

Subscriptions to medical and scholarly journals can be cost-prohibitive. IBCLCs of a certain age will recall when digging up research, even in the early years of lactation consultancy, meant trudging to a physical place. Hopefully one was within driving distance of (and had privileges to use) a decent university or hospital library; with luck, the librarians could help track down articles of interest. The modern age has changed all of that: now the helpful librarian is right inside your computer. Several search engines can be used to find online journals with access to full articles, not just the abstracts. **Figure 4-2** provides a summary of excellent resources available from your closest computer keyboard.

Get Connected Online with Other IBCLCs

Many virtual communities for IBCLCs exist, independent of professional associations. Lactnet is probably the most well known. Started in 1995, it is an award-winning

> email list for anyone involved in providing support to mothers who breastfeed their infants and young children. Lactnet's members include lactation consultants, lay breast-feeding counselors, nurses, doctors, midwives, public health advocates, pharmacologists, marketing experts, writers, journalists, scientists, dietitians and doulas (natural birthing assistants). (Lactnet, n.d.)

The list has approximately 4000 subscribers from 38 countries, covering every continent except Antarctica (Bruce, Myr, Koch, Gribble, & Pohl, 2010; Lactnet, n.d.). Posts cover clinical and policy and public health aspects of breastfeeding advocacy, and extensive archives allow access to years' worth of posts. Be cognizant that, while posts are full of experience, expertise, and wit, they are the mere opinion of each author. Although it does not constitute evidence-based practice, Lactnet posts may send you to sources to substantiate recommendations with the evidence base.

Yahoo Groups are self-created and monitored; some have more restrictive access rules than others; anyone may seek information or access using the simple steps described on the Yahoo Groups webpage (groups.yahoo.com). A search in early 2012 using *breastfeeding* as the term of interest found 2021 groups; *breastfeed* brought up 273 groups; *lactation* garnered 285 groups; *lactation consultant* pulled up 136; under *IBCLC* there were 52 Yahoo Groups. These groups meet the needs of people located in different countries, or serving diverse interests of private practitioners, as well as students taking the IBLCE exam, mentors offering clinical training, hospital-based IBCLCs, and so on (Yahoo, 2012).

Network at Your Workplace

Yes, of course you know you should huddle with other IBCLCs. But the IBCLC, of all people, should realize that breastfeeding and human lactation crosses disciplines.

Figure 4-2 Free Full-Text Resources

Open Access Journals: As the name implies this type of journal allows free and open access to the content online. These journals use a publishing model that does not require users to pay or subscribe to journals to view the content.

1. **PubMed (http://www.ncbi.nlm.nih.gov/pubmed):** Links to free full-text are available for some items. Check with your local library (public, academic, and/or state library) to find out what you can access and what options are available through interlibrary loan (borrowing items from another library for a low fee or sometimes without a fee depending on library policies).

   • **LinkOut (National Library of Medicine):** Free access to over 650 journals.

   • **Take advantage of database features.** You can receive email updates with new articles on a topic or the table of contents for a new issue of a journal you want to follow. To get started check out this link to set up email alerts in PubMed: http://www.ncbi.nlm.nih.gov/books/NBK53592/#savesearch.Setting_up_Automatic _Email_Up

2. **PubGet (http://www.pubget.com):** This is an alternative way to search PubMed. The goal is to get to the full-text quickly.

3. **Google Scholar (http://scholar.google.com):** Google Scholar connects you to academic and scholarly literature with the ease of a Google search. Check out the "advanced" link to limit your results to only the health sciences. When full-text access is available links to full text are listed on the results page. (Also check out the "Library Links" under preferences to connect to your library resources in Google Scholar.)

4. **Centre for Reviews and Dissemination (http://www.crd.york.ac.uk/crdweb):** This U.K.-based site provides access to search several evidence-based resources including Cochrane content.

5. **Check with your state and local public libraries.** For example, the State of Kansas Library provides access to ProQuest Nursing and Allied Health Source database to all users in Kansas (http://www2.kumc.edu/SLK/resource.asp?myses=7388322&cuid =ksuc&cusrvr=muses). Many state and local libraries offer access to databases online. **Get to know your librarian to learn about options available to you!**

Online Journals

• **JAMA (https://subs.ama-assn.org/ama/exec/guest?url=):** Free online access (with registration) older than 6 months after publication.

• **DOAJ (Directory of Open Access Journals; http://www.doaj.org):** Free access to over 4,000 scientific and scholarly journals.

• **BioMed Central (http://www.biomedcentral.com):** Over 150 peer-reviewed online open access journals.

• **On-line Journal of Nursing Informatics (http://www.hhdev.psu.edu/nurs/ojni/dm):** Free access to content from 1996 to present.

(continued)

Figure 4-2   Free Full-Text Resources (continued)

- **Online Journal of Rural Nursing and Health Care (http://www.rno.org/journal):** Online journal with peer-reviewed content.
- **International Breastfeeding Journal (http://www.internationalbreastfeedingjournal. com):** Open access journal focusing on breastfeeding.
- Lastly, many professional organizations include access to online journals they publish to members. Check out what is available to you.

Source: Created by Kristin Whitehair, MLIS, University of Kansas School of Nursing, Dykes Library, Librarian Liaison for ILCA (kwhitehair@kumc.edu) and Karen Wambach, PhD, RN, IBCLC, ILCA Director of Research and Special Projects (karenwambach@ilca.org). Used with permission.

You may have been savvy enough to ask about contributing at staff meetings for practice groups that traditionally see mothers and children: pediatrics, parent education/childbirth preparation classes, nursing or obstetrics departments. Have you considered the emergency department (which may not know how to handle engorged breasts, or drugs/tests for the injured-but-lactating woman), the pharmacy (which may not be using texts or resources specific to lactation when offering advice to breastfeeding women), the x-ray or medical imaging departments (which may be erroneously advising that women "pump and dump" for test procedures)? What about the emergency preparedness department within your city or county, or first-responder agencies like the Red Cross? Emergencies hit at any time; an apartment building fire will be every bit as devastating to its residents as a flood or tornado affecting an entire city or country. In large-scale natural or human-caused emergencies there is immediate need to support breastfeeding women, as their children are the most vulnerable to disease and privation. Lactation advocates understand why those "well-meaning" gifts of infant formula and feeding bottles can wreak havoc on life-saving breastfeeding practices, but those outside lactation consultancy may not (Emergency Nutrition Network, 2012).

Other nonclinical departments in the workplace may have interesting resources to bring to bear. Start with the Risk Management Department. One large U.S. city government describes their risk management as follows:

> [The Office of Risk Management] analyzes the City's insurance and other risk exposure issues, including managing claims, workers' compensation, and service-connected disabilities. Provides safety and loss prevention programs." (Office of Risk Management, Finance Department, City of Philadelphia, 2012, para. 1)

It doesn't take much creativity to foresee a case where a breastfeeding mother, forced to prematurely wean due to incorrect and outmoded advice, wants to sue the doctor or hospital that offered poor advice. But what if she was shamed into leaving a public building where she was trying to nurse her infant? City governments and health departments have deep pockets, too, and are as much a target for litigation as a clinician. Hence, a risk management policy.

Some institutions will have an ethics department or review panel. It may be called into action on a case-by-case basis; it may enforce institution-wide policies geared to encourage ethical behaviors.[1] There may already be policies in place disallowing the commercial influences that remain prevalent in maternal and child health, or encouraging public health practices such as breastfeeding promotion.

Quality improvement, patient relations, or customer/patient satisfaction are other options of departments to explore. Health care is a consumer driven (and funded) process in most countries of the world. Many facilities have huge contracts with outside organizations, designed to conduct surveys on how well they are meeting patient needs (Press Ganey, 2012). Breastfeeding mothers value skilled lactation care; whether such services are offered, and provided efficiently and compassionately, should be measured along with other traditional areas of customer satisfaction.

Look at Other Professions

As a profession barely 26 years old, there is not a great deal out there in the journals and institutions of higher learning that address our profession specifically. In some cases, it has been necessary to extrapolate: we take concepts that have been long accepted in other disciplines, and try them on for size. Sometimes that makes sense; the nursing profession is much like the lactation consultant profession in that

> Both are part of self-regulated specialties with members accountable to a registering/certifying body. In both cases, practitioners are predominantly female professionals providing "bedside" or "hands-on" care. The members of both specialties rarely work as primary care providers and report to or take their directives from primary medical supervisors. (Noel-Weiss & Walters, 2006, p. 205)

---

[1] There is even an organization that caters to this subject matter. The Health Care Compliance Association (HCCA) "exists to champion ethical practice and compliance standards and to provide the necessary resources for ethics and compliance professionals and others who share these principles" (Health Care Compliance Association [HCCA], 2012, para. 2). With 7500 members in the United States, it "is a new forum for healthcare professionals involved in compliance serving all segments of the healthcare industry: hospitals, group practices, laboratory, academic institutions, home health, hospice, skilled nursing facilities, durable medical equipment, payor/managed care, third-party billing, rehabilitation facilities, behavioral health, pharmaceutical manufacturers" (HCCA, 2012, para. 4). An IBCLC practicing her allied healthcare profession might find herself or her patients/clients in every single "segment of the healthcare industry" described here.

Thus, an examination of ethical principles and guidelines from the nursing profession will, if nothing else, get the IBCLC's mental cogs starting to move. While a code of ethics or professional conduct for a *nurse* in Brazil may not be enforceable against an *IBCLC* in Brazil, certainly reviewing such salubrious practice-based information doesn't harm IBCLCs any more than offering evidence-based information harms the mothers we serve. An IBCLC may look to such literature from other professions for insight (Gottems, Alves, & de Sena, 2007).

Summary

Every IBCLC will find herself, one day, facing a legal or ethical situation that raises the little hairs on the back of the neck. She must analyze whether she must act: now, or at all. If she feels action is warranted, her approach (whether formal, or informal) will be guided by factors such as the time-sensitive nature of the issue and her position within the hierarchy of decision making and policy setting. Consideration of the four practice-guiding documents for IBCLCs, the workplace policies in place, and the laws of the land will focus the IBCLC's analysis of what really matters, and what does not, in this dilemma. Often this analysis permits the IBCLC to see that the uncomfortable situation is limited and manageable. Valuing and striving for best professional practices (along with simple experience on the job) will help the IBCLC steer clear of ethical or legal jams. Consideration of ethical precepts practiced by other professions may offer insight and practice tips.

REFERENCES

Academy of Breastfeeding Medicine. (2008). *About ABM*. Retrieved from http://www.bfmed.org/About /Mission.aspx

Baby Friendly USA. (2010). *Does the BFHI enhance breastfeeding?* [Frequently Asked Questions]. Retrieved from http://www.babyfriendlyusa.org/eng/06.html

Barney, A. (2008, October 14). Northwestern cuts lactation consultants, trains staff. *Medill Reports*. Retrieved from http://news.medill.northwestern.edu/chicago/news.aspx?id=100647

Bartick, M. (2011, November 10). *UMass Memorial cuts lactation staff* [letter from Massachusetts Breastfeeding Coalition]. Retrieved from http://massbreastfeeding.org/index.php/2011/umass-memorial -cuts-lactation-staff/

BioMed Central Ltd. (2012). *International Breastfeeding Journal* [Home page]. Retrieved from http://www .internationalbreastfeedingjournal.com

Brooks, L. (2007, November). Association News. *Journal of Human Lactation, 23*(4), 371–372. doi:10.1177 /0890334407308015

Bruce, K., Myr, R., Koch, K., Gribble, K., & Pohl, L. (2010, October 31). *To manage your subscription* [Online forum message]. Retrieved from http://community.lsoft.com/archives/lactnet.html

Dailard, C., & Nash, E. (2000, December). State responses to substance abuse among pregnant women. *Guttmacher Report on Public Policy, 3*(6), 3–6. Retrieved from http://www.guttmacher.org/pubs/tgr/03/6 /gr030603.html de Carvalho, M., Robertson, S., & Klaus, M. (1984, June). Does the duration and frequency of early breast-feeding affect nipple pain? [Abstract] *Birth, 11*(2), 81–84. Retrieved from http://onlinelibrary.wiley.com/doi /10.1111/j.1523-536X.1984.tb00754.x/abstract

Duty of care. (n.d.). In L. Duhaime (Ed.), *Duhaime legal dictionary.* Retrieved from http://www.duhaime.org /LegalDictionary/D/DutyofCare.aspx

Emergency Nutrition Network. (2012). *Infant and young feeding in emergencies* [Resources page]. Retrieved from http://www.ennonline.net/resources/tag.aspx?tagid=121

European Lactation Consultants Alliance (ELACTA). (n.d.). *About us* [Home page]. Retrieved from http:// www.velb.org/english/aboutus/about_us.html

Garfield, E. (2012/1994). *The Thomson Reuters impact factor* [Essay]. Retrieved from http://thomsonreuters.com /products_services/science/free/essays/impact_factor

Genna, C. W. (2009). *Selecting and using breastfeeding tools.* Amarillo, TX: Hale Publishing.

Gottems, L., Alves, E., & de Sena, R. (2007, September/October). Brazilian nursing and pro-fessionalization at technical level: A retrospective analysis. *Revista Latino-Americana de Enfer-magem* [Latin American Journal of Nursing]. Retrieved from http://www.scielo.br/scielo.php?pid =S0104-11692007000500023&script=sci_arttext

Health Care Compliance Association. (2012). *About HCCA; HCCA mission* [Home page]. Retrieved from http://www.hcca-info.org/AM/Template.cfm?Section=About_HCCA&Template=/TaggedPage/Tagged PageDisplay.cfm&TPLID=23&ContentID=10393

Higgins, D., Bromfield, L., Richardson, N., Holzer, P., & Berlyn, C. (2010, August). *Mandatory reporting of child abuse.* Retrieved from http://www.aifs.gov.au/nch/pubs/sheets/rs3/rs3.html

International Baby Food Action Network (IBFAN). (n.d.). *Forms for reporting violations-monitoring the code.* Retrieved from http://www.ibfan.org/code_watch-form.html

International Board of Lactation Consultant Examiners. (2003). *Code of ethics for international board certified lactation consultants.* Retrieved from http://www.iblce.org/upload/downloads/CodeOfEthics.pdf

International Board of Lactation Consultant Examiners. (2008, March 8). *Scope of practice for international board certified lactation consultants.* Retrieved from http://www.iblce.org/upload/downloads/ScopeOfPractice.pdf

International Board of Lactation Consultant Examiners. (2011a, September 24). *Disciplinary procedures for the code of professional conduct for IBCLCs for the international board of lactation consultant examiners (IBLCE).* Retrieved from http://www.iblce.org/upload/downloads/IBLCEDisciplinaryProcedures.pdf

International Board of Lactation Consultant Examiners. (2011b, October 31). *Frequently asked questions (FAQs) regarding the code of professional conduct for IBCLC.* Retrieved from http://iblce.org/upload/downloads /CodeOfConductFAQs.pdf

International Board of Lactation Consultant Examiners. (2011c, November 1). *Code of professional conduct for IBCLCs.* Retrieved from http://iblce.org/upload/downloads/CodeOfProfessionalConduct.pdf

International Lactation Consultant Association. (2006). *Standards of practice for international board certified lactation consultants.* Retrieved from http://www.ilca.org/files/resources/Standards-of-Practice-web.pdf

International Lactation Consultant Association. (2012a). *National/multi-national affiliates and international affiliates.* Retrieved from http://www.ilca.org/i4a/pages/Index.cfm?pageID=3370

International Lactation Consultant Association. (2012b). *Welcome to ILCA* [Home page]. Retrieved from http://www.ilca.org/i4a/pages/index.cfm?pageid=1

International Lactation Consultant Association, Spatz, D., & Lessen, R. (2011). *Risks of not breastfeeding* (Monograph). Morrisville, NC: International Lactation Consultant Association.

Joint Commission Resources. (2012). *Joint Commission requirements.* Retrieved from http://www.jcrinc.com/Joint -Commission-Requirements

Kandall, S. (Ed.). (1993). *Treatment improvement protocol 5: Improving treatment for drug-exposed infants* (Rep. No. 5). Retrieved from http://www.ncbi.nlm.nih.gov/books/NBK64750

Kendall-Tackett, K. (2009). *Antidepressant usage during pregnancy and breastfeeding*. Retrieved from http://www.infantrisk.org/content/antidepressant-usage-during-pregnancy-and-breastfeeding

Lactnet. (n.d.). *L-Soft listserv grand prize winner: Lactnet* [Press release]. Retrieved from http://www.lsoft.com/customers/lactnet.asp

Merewood, A. (2012, February). Newly positioned. *Journal of Human Lactation, 28*(1), 9.

Metzger, M., & McDade, T. (2010, May/June). Breastfeeding as obesity prevention in the United States: A sibling difference model [Abstract]. *American Journal of Human Biology, 22*(3), 291–296. Retrieved from http://www.ncbi.nlm.nih.gov/pubmed/19693959

Miller, R. (2006). *Problems in health care law* (9th ed.). Sudbury, MA: Jones & Bartlett.

Noel-Weiss, J. (2009, July 24). *Ethics and lactation consultants: A needs assessment*. Lecture presented at ILCA Annual Conference, Orlando, FL.

Noel-Weiss, J., & Walters, G. (2006). Ethics and lactation consultants: Developing knowledge, skills, and tools. *Journal of Human Lactation, 22*(2), 203–212. doi:10.1177/0890334406286955

Office of Risk Management, Finance Department, City of Philadelphia. (2012). *Office of Risk Management*. Retrieved from http://www.phila.gov/finance/units-RiskManagement.html

Omission. (2012). In *'Lectric Law Library's Lexicon*. Retrieved from http://www.lectlaw.com/def2/o037.htm

Press Ganey. (2012). *Creating high-performance health care organizations* [About Us page]. Retrieved from http://www.pressganey.com/aboutUs.aspx

Riordan, J., & Wambach, K. (2010). *Breastfeeding and human lactation* (4th ed.). Sudbury, MA: Jones & Bartlett.

Sage Publications. (2012). *Journal of Human Lactation* [Publication description]. Retrieved from http://www.sagepub.com/journals/Journal201341

Scott, J. W. (Speaker). (2005, July 5). *From code to consultation: applying IBCLC ethics to practice* [MP3]. ProLibraries.com, for La Leche League International. Retrieved from http://www.prolibraries.com

Social, Health & Family Affairs Committee, & Rupprecht, M. (2010, September 20). *Child abuse in institutions: Ensure full protection of the victims* [Document No. 12358]. Retrieved from http://assembly.coe.int/Main.asp?link=/Documents/WorkingDocs/Doc10/EDOC12358.htm

Taylor, J., Brownstein, D., Christakis, D., Blackburn, S., Strandjord, T., Klein, E., & Shafii, J. (2004, September). Use of incident reports by physicians and nurses to document medical errors in pediatric patients. *Pediatrics, 114*(3), 729–735. Retrieved from http://pediatrics.aappublications.org/cgi/reprint/114/3/729.pdf

UNICEF. (n.d.). *The baby-friendly hospital initiative*. Retrieved from http://www.unicef.org/programme/breastfeeding/baby.htm

United States Lactation Consultant Association (USLCA), Clegg, S., Francis, D., & Walker, M. (2010, July). *Five steps to improving job security for the hospital-based IBCLC* [Monograph]. Morrisville, NC: United States Lactation Consultant Association.

United States Lactation Consultant Association (USLCA), Gutowski, J., Walker, M., & Chetwynd, E. (2010, July). *Containing health care costs: Help in plain sight* [Monograph]. Morrisville, NC: United States Lactation Consultant Association.

U.S. Dept. of Health and Human Services Administration for Children & Families Child Welfare Information Gateway. (2009). *Parental drug use as child abuse: Summary of state laws*. Retrieved from http://www.childwelfare.gov/systemwide/laws_policies/statutes/drugexposed.cfm

U.S. Dept. of Health and Human Services Administration for Children & Families Child Welfare Information Gateway. (2010). *Mandatory reporters of child abuse and neglect: Summary of state laws*. Retrieved from http://www.childwelfare.gov/systemwide/laws_policies/statutes/manda.cfm#backfn1

Walker, M. (2011). *Breastfeeding management for the clinician: Using the evidence* (2nd ed.). Sudbury, MA: Jones & Bartlett.

Weissman, A., Levy, B., Hartz, A., Bentler, S., Donohue, M., Ellingrod, V., & Wisner, K. (2004, June). Pooled analysis of antidepressant levels in lactating mothers, breast milk, and nursing infants. *American Journal of Psychiatry, 161*(6), 1066–1078. Retrieved from http://ajp.psychiatryonline.org/cgi/reprint/161/6/1066.pdf

Wight, N. E., Morton, J. A., & Kim, J. H. (2008). *Best medicine: Human milk in the NICU.* Amarillo, TX: Hale.

World Health Organization. (1981). *International code of marketing of breast-milk substitutes.* Retrieved from http://www.who.int/nutrition/publications/code_english.pdf

Yahoo. (2012). *Find a Yahoo! group.* Retrieved from http://groups.yahoo.com

Chapter 5

Conflicts Are Interesting. Why Are They Bad?

The International Board of Lactation Consultant Examiners Code of Professional Conduct (IBLCE CPC) addresses conflicts of interest (COIs) in Principles 1.4, 5.1, and 6.1. The notion of avoiding conflicts of interest is also emphasized in the International Board of Lactation Consultant Examiners Scope of Practice (IBLCE SOP) at paragraph 8 and the International Lactation Consultant Association Standards of Practice (ILCA Standards) at Standard 1.3. One could argue that the entire *International Code of Marketing of Breast-milk Substitutes* and subsequent relevant World Health Assembly resolutions (International Code or WHO Code) (International Code Documentation Centre, 2007) is a plea to avoid COIs in matters of maternal and child public health.

Obviously, COIs are a very big deal, and the International Board Certified Lactation Consultant (IBCLC) who seeks to avoid legal and ethical dilemmas is well advised to understand what they are so as to avoid them. The 21st century has brought increased scrutiny of the nexus between the medical profession and the commercial interests (pharmaceuticals and medical devices) that are a customary and necessary part of health care. Individual healthcare professionals (HCPs) are admonished to avoid COIs (Lo & Field, 2009); their medical associations are similarly cautioned (Council of Medical Specialty Societies, 2011; Rothman et al., 2009); and books and articles expose cozy relationships (Elliot, 2010; Kassirer, 2005). Some review of, and expansion on, the concept of conflicts of interest as they affect the IBCLC may be helpful.

Conflicts of Interest Involving Personal Benefit

Conflict of interest is a phrase that gets thrown around a lot, often erroneously: "She can't open a private practice as an IBCLC across the street from the hospital. That would be a conflict of interest!" Or, "You can't stock and sell that brand of product. They violate the WHO Code. It would be a conflict of interest!" Or, "You can't contradict the physician and tell the mother her medications are compatible with breastfeeding. That is a conflict of interest!" If the intent is to alarm the listener, the mission is customarily accomplished, but it is at the expense of a true understanding and application of COI principles. A conflict of interest can happen to any person, in any context. We just need the right set of facts.

What Is a Conflict of Interest Involving Personal Benefit?

Conflict conjures all sorts of imagery, from your schedule putting you in two places at once, all the way up to violent warfare (Axt, Milososki, & Schwarz, 2006). Many ethical analyses look at it from a financial perspective: that you will reap some kind of financial reward as a result of an unsavory conflict of interest (Sample et al., 2001). Harder to grasp, but probably more pertinent to the medical professions (like lactation consultancy) is the notion that your professional clinical integrity can somehow be compromised because of a conflict of interest (Lo & Field, 2009).

Simply put, a conflict of interest occurs when you have a personal stake in the outcome of something over which you can exert some influence. There are direct COIs, in which the conflict is clear and obvious. There are indirect COIs (also referred to as a "perceived COI" or "the appearance of a COI"), in which it *seems* like there is a COI, but none may exist. Or, the COI was appropriately recognized and corrected, yet it *seems* like it is still there. *Simply identifying a COI does not end the analysis.* From there, you examine whether or not the COI matters; and if it matters, whether the COI can be cured or excused.

Let's use a very manageable example. You want your child to be picked for the lead in the school play. No conflict of interest there; you are just being a proud parent. The activity to be scrutinized for any COI, then, is the decision of who is to be cast in the lead role, and the influence you can exert (if any) on that decision. As the facts change, the tension changes, and so does the COI. **Table 5-1** offers an analysis of conflicts of interest, starting off easy with the school play.

Do I Have a COIN? Part 1

A simple mnemonic (COIN) may help you to analyze whether or not there is a conflict of interest. If you think you may have a conflict of interest, the next question you ask is: does it matter? If it matters, then ask whether the conflict can be cured, or explained away. Using the IBCLC profession as our backdrop, let's hone this a bit. Starting with our definition above,

> A conflict of interest occurs when you have a personal stake in the outcome of something over which you can exert some influence.

> (in other words ↓)

> A conflict of interest occurs when your personal interests come into conflict with your "public" obligation as an IBCLC. Your IBCLC certification is a warrant—a promise—that your excellent care for breastfeeding dyads is the manner by which you protect the *public* health and safety.

> (in other words ↓)

> A conflict of interest occurs if a decision you must make, in your job, is going to benefit you personally. How might you reap personal benefits?

Table 5-1 Examples Analyzing Conflicts of Interest (COIs)

Basic Facts: What Is the Decision to Be Analyzed?	Tweaking the Facts	Conflict of Interest *for You?*	Explanation	Does the COI Matter?	Can the COI Be Cured?
You want your child to be picked for the lead in the school play. Decision to be analyzed: Casting of the lead role.	The teacher is the director of the play	No	The teacher is in control of the decision-making process (to pick the cast), *not you. End of COI analysis.*		
	You are the director of the play	Yes: direct COI	The director customarily makes all casting decisions	Yes, if more than one actor is trying out for the role. Everyone wants a shot at the role. No, if your child is the only one trying out for the role. Then, it doesn't matter even if there is favoritism. *End of COI analysis.*	Yes: Have casting director decide all roles; remove yourself entirely from the decision-making process. *End of COI analysis.*
	Your sister is the director of the play	No	Your sister is in control of the decision-making process (to pick the cast), *not you. End of COI analysis.*		
	Your sister is the director of the play	Yes: *for your sister*, an appearance of a COI	*For your sister* there is an appearance of a COI, if the other actors assume she will favor and pick her niece (your child).	Yes, if more than one actor is trying out for the role. Everyone wants a shot at the role. No, if your child is the only one trying out for the role. Then, it doesn't matter even if there is the appearance of favoritism giving	Yes: The director (your sister) explains to every aspiring actor that she impartially auditions and casts on merit only. *End of COI analysis.* No: The other aspiring actors don't believe your sister when she says she is impartial. *End of COI analysis.*

(continued)

Table 5-1   Examples Analyzing Conflicts of Interest (COIs) (continued)

Basic Facts: What Is the Decision to Be Analyzed?	Tweaking the Facts	Conflict of Interest *for You?*	Explanation	Does the COI Matter?	Can the COI Be Cured?
				rise to an appearance of COI. *End of COI analysis.*	
You are planning an office holiday party. Decision to be analyzed: payments made from department party budget.	You hire the regular catering service	No	You have no stake in the outcome; this was a simple planning/business decision		
	You moonlight as a caterer. You hire yourself to cater the party.	Yes: direct COI	You have a direct stake in the decision of who is hired, and you are doing the hiring.	Yes: Putting department funds into your pocket, without valid explanation, is a classic COI.	Yes: If you give *full and prior disclosure* to the department chair of your plans, and receive her *prior consent,* to hire your catering company. *End of COI analysis.* No: If the department chair does not like the appearance of an employee getting a sweetheart deal, she asks you to hire someone else. *End of COI analysis.*
You are an IBCLC in private practice. You consult mothers with lactation problems. You rent and sell breast pumps. Decision to be analyzed: the rental of a breast pump to a mother.	You sell a breast pump to someone planning to use it as a baby shower gift.	No	You are an IBCLC with a legitimate retail/sales operation as part of your business. No COI to make money doing what you do. *End of COI analysis.*		

You rent a breast pump to a mother who came in, explaining she needs one to build supply. She asks your advice on which kind to rent.	No	You are an IBCLC with a legitimate retail/rental operation as part of your business. Your expertise in your product lines makes it appropriate to discuss different features this COI to make money doing what you do. *End of COI analysis.*	
You have a lactation consultation with a mother. You realize she needs to rent a hospital-grade breast pump.	Yes: *direct* commercial COI	You rent and sell pumps. This client needs a pump. You are in a position to exert influence over her decision of where to spend her pump rental dollars.	Yes: IBCLCs are admonished to avoid any COIs, esp. involving commercial products (IBLCE CPC Principles 1.4, 5.1, 5.2, 6.1; IBLCE SOP para. 8; ILCA Standard 1.3; WHO Code Preamble and Articles 4, 5, 6, & 7).	Yes; several options: 1. Inform clients *before* the consult starts that any recommendation to use products will be based on clinical need (ILCA Standard 3.3.6). 2. You can opt *not* to engage in retail or rental transactions with any active clinical clients. 3. Have a list to give clients, showing several options to rent a pump. It is OK to show your shop on the list: it is a simple resource list. *End of COI analysis.*
You have a lactation consultation with a mother. You realize she needs to rent a hospital-grade breast pump.	Yes: *appearance* of a COI	You rent and sell pumps. This client needs a pump. "Outsiders looking in" may assume that you will exert influence over her decision of where to spend her pump rental dollars.	Yes. IBCLCs are admonished to avoid any COIs, esp. involving commercial products (IBLCE CPC Principles 1.4, 5.1, 5.2, 6.1; IBLCE	Yes; several options: 1. Have a posted and public notice that, when consulting with mothers, any recommendation to use products will be based on clinical need (ILCA Standard 3.3.6).

(*continued*)

Table 5-1   Examples Analyzing Conflicts of Interest (COIs) (continued)

Basic Facts: What Is the Decision to Be Analyzed?	Tweaking the Facts	Conflict of Interest for You?	Explanation	Does the COI Matter?	Can the COI Be Cured?
				SOP para. 8; ILCA Standard 1.3; WHO Code Preamble and Articles 4, 5, & 6).	2. You can opt *not* to engage in retail or rental transactions with any active clinical clients. 3. You do not need to have a posted and public list showing other options to rent a pump. You have no duty, generally, to advertise competitors. *End of COI analysis.*
You work as an IBCLC on the postpartum floor. There is a sign-up sheet to buy cookies for a youth group fundraiser. Decision to be analyzed: Whether to buy cookies.	The cookies are being sold by your supervisor's child. You are due for a job performance evaluation next week.	Yes: COI based on inappropriate influence	You will feel pressured to buy cookies to stay on boss' good side in light of upcoming job performance evaluation. Boss is exerting *inappropriate influence* on you.	Yes: If you buy from this person, you will feel pressured to buy for every colleague's favorite cause. No: You figure a box of cookies here, a bar of chocolate there, is just a "business-related expense." Your kid has a sale coming up, too. *End of COI analysis.*	Yes: If there is *no* existing policy on fundraising efforts to benefit outside groups, offer to draft one that prohibits all solicitations. *End of COI analysis.* No: If policies permit solicitations of nominal value, even between supervisors and employees, you can opt to buy or not, but you can't alter the inappropriate influence. *End of COI analysis.*
You are an IBCLC working in a clinic that employs IBCLCs. An important holiday is coming up; you will	A promotion is available. Your boss has let it be known that she will give the promotion to the "best"	Yes: COI based on coercion.	You want the upcoming promotion, and feel pressured to demonstrate your "team spirit" by being the first to "volunteer" for	Yes: The promotion appears not to be based on merit, but rather as a prize after pitting IBCLC	Yes: Offer to draft up an equitable scheduling policy for No: Realistically, there is little you can do to correct this

have out-of-town visitors and family. Your boss said she needs a "volunteer" to work that day since all IBCLCs have sought the day off. Decision to be analyzed: Whether to come in and work the holiday.

team player."

work on a holiday.

colleagues against one other.
No: Your guests all arrive in the afternoon, and your shift can be done by then. *End of COI analysis.*

popular holidays…and hope you get the day off. *End of COI analysis.*

situation in the near term. Some bosses just use peculiar systems to make decisions. *End of COI analysis.*

1. By receiving greater recognition or praise; perhaps a promotion
2. By receiving more money

(in other words ↓)

Receiving greater recognition and praise can be summed up as: receiving "congratulations."

(and ↓)

Receiving more money can be summed up as: receiving "income."

(which means ↓)

A COnflict of INterest occurs when a decision you have to make, in your job, will give you COngratulations or INcome.

(in other words ↓)

COnflicts of INterest involve COngratulations or INcome = COIN

We said that identifying the COIN is just the first step. Next ask: does it matter? Sometimes an identifiable conflict of interest doesn't give rise to any problems that require fixing. In the example of our school play, if your child was the only person expressing an interest in the lead role, it really doesn't matter if you are the director. If no one else tries out for the role you can happily cast your child, because there are no tensions or repercussions as a result of your decision.

Someone coming along and reading the cast list on opening night may see your name and the lead actor's name and assume that some kind of favoritism allowed the child to get the plum role. This is a perceived COI (or, the appearance of a COI) because that theater patron is unaware of any of the circumstances surrounding the auditions and casting for the play. He is simply drawing a conclusion based on the facts in front of him. That is the price you pay for perceived COIs: you can't control what others will assume, given the basic facts. If you want to avoid even the appearance of a COI, you will tell your child she cannot have the lead role, period.

Conflicts of Interest Involving Personal Benefit, Refined

A conflict of interest may be triggered in subtle ways. You may find yourself in a situation where you are being pressured into making certain decisions, even if you will not have any COngratulations or INcome steered your way.

Do I Have a COIN? Part 2

Using our mnemonic:

A conflict of interest occurs if a decision you must make, in your job, is under force or pressure to be decided a certain way, even if you will reap no personal gain.

(put another way ↓)

Being forced to decide something a certain way can be summed up as "coercion."

(or ↓)

Being pressured to decide something a certain way can be summed up as "inappropriate influence."

(which means ↓)

A COnflict of INterest occurs when a decision you must make, in your job, is under COercion or INappropriate INfluence to be decided a certain way.

(in other words ↓)

COnflicts of INterest involve COercion or INappropriate INfluence = COIN

Quiz Questions

Equipment: Case 1
You're working as an IBCLC at the hospital. You operate a pump rental station as a second business. A patient asks you, before she is discharged, what pump she should use when she returns to work in 2 months, and where she should get it.

Question: Yes or no, is it a conflict of interest to tell the patient about your pump rental station?

Answer: Yes, COI. You have the potential to receive INcome from this possible customer. You can "cure" the COI by showing her a list of all local retail options, even if it contains contact information for your second business (assuming the policies of your institution permit this). You *always* have the right to discuss with the mother, generally, the pros and cons of products or equipment, and the therapeutic indications for their use. You should be sensitive to any commercial conflicts of interest you may have (IBLCE, 2011, CPC Principles 1.4, 5.1, & 5.2; IBLCE, 2008, SOP para. 8; ILCA, 2006, Standards 1.3 & 3.3.6).

Equipment: Case 2
You're working as an IBCLC at the hospital. You don't operate a pump rental station. But you do happen to like one brand of pump over the others. A patient asks you, before she is discharged, what pump she should use when she returns to work in 2 months, and where she should get it.

Question: Yes or no, is it a conflict of interest to promote this brand to the mom?

Answer: No COI. If you have no financial interest in the outcome, it is not a conflict of interest to discuss a product when the mother has asked about one. But be cautious. You're an IBCLC, working in a hospital, talking to one of your patients before discharge. The mother may misinterpret your enthusiasm for this one product as a clinical recommendation. Your HCP role is to promote good health and informed decision making, not act as a sales person (unpaid, at that) for a particular product (IBLCE, 2011, CPC Principles 1.2, 1.3, 1.4, 5.1, & 5.2; IBLCE, 2008, SOP para. 8; ILCA, 2006, Standards 3.3.6 & 4.1).

Private Practice: Case 1

You have two jobs: you work as an IBCLC at the hospital, and you have a small private practice seeing mothers in their homes. You want the hospital to include your private practice on the list of community resources given to discharging mothers.

Question: Yes or no, is it a conflict of interest to have your business listed by the hospital on its community resources sheet?

Answer: No COI. The decision rests with the hospital; it gains neither COngratulations nor INcome to have you (or anyone else) on the list. The hospital is providing continuity of care; you are merely seeking to promote your other business, of potential interest to patients at the facility. However, be wise. Double-check the hospital's own policies. They may have rules against promoting outside business interests of staff members, even if they are not a classic COI.

Private Practice: Case 2

You work as an IBCLC with a small private practice seeing mothers in their homes. You want the hospital to include your private practice on the list of community resources given to discharging mothers.

Question: Yes or no, is it a conflict of interest to have your business listed by the hospital on its community resources handout?

Answer: No COI. The decision rests with the hospital; it gains neither COngratulations nor INcome to have you (or anyone else) on the list. The hospital is providing continuity of care; you are merely seeking to promote your private practice. There are no COI tensions here between you and the hospital because you are an outsider, entirely. You may find you have a hard time getting your foot in the door; you are, in the eyes of the hospital, just another vendor or solicitor. But that is irrelevant to an analysis of COI.

Private Practice: Case 3

You have two jobs: you work as an IBCLC at the hospital, and you have a small private practice seeing mothers in their homes. You want the hospital to include your private practice on the list of community resources given to discharging mothers. You are best friends with the hospital staffer who compiles the community resource list. You tell her you'll take her out to lunch at a swanky restaurant if she will list your private practice first, in large font and bold type, on the handout.

Question: Yes or no, is it a conflict of interest for the IBCLC to take her friend to lunch and ask this favor?

Answer: Yes, COI. The IBCLC is trying to maneuver an advantage by exerting INappropriate INfluence on her friend with the lunch-for-better-font scheme.

Doula Doula

You work at the hospital. Your best friend left her job in the hospital, and now works as a postpartum doula. She is fabulous, and you tell all your lactation patients to give her a call when they get home. The doula doesn't know you are promoting her great services.

Question: Yes or no, is it a conflict of interest for the IBCLC to recommend the doula services of one practitioner?

Answer: No COI. You may be offering a fervent recommendation, but *you* will receive no COngratualtions or INcome. But be cognizant of IBLCE CPC Principles 2.1 and 2.2. Does this mother think she is receiving a clinical referral? And even if you are making a referral or suggestion upon inquiry of the mother, should you be offering just one name? The more prudent course would be to provide a range of options to the mother, explaining the pros and cons of each (IBLCE, 2011, CPC Principles 6.1, 2.1, & 2.2; IBLCE, 2008, SOP para. 8; ILCA, 2006, Standards 3.2.3 & 3.3.5).

Leadership Role

You serve as the president of your local IBCLC professional association, and you happen to be a recognized expert on breastfeeding multiples. The group needs a speaker for its next meeting.

Question: Yes or no, is it a conflict of interest for you to offer to the group that you speak on the topic of breastfeeding multiples? You'll do it for free.

Answer: Yes, COI. You will receive recognition (COngratulations) for the talk even if you receive no stipend. Further, your president's role may put INappropriate INfluence on the speaker organizer to choose you.

Remember, however, the next step of the COI analysis. Does it matter? In this scenario, in all likelihood, the answer is no. Who is likely to care? You are a good speaker, and your group of colleagues will get a free talk, perhaps earning continuing education credits (IBLCE, 2011, CPC Principles 1.2 & 2.3; IBLCE, 2008, SOP paras. 3, 4, & 8; ILCA, 2006, Standard 1.6). To be fastidious, you can cure the COI by full and prior disclosure to the speaker selection committee. It is unlikely any will object; with consent of all parties involved, the COI is cured.

Conflicts of Interest Involving Professional Duties

Healthcare providers of all stripes, IBCLCs, doctors, nurses, midwives, physical therapists, psychologists, geriatrists, surgeons—all of them—are entrusted with the health, care, and safety of their patients/clients. As we learned in earlier chapters, a great deal of education and training goes into acquiring the license or certification to practice in a chosen field. The goal of the licensing board or certifying agency is to provide some measure of safety and security to the members of the public who want to use that HCP for their health care. The license or certification is a warrant—a promise—that this practitioner acquired necessary education, from an accredited institution or program. This practitioner has passed exams attesting to her skill; she is duly licensed or certified to practice in this field; she fulfills the requirements (paying annual fees, obtaining continuing education, etc.) to maintain her license/certification. If the HCP fails in these obligations, or offers substandard or negligent care, discipline procedures with sanctions may be brought to bear.

Simply put: if the patient/client is willing to entrust her physical and mental well-being to an HCP, the HCP's obligation is to provide that healthcare with the patient's best interests as the primary objective. The HCP may be paid for the service (directly by the patient/client, through third-party reimbursement [insurance], or via government health ministry policies and regulations). Even if there is no fee involved (e.g., volunteering in emergencies, or *pro bono* work offered through a charitable organization), the HCP's primary professional objective is to provide optimal evidence-based health care, after discussion of treatment options with the patient, in aid of the patient's informed decision making.

Issues arise when the HCP is seen to have a bias of some sort in providing healthcare options with the patient. Imagine Dr. Smith was wined and dined last week by the pharmaceutical sales representative for Brand X asthma drug. He got a lavish lunch, some free samples of Brand X, and a pocket full of pens and notepads emblazoned with the Brand X logo. Now the doctor is seeing a patient about his asthma flare-up. And he is writing out a prescription, using his Brand X pen, on his pre-printed Brand X prescription pad, for—you guessed it—a round of Brand X. Refillable several times. No generic alternatives allowed.

It is entirely fair to ask, did the doctor prescribe Brand X because that really, truly is the best clinical option for the asthma patient? Or is he prescribing Brand X because that lovely lunch with that nice young man from Brand X company is fresh in his memory? Could it be that he is ordering Brand X because he found his lunch partner an agreeable fellow, one whom he trusts and has generally positive feelings about (Campbell et al., 2007)?

The flip side to this examination is the purveyor of Brand X, or any pharmaceutical, medical device, product, or gadget that is used in providing health care. Whereas the HCP has professional and ethical obligations—first, foremost, and only—to care for his patient/client, the salesman's obligation is to increase profits for the company. He does this by selling (or generating sales of) his product, drug, or gadget. His motives and obligations are entirely commercial in nature. That, in and of itself, is not unethical. To be sure, the motive to invent drugs and medical devices can be magnanimous (even philanthropic) in nature, but the only way those products can be developed and mass-marketed is by aligning with a commercial enterprise at some point along the way. This is simply the way the free market system works: materials cost money; research and testing costs money; development and marketing costs money; quality control costs money. Even when the company offers up free drugs or gadgets as part of a goodwill and humanitarian gesture, the cost of providing those "freebies" is simply absorbed by other parts of the business (usually the marketing department) that show the costs on their portion of the account ledger (Katz, Caplan, & Merz, 2003).

We know healthcare providers are heavily marketed to by industry. And the method enjoys great success. Even the physicians admit it: 1662 physicians in six practice areas (in the United States) were surveyed:

> Most physicians (94%) reported some type of relationship with the pharmaceutical industry, and most of these relationships involved receiving food in the workplace (83%) or receiving drug samples (78%). More than one third of the respondents (35%) received reimbursement for costs associated with professional meetings or continuing medical education, and more than one quarter (28%) received payments for consulting, giving lectures, or enrolling patients in trials. (Campbell et al., 2007, p. 1742)

Noteworthy, too, are the researchers' comments that these results may not reveal enough: "Respondents may have underreported their associations with industry, a phenomenon known in the survey literature as social desirability bias" (Campbell et al., 2007, p. 1748).

The pervasive influence of marketers upon the healthcare profession is all the more disconcerting because even gifts of negligible value (those "harmless" pens, notepads, and coffee mugs) can influence HCP behaviors; and insidiously, the HCPs may not even realize it is happening. Indeed, the more gifts a physician receives, the more likely he is to believe that they do not influence professional behavior (Katz et al., 2003).

We are humans. While we live in different cultures and societies all over the world, there are some elements of human interaction that are universal. Receiving a gift or a kind gesture, no matter how small, instills a sense of indebtedness, of reciprocity, of the need to acknowledge and return the favor. "Food, flattery, and friendship are all powerful tools of persuasion. [F]ood is 'the most commonly used technique to derail the judgment aspect of decision making'" (Katz et al., 2003, p. 8; Razran, 1940). Compounding the scenario is the notion that failure to reciprocate is tinged with negative associations ("mooching") (Cialdini, 1993; Katz et al., 2003, p. 9). While some efforts have been made to curb these influences (such as guidelines by medical professional associations allowing acceptance only of *de minimus* gifts),

> Guidelines establishing thresholds, such as the arbitrary amount of [US]$100, are based on the belief that there is a direct "dose response"—that the risk of bias increases as the value of the item increases. There is no level, however, below which it is guaranteed that marketing wares have no effect on the recipient. (Katz et al., 2003, p. 12)

While much of the published research in this area of bioethics studies physician behavior, the IBCLC can certainly be as influenced by notions of reciprocity as doctors—as can nurses, specialists, and allied healthcare providers, all of whom are as heavily marketed as the physicians. Thus, the IBCLC who attends a luncheon paid for by a medical device manufacturer (like a breast pump) can be every bit as influenced as the physician who attends a luncheon paid for by a pharmaceutical manufacturer.

Do I Have a COIN? Part 3

Perhaps our mnemonic will work to sort out this murky area as well.

A conflict of professional interest occurs if your duty of care to the patient/client is influenced (whether you consciously realize it or not) by a commercial interest, even if you will reap no personal gain.

(in other words ↓)

Care of your patient/client, if it is influenced (whether you realize it or not) by your prior contacts with vendors, can be summed up as "commercial influences."

(and ↓)

Your professional, ethical responsibilities to offer evidence-based care, so the patient/client can make informed decisions, can be summed up as "conduct in providing care."

(in other words ↓)

A COnflict of professional INterest involves COmmercial INfluences driving your COnduct IN providing care.

(in other words ↓)

COnflicts of professional INterest . . . COmmercial INfluences . . . COnduct IN providing care = COIN

In obvious cases of conflict of professional interest, the commercial entity may provide direct monies to the HCP, such as paying for the practitioner to speak at a conference, or to do research on their new drug. The amounts of money spent by pharmaceutical companies to directly pay for healthcare providers' education, speaking, and research is staggering (ProPublica, 2012), and the conflicts of interest readily apparent (Lo & Field, 2009).

The salient point here is that the influence being brought to bear by the commercial interest can be very subtle, and have just as much impact. The IBCLC (or any HCP) may *think* that professional clinical judgment cannot possibly be swayed by something so inconsequential as accepting a logo-emblazoned pen from a vendor's exhibit booth at a professional educational conference, but the research tells us otherwise. If these word-tricks and explanations aren't clearing the fog, recall the simple advice offered in earlier chapters: Just say no to freebies and gifts.

More Quiz Questions

Freebies: Case 1

You are an IBCLC working on the maternity floor. The sales representative for a pharmaceutical company wants to give you a free identification holder bearing their cardiac drug logo.

Question: Yes or no, is it conflict of interest for the IBCLC to wear the badge holder with the company brand on it?

Answer: Yes, COI. The IBCLC may think she is "in the clear" because the product being advertised does not fall under the International Code, and is not regularly used on the maternity floor, but this gift is coming from a drug manufacturer. It has nominal value, but the feelings of reciprocity that taking it will engender is the "toe in the door" the salesperson is looking for. You may want to avoid being a billboard for *any* product (IBLCE, 2011, CPC Principles 1.2, 1.4. 5.1, & 5.2; IBLCE, 2008, SOP para. 8; ILCA, 2006, Standard 1.3). You may want to avoid building a relationship with a salesperson that can later be exploited to commercial advantage.

Freebies: Case 2

You are an IBCLC and supervising nurse manager on the maternity floor. A pump manufacturer wants your hospital (under exclusive contract now to another pump company) to switch to their brand. Your hospital uses many pumps with new mothers (you have a neonatal intensive care unit), and you are dissatisfied with the customer service you have been receiving from the current company. The sales representative invites you to lunch at a luxurious country club to talk about the details; your husband can even play golf there.

Question: Yes or no, is it a conflict of interest for the IBCLC/nurse manager to accept this free lunch to discuss options and details of switching to a new pump company?

Answer: Yes, COI, and lots of it. Even though it may be appropriate for the IBCLC/nurse manager to think about switching companies (since the current vendor is not providing satisfactory service for a type of durable medical equipment that is in constant use on her floor, and upon which the hospital relies in order to properly care for patients), the swanky country club is not an appropriate setting. The IBCLC's ability to make a dispassionate decision will be affected by being fed well, and for free. Her husband is playing golf in the bargain, creating more feelings of obligation (and perhaps setting her up for INappropriate INfluences in her decision making). Further, she may be violating hospital policies requiring all commercial bargaining to be made by nonclinical professionals in the purchasing/requisitions department. Lastly, if this pump manufacturer is not meeting its obligations under the WHO Code (World Health Organization [WHO], 1981) (for its inappropriate marketing of bottles or teats; recall that pumps themselves are not covered by the WHO Code), the acceptance of gifts by the IBCLC/nurse manager creates further tensions (International Baby Food Action Network [IBFAN], n.d.; WHO Code Article 7; IBLCE, 2011, CPC Introduction para. 3).

Freebies: Case 3
You are the junior IBCLC on the maternity floor. You do not have authority to order as much as a paper clip. A pump manufacturer wants your hospital (under exclusive contract now to another pump company) to switch to their brand. Your hospital uses many pumps with new mothers (you have a NICU unit). Even though you are the newest hire, you are aware that the hospital's customer service from the current company is lacking. The sales representative for the new pump company invites you to lunch at a luxurious country club to talk, generally, about what their pumps do. Your husband can even accompany you and play golf there.

Question: Yes or no, is it conflict of interest for the newest IBCLC, without any bargaining or purchasing power at the hospital, to accept this free lunch to learn about a pump company and its products?

Answer: Yes, COI. Don't be misled by the IBCLC's new-kid-on-the-block standing. The meal has value, just as INcome has value. The WHO Code tensions (if any) are as real here as for the IBCLC/nurse manager. Our junior IBCLC will still walk away with (perhaps unwitting) feelings of reciprocity. And this is a prime example of an HCP being "courted," perhaps to facilitate future decisions in the company's favor.

We have identified a COI in this example. Can the IBCLC cure the COI, perhaps by prior and full disclosure to her superiors, with permission granted? ("Boss, I have a chance to get a free lunch and a round of golf from this pump company! Our hospital doesn't have a contract with them, so there is no direct conflict of interest! Heck, I can't even order a paper clip! Can I go, please, can I go?")

Let's assume the boss does give the junior IBCLC permission to go to this lunch. While *full and prior disclosure*—with *consent of the parties involved*—customarily cures almost any COI, it just may not pass "the smell test" in this case. Any time an IBCLC's nose starts to wrinkle, she should step back and think again. You can never be wrong with the simple decision of, "No, I am not going to do this." The junior IBCLC's reputation may well suffer among her HCP colleagues for going to this lunch, given the implied (or perceived) COI of a cozy relationship with a commercial vendor. And she will have provided a toe in the door for the salesperson to come back, and build upon that sense of reciprocity created at the first lunch.

Where Is the Conflict of Interest? Situation 1
Question: Which scenario, (a), (b), or (c), presents a conflict of interest for the IBCLC?

(a) You instruct your fellow IBCLCs they must use the newly approved breast-feeding chart you designed, or face discipline.

(b) You offer to (personally) pay the way for your subordinate (1 of 5 IBCLCs you supervise) to attend a lactation conference you are also attending.

(c) You bring dozens of skin-to-skin articles to the obstetrics meeting, telling the doctors they will all get sued for malpractice if they don't read the articles and change their practices.

Answer: (b). It represents an INappropriate INfluence on someone (who must answer to you in the work setting) to arbitrarily pay her way to a conference. It will be very difficult for her to refuse; you're the boss. Imagine when you both have returned from the conference, are in a staff meeting, and must vote on a controversial matter. Your travel companion votes with you; the others oppose. Will the others assume the travel companion voted with you because she agrees with you or because she has feelings of reciprocity, having been given that trip? Does she truly support your position, or is the reciprocity talking, as the others suspect? The far better course would be to devise an equitable system whereby all members of the department can vie for the limited funds for continuing education, rather than cherry-picking someone to go. Option (a) presents no conflicts of interest, though marching into a meeting and barking bossy orders around may not be the best style of management. Similarly, option (c) is not an issue of conflicts of interest, but of poor communication skills when trying to encourage a paradigm shift in thinking.

Where Is the Conflict of Interest? Situation 2
Question: Which scenario, (a) or (b), presents a conflict of interest for the IBCLC?

(a) Your 14-year-old eye-rolling daughter joins you for Bring Your Child to Work Day. You ask the front desk assistant on the floor to supervise her while she assembles information packets for the discharging patients; the packets have materials about where to seek breastfeeding help once at home.

(b) The nurse manager asks you to take her 14-year-old eye-roller on your lactation consultant rounds today.

Answer: Both are examples of COI: It is COercive to put an employee in the uncomfortable position of having to acquiesce to the "request" made by someone higher up on the chain of command (assuming the IBCLC holds a position superior to the assistant, and the nurse manager is superior to the IBCLC). But the real question here is why there isn't greater concern for patients' privacy, under the regulations of the institution, the law of the land (e.g., the privacy sections of the Health Insurance Portability and Accountability Act of 1996 [HIPAA] in the United States), and the IBCLC's practice-guiding documents (IBLCE, 2011, CPC Principle 3.1; IBLCE, 2008, SOP para. 7; ILCA, 2006, Standard 2.4). The patients should be able to assume that anyone with access to their private information has legitimate access, which a 14-year-old non-clinician visitor does not.

Where Is the Conflict of Interest? Situation 3

Question: Which scenario, (a), (b), or (c), presents a conflict of interest for the IBCLC?

(a) Your former IBCLC mentor has retired from clinical work at her hospital. She interviewed recently for an administrative job at your facility, to head up prenatal education. She asks you to put in a good word on her behalf with the supervisors who are making the hiring decision.

(b) A nurse colleague left her identification badge at home, and asks to borrow yours to "swipe in" to the secure NICU nursery.

(c) You have been asked to organize the next staff meeting. You are presenting about Internet-based research tools. The pharmaceutical representative dropped off several small USB-port memory sticks ("thumb drives") yesterday; all have the logo for a blood pressure medicine on them. That gave you an idea. You arranged to *purchase* them from the drug company, to avoid receiving gifts from a vendor.

Answer: (c). Option (a) represents good old-fashioned networking. You aren't doing the hiring; it is not a conflict of interest for you to discuss your friend's professional merits to a group with a keen and legitimate interest in hiring a capable person. Option (b) represents a number of security policy violations; you and your forgetful colleague could be subject to disciplinary action in which COIs are the least of your worry. Option (c) is an example of the tensions of a conflict of professional interest. Yes, you purchased the thumb drives, at a fair market price, but why are you going to a pharmaceutical manufacturer to purchase an item available from thousands of office supplies stores or websites? The thumb drive has a nonlactation-related pharmaceutical logo on it, but why should HCPs in your facility be walking billboards for any product from any medical company? In this hypothetical case, your conversation with the drug representative involved some kind of give and take. In the end both parties walked away "feeling good" (you got a good price for the thumb drives; he made in-roads with clinical staff). This could be used by him in the future to solicit more contacts, meetings, and discussions. All of which benefits the pharmaceutical company and not the IBCLC.

Summary

The IBCLC must be aware of, and either avoid or cure, conflicts of interest (COI) in her profession (IBLCE, 2011, CPC Principles 1.4, 5.1, 5.2, & 6.1; IBLCE, 2008, SOP para. 8; ILCA, 2006, Standards 1.3 & 3.3.6; IBFAN, n.d., WHO Code, Preamble and Articles 4, 5, 6, & 7). Conflicts of interest involve:

• Decisions that bring you COngratulations or INcome
• Decisions that subject you to COercion or INappropriate INfluence

- Professional decisions where COmmercial INfluences drive your COnduct IN providing care.

The topic can seem difficult to master, but the simple mnemonic COIN may assist the IBCLC in identifying a COI, and whether it can be cured or excused. Another simple tactic to avoid legal and ethical tensions is simply to refuse any gifts or favors from commercial manufacturers of any products or services (such as medical devices, pharmaceuticals, and supplies) that are used in clinical practice. Negotiate business transactions at arm's length, and have meetings in a professional setting, without extraneous gifts and food involved.

REFERENCES

Axt, H.-J., Milososki, A., & Schwarz, O. (2006, February 23). *Conflict: A literature review.* Retrieved from http://www.europeanization.de/downloads/conflict_review_fin.pdf

Campbell, E., Gruen, R., Mountford, J., Miller, L., Cleary, P., & Blumenthal, D. (2007, April 26). A national survey of physician–industry relationships. *New England Journal of Medicine, 356*, 1742–1750. Retrieved from http://www.nejm.org/doi/full/10.1056/NEJMsa064508#t=articleTop

Cialdini, R. (1993). *Influence: The psychology of persuasion.* New York, NY: Quill William Morrow.

Council of Medical Specialty Societies. (2011, March). *Code for interactions with companies* [Model policy]. Retrieved from http://www.cmss.org/uploadedFiles/Site/CMSS_Policies/CMSS%20Code%20for%20Interactions%20with%20Companies%20Approved%20Revised%20Version%203-19-11CLEAN.pdf

Elliott, C. (2010). *White coat black hat: Adventures on the dark side of medicine.* Boston, MA: Beacon.

Health Insurance Portability and Accountability Act of 1996 [HIPAA], 45 C.F.R. § Parts 160, 162, & 164 (1996), http://www.access.gpo.gov/nara/cfr/waisidx_07/45cfr160_07.html.

International Baby Food Action Network (IBFAN). (n.d.). *The full code and subsequent WHA resolutions.* Retrieved from http://www.ibfan.org/issue-international_code-full.html

International Board of Lactation Consultant Examiners. (2008, March 8). *Scope of practice for international board certified lactation consultants.* Retrieved from http://www.iblce.org/upload/downloads/ScopeOfPractice.pdf

International Board of Lactation Consultant Examiners. (2011, November 1). *Code of professional conduct for IBCLCs.* Retrieved from http://iblce.org/upload/downloads/CodeOfProfessionalConduct.pdf

International Code Documentation Centre (Ed.). (2007, May). *International code of marketing of breastmilk substitutes and relevant WHA resolutions (annotated)* (2nd updated edition). Penang, Malaysia: IBFAN Penang.

International Lactation Consultant Association. (2006). *Standards of practice for international board certified lactation consultants.* Retrieved from http://www.ilca.org/files/resources/Standards-of-Practice-web.pdf

Kassirer, J. (2005). *On the take.* New York, NY: Oxford University Press.

Katz, D., Caplan, A., & Merz, J. (2003, July 1). All gifts large and small. *University of Pennsylvania Center for Bioethics Papers Repository.* Retrieved from http://repository.upenn.edu/cgi/viewcontent.cgi?article=1050&context=bioethics_papers

Lo, B., & Field, M. (Eds.). (2009). *Conflict of interest in medical research, education, and practice.* Retrieved from http://www.ncbi.nlm.nih.gov/bookshelf/br.fcgi?book=nap12598

ProPublica. (2012). *Dollars for docs: How industry dollars reach your doctors* [Database of pharmaceutical funding to healthcare providers]. Retrieved from http://projects.propublica.org/docdollars/

Razran, G. (1940). Conditioned response changes in rating and appraising sociopolitical slogans. *Psychology Bulletin, 37*, 481.

Rothman, D., McDonald, W., Berkowitz, C., Chimonas, S., DeAngelis, C., Hale, R., . . . Osborn, J. (2009, April 1). Professional medical associations and their relationships with industry: A proposal for controlling conflict of interest [Special section]. *Journal of the American Medical Association, 301*(13), 1367–1372. doi:10.1001/jama.2209.407

Sample, S., Smith, L. D., Berry, S., Brenner, M., Chadwick, G., Dynes, R., . . . Grant, G. (2001, October). *Report on individual and institutional financial conflict of interest.* Retrieved from http://ccnmtl.columbia.edu /projects/rcr/rcr_conflicts/misc/Ref/AAU_CoI.pdf

World Health Organization. (1981). *International code of marketing of breast-milk substitutes.* Retrieved from http://www.who.int/nutrition/publications/code_english.pdf

Chapter 6

The IBCLC in the Courtroom: As Expert, Witness, or Party

Just as women are found in every walk of life, *lactating* women are found in every walk of life—and that can include the courtroom. If breastfeeding and human lactation are directly or indirectly involved in the issues before the court, an International Board Certified Lactation Consultant (IBCLC) may well have a role to play. Sometimes she is in the courtroom herself, testifying as a fact or expert witness; sometimes she is hired as an advisor to the mother or the lawyers, offering them background information and advice to assist in the litigation. Sometimes breastfeeding itself is the focus of the legal action bringing the mother to the courtroom (picture Millennial Mom, suing a facility that shamed her for breastfeeding in public, as was her right in that location). Breast-feeding may be a related matter (imagine a divorce court hearing at which overnight custody is sought by father, at a time when Millennial Mom's 4-month-old baby is still breastfeeding at night). Breastfeeding may also be a "red herring" when a litigant is in court on matters unrelated to breastfeeding, yet lactation is being raised to divert attention from other issues at hand (imagine a divorce court hearing at which overnight custody is sought by father, at a time when Millennial Mom's 4-year-old child is nearly entirely weaned, and regularly sleeps through the night).

The goal of this chapter isn't to imagine every kind of lawsuit that may involve breastfeeding but rather to describe how the IBCLC might prepare herself if she is called to the courtroom, formally or informally, in a matter that will require her exper-tise as an allied healthcare provider. To state the obvious, we will examine the IBCLC's presence in her healthcare provider (HCP) role. IBCLCs are in every walk of life, too: getting sued (or suing) over broken contracts, injuries to person, or infringed property rights; even getting arrested for crimes petty and felonious. While our sympathies may rest with our colleagues embroiled in such legal matters, this chapter will not.

Law for IBCLCs: What Concepts Apply (Nearly) Everywhere?

IBCLCs have an internationally recognized certification for their training and skills, as allied healthcare providers, in the field of breastfeeding and human lactation. We practice all over the world. As such, we are—depending on our country of residency and our citizenship(s)—subject to as many legal systems as there are nations, provinces, states, territories, principalities, counties, cities, townships, boroughs, and municipalities. All of these levels of government may exert some authority over us when we are within their borders. No one can know all of this law. Indeed, one of major tasks for a freshly retained attorney (practicing in any area of law, in any location in the world) is to "look it up": Find the law in the jurisdiction, given the facts of the controversy at hand. Armed with the results of this legal research, the lawyer can advise the client on available options to address (or avoid or answer) the controversy.

Some general concepts of law apply almost everywhere. There will be variations in process and procedure in different parts of the world, but a review of these concepts will help to set the stage for our exploration of the IBCLC in the courtroom.

Rule of Law

Cultures and societies throughout the world use systems, simple and complex, to enforce the basic rules of living within that group. Any misbehaving 5-year-old knows what "that look" from a parent or teacher means, and the consequences that will follow if behaviors are not altered. Similarly, any person caught speeding on the highway knows that the trooper approaching his car can write him a ticket for a hefty fine. When a society agrees to use a system of laws, law enforcers, courts, administrative regulations, and judicial opinions to keep order within the group, it embraces "the rule of law," meaning:

> Sometimes called "the supremacy of law," [the rule of law] provides that decisions should be made by the application of known principles or laws without the intervention of discretion in their application. (Rule of law, 1979, p. 1196)

or

> Individuals, persons and government shall submit to, obey, and be regulated by law, and not arbitrary action by an individual or a group of individuals. (Rule of law, 2010, para. 1)

As IBCLCs, it is very easy to get swept up by our passion for the cause. We consult with breastfeeding mothers who have the simple goal to breastfeed their children; yet, they must slog away against enormous odds, in the medical system, in their workplaces, in their communities and even families, to accomplish what ought to occur naturally, happily, and without fuss. An IBCLC's desire to be an advocate for a breastfeeding mother in a legal matter will go unrealized, however, unless the IBCLC has an official role in the proceeding, no matter how strong, compassionate, articulate and zealous the IBCLC may be on behalf of the mother. Unless you (or your message) have a right to be heard, you may as well go bloviate in the mirror.

The rule of law is built on the notion that justice should be dispensed in an equitable and predictable manner. It requires that we will all abide by the decision, or use legitimate procedures to try to change the result. Lofty legal principles do underpin the seemingly arcane rules having to do with filing deadlines, and length and formatting of documents, proofs that people got their copies, and requirements for the strongest evidence even if it is hard to get. It assumes that laws have been passed for the benefit of all, by those with authority to do so. It can be frustrating for those unfamiliar with the rigors of process and procedure demanded by the legal system to find that their eagerness to "do right" by the mother can be squelched, perhaps from the start. We can all, of course, point to individual instances where justice was not meted out fairly (or at all). But the rule of law is designed to provide a sense of consistency and predictability in our culture. Surely it would be alarming if every person who was caught speeding on the highway had to guess at the consequences. If one person gets a ticket, the next is asked to fork over the keys to the car, the third is led away in chains, the fourth is punched in the nose, and the fifth is told to cough up $5000, cash, on the spot, chaos would reign. The rule of law is a system of justice by which all persons, businesses, organizations, the government, and law enforcement agree to live.

Therefore, for the IBCLC to make any meaningful contribution in a courtroom matter involving breastfeeding and human lactation, she needs more than her passion. She must employ tactics that earn her, or her message, a place at the table (or, rather, bar of the court). The rule of law requires that she fit into the framework of procedures that have been set up to have a matter appropriately heard and decided.

Hierarchy of the Legal System

Legal and non-legal systems alike have a pyramid of authority to which a person may appeal (or be subjected) for justice. That child who ignored "the look" from the teacher may next find himself in the principal's office. If the sanctions meted there are deemed onerous, the child's family can next appeal "up" to the school administrator who is the principal's supervisor. And so it is with legal systems. Using the United States as an example, the following describes the hierarchy of legal authority on federal matters.

U.S. Constitution

At the top of the pyramid is the U.S. Constitution. The written document "constitutes" the system of governance agreed to by the people who wrote and enacted it. It describes a system of federalism by which the federal government is granted limited authority, with all remaining authority left to the 50 states. This is accomplished by three separate but equal branches of federal government (judicial, legislative, and executive). The U.S. Constitution is called a living document because it continues to be interpreted through the lens of modern day culture and society, with respect for prior cases, via written opinions of the U.S. Supreme Court.

Law-Making Powers of Three Branches of Government

Laws can be "made" by all three branches of government. Most of us know that the legislative branch (the United States Congress, comprising the U.S. Senate and U.S. House of Representatives) passes federal laws (meaning they apply to every U.S. citizen). But the executive branch (through the federal administrative agencies or the military arms) writes regulations that also have the force of law. These agencies are customarily given the authority to do so under the enacting statutes passed by Congress.[1] The judicial branch (through the Supreme Court, the federal court system beneath it, and some "special courts" on the side governing matters like bankruptcy or claims against the federal government) decides lawsuits and/or writes judicial opinions, and these carry the weight of law. It is called "case law" or sometimes "common law" when a judge's reported decision, in the form of a written opinion, is issued (Case law, 1979, p. 196; Common law, 1979, pp. 250–251).

The higher the court, the more weight and authority its written decisions will have, setting "legal precedent":

> A case which establishes legal principles to a certain set of facts, coming to a certain conclusion, and which is to be followed from that point on when similar or identical facts are before a court. (Precedent, 2010, para. 1)

Going hand in hand with the concept of precedent is *stare decisis*, which is:

> To abide by, or adhere to, decided cases. Policy of courts to stand by precedent and not to disturb settled point [case citation omitted]. Doctrine that, when court has once laid down a principle of law as applicable to a certain state of facts, it will adhere to that principle, and apply it in all future cases, where facts are substantially the same; regardless of whether the parties and property are the same [case citation omitted]. (Stare decisis, 1979, p. 1261)

One can see why a lawyer would be so eager to "look up" the law. If she can find statutory language or a judicial opinion (case law) that fits the facts of the controversy

---

[1] For example, the Fair Packaging and Labeling Act was enacted by the U.S. Congress in 1966 because, "Informed consumers are essential to the fair and efficient functioning of a free market economy. Packages and their labels should enable consumers to obtain accurate information as to the quantity of the contents and should facilitate value comparisons. *Therefore, it is hereby declared to be the policy of the Congress to assist consumers and manufacturers in reaching these goals in the marketing of consumer goods*" (Fair Packaging and Labeling Act, 1966) (emphasis added). A portion of the enacting legislation also reads, "*The authority to promulgate regulations under this chapter is vested in* (A) the Secretary of Health and Human Services (referred to hereinafter as the 'Secretary') with respect to any consumer commodity which is a food, drug, device, or cosmetic, as each such term is defined by section 321 of title 21; and (B) the Federal Trade Commission (referred to hereinafter as the 'Commission') with respect to any other consumer commodity" (Fair Packaging and Labeling Act, 1966) (emphasis added). Those regulations appear in part at Title 16 of the Code of Federal Regulations, Parts 500–503, which contains the "Regulations Under Section 4 of the Fair Packaging and Labeling Act," *issued by the Federal Trade Commission* (Fair Packaging and Labeling Act, 2000).

before her, she will have a fairly good predictor of how the judge will decide the case. If that suits her client's cause, she will argue that the prior opinion is binding under the principle of stare decisis. If she doesn't like what her research has revealed, she will have to argue that the current controversy is different, somehow, from the facts in the precedent-setting case. If she is persuasive, today's judge can create a new precedent with a new written opinion, based upon the slightly different facts before the court.

Types of Cases

There are several types of cases; they are decided within court systems designed to address that body of law. The law types most people are familiar with include civil cases and criminal cases.

Civil cases (or actions) generally address the rights of a citizen (Civil law, 1979, p. 223), and grievances between two parties, be they person-versus-person, person-versus-corporation/organization, or person-versus-governmental authority. Actions can be brought under statutes or common law (judge-made case law). Civil cases come in many flavors (tort, contract, wills and trusts, etc.), and remedies are usually confined to money damages or a requirement that a certain action be performed (or ceased).

Most court actions involving an IBCLC will fall into the very broad category of civil law, which covers torts (such as negligence, a common theory in medical malpractice), family law (separation, divorce, and custody matters involving breastfeeding mothers and children), employment or labor law (conditions owed to a breastfeeding mother who works outside the home), and civil rights (infringements of conditions and rights to breastfeed [for the mother]) or to be breastfed [for the child]).

Criminal cases involve disregard for laws passed by governments for the protection of the public safety (Criminal law, 2010, para. 1). Prosecutorial authority is vested in the government, and sanctions can involve fines and incarceration.

Other types of cases that will be decided in court systems set up for that purpose include:

- Administrative law, which covers the rules and regulations, orders, and decisions written under statutory authority by the administrative branches of government, as in our example of the Fair Packaging and Labeling Act above (Administrative law, 1979, p. 43).
- Military justice, employed for disputes involving military personnel or property. Within such a system there are procedures to handle civil, criminal, and purely military matters (Military law, 1979, p. 896).
- International law, involving "the intercourse of nations; the law of nations" in times of peace and war (i.e., treaties and trade pacts) (International law, 1979, p. 733).
- Martial law for those situations where customary civil authority has broken down (perhaps due to natural disaster or war), and the military system is used to enforce day-to-day governmental authority (Martial law, 2010, para. 2).

Different Levels of Court Authority

Generally speaking, all the types of cases described above will be decided in a tiered system of court authority. We'll use the U.S. federal system as an example.

- Trial level—At the first (or bottom) tier is the entry level or trial stage. These are the federal district courts. This is where the case is tried. Evidence is introduced and witnesses are heard under strict rules of procedure and evidence. The case is decided by a jury, judge, officer, administrative law judge, or mediator, depending on the type of case at hand.

- Intermediate appeals level—After the trial stage verdict or decision, there may be grounds to appeal by the losing party. If so, the case goes to the second tier (or intermediate appeals) court, called the U.S. Circuit Court of Appeals. Here, the matter is reviewed "on the record" by one or more judges, meaning the errors alleged at the first tier are reviewed and analyzed by the intermediate appeals court. They will read the written record, and review the evidence that was entered below. Lawyers will file written briefs (citing precedential case law) and offer oral arguments that the trial level decision should remain or be overturned (in all or part). New witnesses and evidence are *not* called at the appeals stage. An appeal is to examine whether the *trial* court did everything correctly, and so review is confined to the actions of the trial court proceedings.

- Final appeals level—The last level to which appeal may be made, the court of last resort, is the U.S. Supreme Court. The lawyers will first have to convince the court to hear the case (to "grant *certiorari*"), arguing that there is a split of authority between the circuit courts, or this matter involves important unsettled principles of constitutional law, or conflicts between state and federal courts (Fine, 2008, p. 3). Only a very few cases get through the system, to be argued before the justices, and for which written opinions (some with dissenting sections) will be issued.

State Laws and Courts; Municipal Authority

In the United States, there is the similar system set up in each of the states (territories, and the District of Columbia): a separation of powers into legislative, executive, and judicial branches; a system defining the types of cases (under civil law, criminal law, etc.) and a tiered court system to hear lawsuits and allow for their appeal. The IBCLC in the courtroom will most likely find herself in a state-based judicial system, as tort law and family law are primarily defined and enforced under state authority.[2]

---

[2] This is why there can be different laws for marriage/divorce in different states of the union. Marriage customarily involves legal requirements in addition to a religious ceremony. "The Supreme Court has held that states are permitted to reasonably regulate the institution by prescribing who is allowed to marry and how the marriage can be dissolved. Entering into a marriage changes the legal status of both parties and gives both husband and wife new rights and obligations. One power that the states do not have, however, is that of prohibiting marriage in the absence of a valid reason. For example, prohibiting interracial marriage is unconstitutional because it violates the Equal Protection Clause of the Constitution" (Cornell University Law School, 2010c, para. 3).

In the smallest geographical jurisdiction, there are local or municipal regulations governing the place where one lives (for example, to regulate how and where businesses may operate [zoning], or how local taxes will be structured to support the public school system). There may not be a multi-tiered court system at the local level, but there will be a process by which one can appeal decisions imposed by a local authority (Fine, 2008).

How Do Laws and Ethics Differ?

Recall the discussion in earlier chapters describing the four practice-guiding documents for IBCLCs, and how they fit with the rules of the workplace, and the laws of the land, which also govern lactation consultancy. It is worth repeating the general premise here: Laws are constitutions, statues, regulations, or case law (judicial decisions or opinions) that are written down somewhere, having been enacted or produced by those with authority to do so. Laws are enforced using a defined court/ judicial process, and final decisions rendered after all appeals have been exhausted are to be respected by all.

Ethical codes are also written down somewhere, such as our International Board of Lactation Consultant Examiners Code of Professional Conduct (IBLCE CPC) (IBLCE, 2011b), but they are not a constitution, a statute, a regulation, or case law, and that is one "bright line" test between law and ethics (Hall, 2002). Ethics codes may have a trial-like disciplinary or sanctions process to adjudicate infractions of an ethical code (such as our IBLCE Disciplinary Procedures for the Code of Professional Conduct for IBCLCs [IBLCE, 2011a]), but they are not enforceable in the court system, using the same means and methods as for laws. While a conflict in the *law* may be resolved in court, with a decision binding on the parties and forming precedent for all later litigation, a conflict in *ethics* may be resolved differently each and every time a quandary occurs. Ethics involve the internal tug-of-war between right and wrong (that feeling we described elsewhere as "the hairs going up on the back of the neck" when something occurs that isn't quite right), and may be resolved differently according to the situation of each case.

Concepts in law and ethics may overlap, and specific conflicts or quandaries may involve aspects both of law and ethics, but the two principles are distinct from one another. Law is black and white, and ethics is always gray. To use a simplified example: Ethics tells us that if you are being chased on foot by a robber and fear for your life, you are justified in stealing a car to get away. The act is considered a crime (since the law against stealing cars applies equally to all), but your action is ethically justified, given the terrifying circumstances. If you are about to be arrested for the crime of stealing the car, you may be able to argue to the police officer that the circumstances exonerate you from the admittedly illegal act (since ethics examines all the circumstances of the conflict). Another oft-used example: the quandary of whether the parent would steal bread (a crime) to feed his starving family (an ethical obligation).

Typical Actions Involving Lactation Issues

That quick explanation of common legal structures used the United States as an example, but the basic notions in democratic societies will be very similar. Indeed, much of the common law in the United States comes from historic legal concepts originating in England and France. Let us now turn to the IBCLC in particular, and discuss how she might find herself as an expert or witness in a courtroom, deferring for now her role as a party in a lawsuit. We'll use an American jurisprudential model, but many of the concepts will be applicable to IBCLCs from other countries of the world.

Tort Actions

Lawsuits in tort can be grounded in federal statutory or common (case) law, or in state statutory or common (case) law, and which court system hears the lawsuit depends on which law it is brought under. Generally, a tort involves a non-contractual duty from one party to another, a breach of that duty, and damage as a proximate result (Tort, 1979, p. 1335). Some of the theories of a cause of action, in tort, will sound familiar to anyone who is a healthcare practitioner.

Medical Malpractice (Negligence)
Negligence is the theory of law underpinning most medical malpractice lawsuits, and thus it is no surprise that negligence forms the most frequent basis for liability by HCPs (Miller, 2006).

Unintentional negligence involves an examination of fault: the practitioner didn't meet the basic standards of care, or wasn't paying enough attention, and the mistake caused injury. The negligence can be due to commission (actively doing something, such as administering the wrong medication or dosage), or omission (failing to act when one should, such as giving medication at the proper time) (Pozgar, 2005). The negligent act may be characterized as misfeasance (improper performance of an act, such as surgery on the wrong limb) or nonfeasance (failing to act, such as failure to order diagnostic tests). The legal case will examine the basic elements of a tort action: a non-contractual duty, breach of the duty, and damage or injury as a result.

A medical malpractice suit may also be brought under a theory of intentional tort, where an evaluation of fault need not be examined, and a standard of care needn't be established. All that need be shown are the wrongful act and resultant injury. Intentional torts can involve either commission or omission. These acts are sometimes called mal-feasance; "the commission of some act which is positively unlawful . . . a wrongful act which the actor has no legal right to do" (Malfeasance, 1979, p. 862). Examples of causes of action for intentional tort are assault and battery, defamation, invasion of privacy, and intentional infliction of emotional distress (Miller, 2006). The IBLCE CPC offers its own definitions of "misfeasance," "malfeasance," and "due diligence" as they apply to IBCLC practice (IBLCE, 2011b, CPC Definitions and Interpretations 3 & 6).

It is easy to imagine any number of scenarios where a lactating mother sues for medical malpractice under a theory of negligence on the part of her caregivers. A mother is told by her primary healthcare provider that she cannot breastfeed while on medication for depression; she stops taking her medication and spirals downward into severe depression bordering on psychosis. She sues her healthcare provider for negligence (for failing to meet his basic standard of care to know which medications were compatible for his lactating patient). She may even add an allegation of intentional infliction of emotional distress (for putting her through that miserable experience). Or, a mother's baby is erroneously brought to another patient, who then breastfeeds the infant. Mother No. 1 sues the hospital for negligent infliction of emotional distress, as well as the intentional torts of invasion of privacy, battery, intentional infliction of emotional distress (Bornmann, 2008).

Breach of Warranty

A warranty is a promise. Most of us are familiar with the piece of paper that comes with a consumer good we've purchased, promising that the product will be replaced or repaired if it breaks. Similarly, a warranty in the area of tort law involves a promise that a certain outcome will result if a product or service is used, and the breach happens when that promised result does not occur (Bornmann, 2008). If a mother is told that her milk supply *will* increase through the use of various medications or products, she may well have grounds to allege breach of warranty if her supply does not improve. IBCLCs are well advised never to make any promises to a mother, other than a general promise as an allied healthcare professional to provide evidence-based information and support to the mother, so that she may make an informed decision about lactation matters.

Assault and Battery

Assault and battery were described above as intentional torts; there may also be criminal laws in some jurisdictions that proscribe assault and battery. As a cause of action in tort, battery is "offensive and intentional contact, direct or indirect, which causes injury" (Battery, 2010, para. 1). Assault is an action (which usually precedes battery) which puts another in fear of offensive or injurious touching (Miller, 2006). We customarily think of assault and battery in the criminal context: a street brawl or domestic violence confrontation. But in the medical arena, it occurs when treatment is attempted or performed without consent or lawful authority. In lactation, a hypothetical example is the mother who sues for assault and battery when her baby is given formula in the nursery, despite explicit instruction against such action (Bornmann, 2008).

Unauthorized (Unlicensed) Practice of Medicine

This tort goes to scope of practice (the activities in which a practitioner may engage) and license (or certification) to practice (under authority granted by a licensing or certifying organization). A cause of action for practicing without a license or outside a scope of practice might not specifically allege patients/clients have been injured; rather, it may allege this *might* occur, because the practitioner has not followed the customary required steps, designed to ensure public safety, of obtaining rights to practice in this jurisdiction. These are often turf battles: scope of practice is all about turf; turf is green; green means money.

Products Liability
This tort involves injuries caused by use of a product that is unreasonably dangerous. Sometimes the manufacturer will be held "strictly liable," which (like intentional torts) means fault needn't be proven, only that an injury resulted from use. With products liability, there is an overlapping concept based on contract law. Implied warranties of (a) "merchantability" and (b) "fitness for a particular use" mean the product was sold with the intent that it would perform as advertised. We expect a radio or television to transmit programming; we expect a blow-up swimming pool to hold water; we expect a coffee pot to make coffee. In the 21st century, for many mothers, the very natural and biologic act of breastfeeding increasingly involves the use of gadgets: pumps, nipple shells and shields, bottles and teats/nipples, contraptions designed to address nipple and breast conditions (such as nipple "everters" and leaking-milk inhibitors). A products liability theory to redress injuries caused by use of the product, or the materials that make it up, is certainly plausible for a breastfeeding mother.[3]

Family Law Actions

Marriage, divorce, separation, custody, visitation, alimony, child support, adoption, foster care, and so on may generally be described as "family law" or "domestic relations" matters. Family law falls under local or state court jurisdiction because traditionally, these matters are considered to reflect the common law of the locality. This is why marriage requirements can differ from state to state (e.g., license fee, blood test, or age or waiting period requirements) (Cornell University Law School, 2010b). Similarly, the laws governing dissolution of a marriage (divorce), and the care and custody of children, will vary from jurisdiction to jurisdiction (Cornell University Law School, 2010a). Some states in the United States, and in the Family Law Courts of Australia, have voluntary arbitration, mediation, or alternative dispute resolution tracks for resolving family law matters, but the end result is that family law matters are being discussed, and IBCLCs may bring their expertise to bear either in preparing a family law case, or in offering testimony or written evidence to the judges or panelists who decide these

---

[3] A federal district court decision, granting several portions of motions to dismiss (for pleadings deficiencies) in a combined lawsuit brought on consumer protection law theories against manufacturers of baby bottles and formula cans containing Bisphenol-A ("BPA") (a toxic substance), indicates that products liability was not asserted by plaintiff but alludes that such a cause of action may have been viable. (In re: Bisphenol-A [BPA] Litigation, 2009).

matters (Family Law Courts of Australia, n.d.). Because these courts are parochial, and guard their jurisdiction fiercely, litigants are wise to find *local* experts (like lawyers and IBCLCs) to assist in the case. Local counsel will be familiar with the local rules of court procedure, the unwritten customs of the court, and the demeanors and peculiarities of the judges who sit in these cases. Such expertise and insight will be invaluable.

Employment or Labor Law Actions

Once again, alternate phrases may be used by different countries to describe this general area of law, but it covers all areas of the employer–employee relationship. For the breastfeeding woman, lactation may present an issue that needs to be addressed at the woman's job upon her return to work after the birth of a baby.

There is a huge range of maternity-based rights and privileges, depending on the country and work setting (Alewell & Pull, 2005). Whether the region has a developed or developing economy, or government provides some (or all) healthcare under ministry regulation, or the mother is in an entry-level or executive position, will all have a bearing on what benefits may accrue. In a large company, the human resources department customarily will be well versed in what benefits the employee of the company is entitled to access, because the infinite variability of birth experiences renders infinite variations on access to benefits. Examples: Is the woman who becomes ill and hospitalized due to complications of her cesarean delivery considered to be on sick leave or maternity leave? Does the mother's health insurance through her employer cover delivery at home by a midwife, or must she deliver at a hospital with an obstetrician?

IBCLCs around the world should be familiar, at least in passing, with the sorts of benefits to which a mother employed outside the home may be entitled. Several areas of the IBCLC's professional responsibility require that she be cognizant of, and work within, the mother's family and economic situation (IBLCE, 2011b, CPC Principles 1.1, 1.2, 1.3, 1.4, 1.5, 5.2, 6.1, & 6.3; IBLCE Scope of Practice [SOP], 2008, paras. 3, 4, 5, 7, & 8; International Lactation Consultant Association Standards of Practice [ILCA Standards], 2006, Preface, Standards 1, 3, & 4). That cannot be done if the IBCLC doesn't know what working conditions the mother will return to, and when.

When Lactation Is "Homeless" in the Law

In the United States, lactation does not neatly fit into the definitions of pre-existing areas of law, carved out to address an employee's rights (springing from pregnancy, childbirth, and maternity/family leave laws), and a citizen's right to equal protection of the law (civil rights). Maternity/family leave parameters are a function of what a nation's laws permit or require (see, for example, Canada Ministry of Labour, 2012). While breastfeeding is linked inextricably with the biologic functions of pregnancy and childbirth, it does not have easily identified start- and finish-dates. It doesn't "end" with the delivery of the baby, as do pregnancy and childbirth. Full-term, uncomplicated pregnancy for humans worldwide is 40 gestational weeks (give or take a few weeks), yet uncomplicated lactation can occur for anywhere from a few days up to several years (Dettwyler, 1995). Mothers (and their attorneys) have had to use clever thinking to "fit" lactation into existing doctrines; sometimes it works, and sometimes it doesn't.

The U.S. Pregnancy Discrimination Act of 1978 (PDA) is an amendment to the Civil Rights Act of 1964, written to require fair treatment for those with pregnancy-related medical conditions (including those that may temporarily "disable" the pregnant woman from performing certain work-related tasks). Courts have not been willing to define breastfeeding, lactation and the need to express milk as "medical conditions" that are protections guaranteed under this federal civil rights law (Christrup, 2001; Marcus, 2011; Orozco, 2010). It would seem that, since only women can breastfeed, they ought to enjoy protection from discrimination based on their sex under Title VII of the Civil Rights Act. Unfortunately, the courts haven't gone in that direction. A fairly steady line of decisions (remember the discussion of precedent and stare decisis, above) considers breastfeeding as distinguished from pregnancy, and inherently part of child rearing. One court opinion stated, "it is a disservice . . . to both men and women to assume that child rearing is a function peculiar to one sex" (Christrup, 2001, p. 485, quoting 1985 federal district court opinion); another court wrote that "Title VII and the PDA do not cover breast feeding or childrearing concerns because they are not 'medical conditions related to pregnancy, childbirth or related medical conditions.'" (Orozco, 2010, p. 1305 quoting 1999 federal district court opinion).

The Americans with Disabilities Act (ADA) requires employers to provide reasonable accommodation (including flexible work schedules) to their employees with disabilities, which would seem a good fit for the accommodations the breastfeeding mother seeks (Americans with Disabilities Act, 1990). However, the ADA has not been interpreted to include lactation, in part because of reluctance to characterize the transient process of breastfeeding as a permanent disability, akin to, say, an employee with permanent hearing or vision loss (Christrup, 2001).

Without question, the Family and Medical Leave Act (FMLA) in the United States covers the mother who is caring for a newborn (including breastfeeding), but it falls short in that breastfeeding can occur for months and even years after the initial guaranteed family leave time has elapsed (a matter of weeks in the United States) and the mother is back at her place of work. Other FMLA provisions allowing employees periodically to be away from work are predicated on the illness or disability of the employee or a loved one. For example, FMLA allows an employee to take unpaid, job-protected leave to care for a seriously ill family member (Family and Medical Leave Act, 1993). But breastfeeding is not an "illness" in the same way that, for example, recovery from surgery is; indeed, breastfeeding is promoted as a public health imperative for both mother and child. Some states have laws that expand FMLA, allowing for a portion of the guaranteed leave to be paid, or increasing the leave time (e.g., the California Family Temporary Disability Insurance [FTDI]) (California Employment Development Department, 2010), but they don't help shoehorn the breastfeeding mother into the application of the law.

Civil rights in the United States (specifically, freedom from discrimination based on sex) is another area of law that has been argued on behalf of breastfeeding women. In the United States, sexual harassment, a workplace-based violation of civil rights based on sex discrimination, requires unwelcome verbal, visual, or physical conduct of a sexual nature; it must be offensive and severe or pervasive enough that it affects working conditions or creates a hostile work environment (U.S. Equal Employment Opportunity Commission, n.d.). Other countries also recognize causes of action for sexual or violent harassment in the workplace (e.g., for the United Kingdom, see Cowling & Sinclair, 2007). But these protections are predicated on *harassment*. The breastfeeding mother who seeks breaks to express her milk or directly feed her infant may find no help under these laws, unless her co-workers have also made crude, lewd comments about her breasts.

These inconsistencies in the United States may reflect an accurate description of how the courts have interpreted federal cases as of early 2012, but they defy common sense understanding by the mothers and their employers who are expected to comply with the law. Legislation has been introduced in recent Congressional sessions to make clear, once and for all, that a woman who is breastfeeding enjoys protections against discrimination in the workplace, and as a civil right (U.S. Breastfeeding Committee, 2011a) but the bills had not progressed to the hearings stage as of March 2012.

When Lactation Is Not "Homeless" in the Law
One recent law very specific to the needs of working breastfeeding mothers was included in major healthcare law reforms enacted by the United States in 2010. This portion of the healthcare reform was an amendment to the Fair Labor Standards Act, providing for unpaid but guaranteed break time, up to 1 year after the birth of the child, for a mother to express her breastmilk (U.S. Dept. of Labor, 2010; U.S. Breastfeeding Committee, 2011c). The law covers hourly wage workers; salaried (often management) workers are not covered, but their (usually more generous) benefits package may provide for workplace accommodations to express milk (U.S. Breastfeeding Committee, 2011b). Employers of less than 50 employees can claim exemption from the law *if* they can first establish that it would be a hardship to provide "a place, other than a bathroom, that is shielded from view and free from intrusion from co-workers and the public, which may be used by an employee to express breast milk" (Patient Protection and Affordable Care Act, 29 U.S.C. § 207(r) (1)(B), 2010). With passage of this legislation, the United States "[joined] 120 other countries whose employed women enjoy protection for lactation breaks at work" (U.S. Breastfeeding Committee, 2010, p. 12).

Civil Rights Actions

We have described how civil rights law in the United States is not, as of early 2012, a surefire means of protection for a breastfeeding mother in the workplace. With the exception of some lovely language in a Fifth Circuit Court opinion,[4] there has been unwillingness to accord breastfeeding the constitutionally protected privacy rights that parenting choices customarily enjoy. Thus, the federal law position offers rather half-hearted support to a breastfeeding mother: while states cannot specifically infringe upon a woman's right to breastfeed, neither are the states required to "legislate, enforce, or mandate any laws specifically protecting that right" (Christrup, 2001, p. 493).

Thus, in the absence of a strong federal legal precedent, many states and municipalities in the United States have passed laws designed to protect breastfeeding as a civil right, just as they stepped in to pass laws to fill the void of protection for breastfeeding mothers under employment law. By mid 2011:

- Forty-five states, the District of Columbia, and the Virgin Islands have laws protecting a woman's right to breastfeed in public or in private.
- Twenty-eight states, the District of Columbia, and the Virgin Islands exempt breastfeeding from public indecency laws.
- Twenty-four states, the District of Columbia, and Puerto Rico have statutes regarding breastfeeding in the workplace.
- Twelve states and Puerto Rico exempt a breastfeeding mother from jury duty.
- Five states and Puerto Rico have implemented or encouraged the development of a breastfeeding awareness education campaign.
- Several individual states have enacted unique breastfeeding-related laws (breastfeeding mothers may do so on any land owned by Virginia; Puerto Rican shopping malls and other public places must have non-bathroom areas for breastfeeding and family care; two states have provisions to prevent discrimination by child-care providers and to ensure safe handling of breastmilk in such places; California requires training of hospital staff in the importance of breastfeeding at facilities with the lowest exclusive breastfeeding rates; Maryland exempts breastfeeding equipment

---

[4] "Breastfeeding is the most elemental form of parental care. It is a communion between mother and child that, like marriage, is intimate to the degree of being sacred. Nourishment is necessary to maintain the child's life, and the parent may choose to believe that breastfeeding will enhance the child's psychological as well as physical health. In light of the spectrum of interests that the Supreme Court has held specially protected we conclude that the Constitution protects from excessive state interference a woman's decision respecting breastfeeding her child." *Dike v. School Board of Orange County, Florida*, 650 F.2d 783, 787 (5th Cir. 1981). This case involved a teacher working in a state-run workplace, who sought break time to breastfeed her baby who was brought to her workplace for that purpose. Though finding breastfeeding to be specially protected under the U.S. Constitution, the opinion remanded the matter to the courts below to determine if the state had a sufficiently important interest to protect that it could interfere with this mother's right to breastfeed, and whether such restrictions on breastfeeding could be closely tailored to meet that narrow state interest. Upon remand the district court below determined: Yes, the state had an important interest to protect (avoiding disruption of the educational process) and, yes, this intervention (not allowing non-school-aged children on campus) was a narrow means to protect that state interest (Christrup, 2001, p. 492). Sadly for this mother, that meant no more breaks for breastfeeding her child.

from sales tax; three states have laws governing procurement, processing, distribution, or use of human milk; New York has a Breastfeeding Mothers' Bill of Rights law) (National Conference of State Legislatures, 2011).

While this appears to be a strong body of law protecting the breastfeeding mother, there are plenty of news stories even in recent years of mothers who have been asked, flat out wrongfully and in violation of federal, state or local law, to stop breastfeeding their babies in the restaurants, museums, and airplanes where they had every right to be. The experience can be traumatizing and embarrassing, leaving the mother feeling ashamed when she was the only one who was acting in accordance with the law. For:

A basic maxim of American law is that a right without a remedy is no right at all. [Footnote omitted.] In plain terms, this means that although you may have a "right" to do anything not otherwise forbidden by law, if you do not also have a legal protection against someone interfering with that right, your ability to exercise it may be limited. (Marcus, 2007, para. 3)

Thus, the mother who has a right to breastfeed in public, and has that right erroneously infringed by another, may not be in a position to do much about it after the fact. Sadly, most laws that uphold the right to breastfeeding in public do not have a corresponding enforcement provision (Marcus, 2007).

IBCLCs frequently are called into this fray, because it is the "court of public opinion" to which the mother and her allies must turn to seek redress, when the law of the land does not provide any remedy or recourse. Some advocates choose to write letters or seek meetings with the owners of the facility that ousted the mother, extracting an apology and some promise that staff training to raise sensitivity and awareness will occur (*Breastfeeding at the Philadelphia Museum of Art*, 2006). Others choose a more public option, staging "nurse-ins" (easily advertised through Millennial Mom's active social media on the cell phone and Internet) to raise awareness and force public discussion of the issue (Rochman, 2011; Silver, 2009). Some will resort to filing lawsuits: even if the law is not heavily weighted to favor the mother's cause of action, the publicity surrounding the lawsuit and the circumstances giving rise to it can be persuasive in effecting change by a corporation (Mittleman, 2009; Rathke, 2012).

Whether and how an IBCLC chooses to participate in such activities depends on how comfortable she is in publicly advocating for breastfeeding mothers, breastfeeding children, and breastfeeding itself. Those who opt not to participate have made as ethical and legal a decision as those who do.

What Really Is at Issue, and Can the IBCLC Be of Help?

A very basic question should be asked before the IBCLC hunkers down to prepare herself for the courtroom. Should she even be there? Is this a battle that only coincidentally involves a breastfeeding mother? Or is there an issue involving breastfeeding and human lactation about which an IBCLC, with her specialized skills and knowledge, can offer relevant information and insight to the trier of fact? (The trier of fact is the jury, or the judge, who will ultimately decide the case; who decides which litigant's version of the facts is correct, justifying a decision of the case in that litigant's favor.)

IBCLCs may find themselves pulled into a case, at the beginning, because of outreach by the mother. Millennial Mom is very good about surfing the Internet and surveying her friends to find a clinician who may be sympathetic to the cause, and then reaching out to the IBCLC by phone or email. Mothers are *parties* to an action, they are not the lawyers. Of course, there are mothers who happen to be attorneys, who might be parties to the action. A corollary is that nonlawyers and lawyers alike can represent themselves in any legal proceeding, without hiring a separate lawyer ("appearing *pro se*" [Pro se, 2010, para. 1]). For purposes of this text, we will assume the more conventional set up: Mother's lawyer is someone else.

Generally speaking, the IBCLC who is going to be involved in a case ought to refrain from in-depth interaction with any party; her contacts should be with the lawyer who aspires to organize and control the preparation of the case. But there will be that fuzzy time period at the start when no one is quite certain, yet, where all of this is going. It is so early on that no lawsuits have been imagined, much less filed. So, the breastfeeding mother may call the IBCLC, weepy and distraught over a situation where her rights have been infringed, or some dastardly deed has been perpetrated on her. All of that may have occurred, but it still begs the question: Does the issue spring from the act of breastfeeding and human lactation, or does the issue spring from a woman who coincidentally is breastfeeding?

Here is an example, drawn from real life. Breastfeeding mother works as a kindergarten teacher. Upon her return to work, she would like to use her break time (when the children are supervised elsewhere, such as gym class) to express her breastmilk. Excellent. She would like to do it in the classroom, when she will be alone, allowing her to multitask at her desk (check emails or listen to phone messages while using her breast pump). Excellent. She would like to cover over the window in the door to the classroom during the breaks, for privacy. Certainly reasonable. The principal (teacher's boss) has no problem with accommodating mom with a place for clean and private pump breaks, but she has denied the request to cover the classroom window. Rationale: Rules in their school district require administrators and parents alike to have an unfettered view of the classroom at all times, to meet child protection and safety guidelines. And that is certainly reasonable, too.

These additional facts change the circumstances, and the analysis. Principal has offered some viable alternatives to the teacher/mother: use of private rooms in the school nurse's office; use of the teacher's lounge; creation of some other private, clean space in the building. Certainly reasonable, again. Mother, however, wants the classroom, or nothing at all. Can the IBCLC please come to her aid? Can she convince the principal that this pumping time is very important to the health of mother and child, and she is entitled to breaks to pump?

At first blush, the IBCLC might want to jump onto her white steed, lance in hand, and charge off in defense of this damsel in breastfeeding distress. But is that really needed here? The mother is breastfeeding, and by her own admission, her boss has agreed that she should have a private and clean space to periodically express her breastmilk every day. The breastfeeding-related interests have been acknowledged, with a promise that they will be met. All that remains at issue is the *nature* of the accommodation, and that is no more remarkable than any accommodation an employer makes for any employee. The mother's stubborn desire to be able to stay in her classroom does not consider the principal's equally valid requirement to meet safety and child protection guidelines disallowing window coverings. Lactation is a red herring here: an irrelevant legal or factual issue (Red herring, 2010, para. 4). The IBCLC isn't needed to establish the need for protection of breastfeeding or pumping, because that has already been recognized and agreed to.

A corollary examination is: can the IBCLC truly be objective, given the facts of any given case? Can she fairly view the case from the standpoint of the baby, both mother and father, and near- or extended relatives, all of whom may have a role in the case? If she cannot, she should not be used as an expert witness on the stand. The IBCLC's testimony should be no different, on the matter of preserving milk supply while *this* baby is separated from *this* mother, whether the infant is being pried from his mother's arms to have weekend visitation with the father from whom mother is unhappily divorced, or baby is happily handed off to doting grandparents so the loving couple can have a second-honeymoon-weekend.

Informal Assistance to the Mother in Trouble

Let us assume Millennial Mom tracked you down somehow, and you are moved by her plight, despite the words of wisdom above advising that your contacts with the mother are better channeled through her lawyer. Maybe the mother doesn't have a lawyer, or thinks she doesn't need one, because her "best friend's brother is going to law school and he said he could help for free." IBCLCs have hearts, and they are entitled to be moved to offer some kind of support. There are some ground rules to remember.

If you do offer support for the mother, be aware that you have removed yourself, forever, from being used as an expert witness. You will be seen as siding with the mother, and rightly so, given your prior connection to her. You may also be tainted as a fact witness: even if you first came to know the mother because you saw her clinically, if you then formed a bond with her by providing emotional support during the travails of the lawsuit with the father, his attorneys may be able to successfully impeach your credibility as a witness.

Help the mother to obtain the legal help she needs: an attorney well-versed in family law in her jurisdiction, who is willing to learn how and why mother's breastfeeding relationship is worthy of consideration. Yes, it costs money, but there are options for low- or no-cost representation by excellent and zealous attorneys. Suggest that the mother contact the local bar association (the professional association for lawyers), and ask for referrals to lawyers knowledgeable in family law. Ask if there are any programs sponsored by the bar to offer low- or no-cost representation for clients in need; cases in which the health and welfare of young children is at stake may provide front-of-the-line eligibility over other people whose legal squabbles go to contract or property issues.

Often, the mother just needs a sympathetic shoulder, and IBCLCs are very good at offering compassionate ears. Be aware (as with your needy lactation clients) that some mothers may take advantage of your kind heart, calling at all hours and without regard to your other obligations. It probably isn't intentional: most mothers who feel their children will be "taken" from them (as divisive custodial arrangements are perceived to be) move into "mother bear" mode, where protection of their child takes precedence over all other concerns (including your sleep).

If things are friendly between the mother and father, suggest that mother take the time and effort to get her custody, support, and visitation orders squared away *now*. It does not take a legal scholar to know that people will discuss and negotiate difficult topics better when tempers are calm and emotions are in check. Suggest that mother offer up plenty of parenting time to the father *now*, not only because that is healthy for both the father and the child, but because it provides a much clearer picture of the stress and time involved in capable parenting. In a custody fight, exclusive time with the children is often used as a "power play" by the parties, not because of any consideration of true parenting requirements, but rather as a means to "win" something over the other parent. And, yes, mothers do this too.

If things are starting to turn sour between the parents, especially if mother has concerns about her own or her child's safety, suggest she keep a simple notebook or diary where she contemporaneously writes down her worries (with date, time and a list of others present). Mother can use this personal journal to freely write her inner-most thoughts and feelings. This is not something she should advertise that she has; it is her private, confidential journal. Just the act of writing can be very cathartic and empowering for a woman who feels increasingly powerless in a deteriorating situation. But it can also be a very helpful tool, later on, if she is trying to reconstruct a series of events, in consultation with her lawyers, about the changing nature of the relation-ship. It is simply a good memory-jogging tool, and anyone who has tried to recreate important events in time and place without aid of a calendar or diary will understand the usefulness of this exercise. The diary will not be accepted as "evidence" that "Dad smelled like alcohol when he brought the baby home late," but it can be used (even at trial) to allow the mother to be reminded of this event, about which she can then testify in person, where her veracity can be assessed through observation and tested under cross-examination.

Assistance as a Legal Consultant

The IBCLC may be approached, at the outset, by the attorney. He may not feel the need to use you as an "expert" on the stand, but may realize he needs to learn a little bit more about lactation and its impact on the strategy of the case, because his client is breastfeeding. In this situation, you are serving as a "legal consultant" in that you are offering information and advice to the attorney. Many mother-to-mother counselors find themselves in this role primarily because, as volunteers who have spent many hours with the mother during the phone calls and meetings for breastfeeding support, they have been privy to the details giving rise to the lawsuit at hand. By the same token, they are often heavily invested in the outcome, on behalf of the mother, and their ability to provide an impartial assessment of the breastfeeding picture may be tainted. This is not to indict lay counselors: this is to make the point that a "fresh set of eyes" in any situation, particularly an emotional one involving mothers and babies, may offer the best information for the lawyers to use.

Charge for Your Time
Just as the attorney is a professional who charges for his time, any IBCLC who is approached to provide her expertise should feel comfortable charging for her time as well (*General Information About Expert Witnesses*, 2012). It is ethical to do so. You aren't "selling" a viewpoint; you are charging for the time it takes to call upon your years of training and clinical experience to formulate a professional opinion about the facts of the case. The lawyer can ponder whether your information is useful to the theory of the case, but the IBCLC's job is merely to offer up the unvarnished information. You can, of course (as with any consultation with a mother) choose to waive some or all of your fee, and provide the legal consultation even on a pro bono publico basis. But you should track your hours nonetheless; don't be shy about letting the attorney or mother know the value of the information they are getting at no cost. Waiving the fee (as with your free consults with mothers) does *not* absolve you of the need to meet all your other professional obligations, such as charting and protection of confidentiality.

Formal Engagement in the Case

The IBCLC may get a phone call or email from an attorney in the case; she may even be served a subpoena because the rules of litigation require such proofs. The non-lawyer's typical response to a subpoena is to feel scared and a little bit guilty ("Oh my goodness! What did I do wrong?"). Stop, take a deep breath, and assess (just as you do when a mother comes before you with clinically challenging breastfeeding problems). If you are served a subpoena at your place of work, there are likely to be rules in place designed to alert the necessary administrators. There is probably a hospital policy that any legal documents served at the institution are to be forwarded to the legal counsel's office for review and action. If you don't know what to do, ask your supervisors: it is certainly their job to know the procedures the hospital should follow. If you work alone, or in a small office without a bureaucratic hierarchy, you should contact your professional liability insurer *even if* the legal papers do not accuse you of doing anything wrong. Part of the service you are purchasing through your professional liability insurance is access to legal advisors. The law firm on retainer to the insurance company will be able to quickly tell you what this subpoena requires.

Let us assume, instead, a less-harrowing introduction to the case: the attorney contacts you. Perhaps the mother gave him your name; perhaps he plucked your name from a local list of community IBCLC resources, and did a quick Google search to verify your credentials. The IBCLC is entitled to do some initial fact gathering of her own. Find out:

1. Basic contact information of the caller, so you can verify who he or she is
2. How they got your name
3. The nature of the concern or proceeding
4. The information sought from you
5. Why the information is needed
6. The desired format for receiving the information:
   a. Written report
   b. Telephone meeting
   c. In-person meeting
7. The time frame to provide the information

These are perfectly reasonable requests that should not alarm the caller (if they do, your own alarms should be going off). You may be required to obtain necessary releases, first, to share confidential information. Your emphasis is not that you are necessarily going to assist this lawyer, but rather that you must follow the ethical rules of your profession, and the legal steps required by your place of employment, before sharing any information (IBLCE, 2011b, CPC Principles 2.1, 2.4, 3.1, 7.2, 7.3 & 8.2; IBLCE, 2008, SOP paras. 3, 4, 6, & 7; ILCA, 2006, Preface, Standards 1, 2, & 3). Do make a promise as to when you can get back, and then keep it.

The lawyer may have a specific idea of how you can help the case: an "advocate expert" will support a certain position based on a particular philosophy. An "impartial expert" provides an independent evaluation of a case (reviewing data, pro and con, and forming an opinion on the basis of the data). An "ivory tower" expert is a recognized expert in a particular field, with no connection or knowledge about the specific facts of the case, but whose opinion will hold sway coming as it does from this source. A "hired gun" is a disparaging term used to describe the expert who will testify on any matter, given the right fee. It is described here only to round out how an expert may be viewed.

Another role for the IBCLC is to act as a legal consultant, an option we alluded to above. This can be very satisfying for the clinician: without the stress of being called to the stand, she is hired to assist in preparation of a case, evaluating evidence, perhaps preparing a technical report explaining clinical terms. She may help formulate questions to ask the witness during discovery or on the stand; she may critique the opinions and evidence from the other party's experts or witnesses (Barsky & Gould, 2004).

Put Your Role and Responsibilities in Writing

If you do decide to be hired to work, formally or informally, with the legal team, get it in writing. Often the IBCLC is called when the attorneys are harried, meeting deadlines, and scrambling to get the case sorted out. That they procrastinated on case preparation is not your problem or fault. You should not have to proceed without the professionalism inherent in describing and agreeing upon mutual expectations, and an agreed timetable and fee arrangement.

Your arrangements are made with the lawyer, *not* the mother. This is no small detail. This means you answer to the lawyer, are directed by the lawyer, and should expect payment to come from the lawyer. If the mother tries to consult with you "behind the lawyer's back" (clients do disagree with their lawyers about tactics), you should explain that the ethics of your profession require that the lawyer be made privy to any conversation you have with the mother. How so? You are in a contractual arrangement, now, to provide expert advice to the lawyer, who works on behalf of the client. The IBLCE CPC Introduction, Preamble, and Principles 2.3. 2.4. 6.1, and 7.2 all address the IBCLC justifying public trust in her professional competence, fulfilling professional commitments in good faith, and conducting herself with honesty, integrity, and fairness. The IBLCE SOP at paragraphs 3 and 6 describe the IBCLC's duty to work within the legal framework of her setting, including the rules of procedure that must be followed in this court case. The ILCA Standards repeat these admonitions at the Preface, and Standards 1 and 2.

Your Contract

You should look for most or all of these elements to be a part of your contract with the lawyer. Draft your own contract, or let the lawyer do so.

1. Clearly define the scope of your engagement as an expert, whether to:
   a. Serve as a legal consultant
   b. Offer assessment or investigation
   c. Provide testimony in court
   d. Perform a literature review
   e. Conduct empirical research
   f. Write a report for counsel or the court
   g. Meet deadlines for materials to be produced
2. Define services you will *not* provide
3. Describe the manner and amount of fees to be paid to you. An expert is paid for her time, not for an outcome. As such, contingency fees (where your fee is a percentage of the award given to the party that hires you) are unethical for an expert witness.
   a. Community standards and your level of expertise will affect your rate.
   b. Consider differing rates for work you can do in your own office, at the lawyer's office, during the discovery phase, and for trial testimony.

    c. Spell out recoverable expenses (travel, phone and copying charges, library access fees, etc.).

    d. Define how your time will be compensated if the proceedings change, or settle, or the attorney decides not to call you as a witness.

4. Describe your method of tracking time and expenses, and billing the attorney. When you submit your bill, if you have waived part of your fee in a kindly gesture, show that credit on the invoice.

In the Courtroom

The preceding pages have provided a snapshot of the legal system, the kinds of lawsuits that may involve lactation issues, and how the IBCLC may find herself involved (formally or informally) in preparation of a court case. Fortunately, the IBCLC does not have to know all of this information, even cursorily. The IBCLC needs to know, simply, that it is up to the lawyers and judges to "look up" the law, to sort out where a lawsuit or administrative action should be brought, and decide what theory of law should be argued. Let us turn, then, to how the IBCLC's special expertise in breastfeeding and human lactation may find itself being used in one of those lawsuits in one of those courtrooms.

Different Kinds of Witnesses

Recall that systems of justice, just about everywhere, follow very exacting rules of procedure in order to conduct their business. This allows controversies to be examined and decided in as fair and dispassionate a setting as possible. Rulings and verdicts should be based on facts and evidence correctly considered, rather than mood or emotion. Witnesses provide evidence of what they saw and heard. Different kinds of witnesses in the courtroom are used pursuant to different rules of evidence and procedure. All witnesses will be sworn to tell the truth; all witnesses will be assessed (and challenged) for their credibility.

Fact Witness

A fact witness is someone who has important information to share about the facts of the lawsuit. An IBCLC could easily fill this role: if a woman is suing the hospital about her treatment there, the IBCLC could certainly be called, as could any clinician, to discuss the interactions she may have had with the patient/litigant. Imagine the mother claims no one told her how to hand express extra breastmilk to give to her sleepy, jaundiced baby. The IBCLC could well be called to refute that allegation; to testify that she had a discussion with the mother about hand expression and rental or use of a hospital-grade pump during the time the baby was undergoing light therapy (Walker, 2011). The IBCLC is offering facts to the court through her eyewitness testimony; she may also validate and thus allow for entry of written evidence (e.g., her lactation chart and notes). Like any witness before the court, the IBCLC's evidence will be evaluated and even challenged: her demeanor and truthfulness will be silently assessed by the "trier of fact" (the judge or jury, whomever renders the final verdict in the case); the validity and weight of the evidence offered can be tested (her direct eye witness observations will count; reporting what she heard another nurse say will be rejected as inherently less reliable hearsay evidence); the truthfulness of her testimony upon direct examination can be challenged on cross-examination (and even "rehabilitated" on redirect examination).

Expert Witness

An expert witness before the court has a different role from a fact witness, and it is as an expert that the IBCLC may find herself utilized. The pages above describe how the IBCLC may be hired in that capacity; let us explain here the legal significance of an expert witness.

An expert is the only kind of witness before a court who is allowed to offer *opinion* testimony. Experts are called because they are deemed to have specialized knowledge, beyond the ken of an ordinary citizen (or judge) that can shed some light on the facts and controversy at hand. Imagine someone filing a lawsuit over the construction of a bridge. Unless you have an expert (an engineer) who can explain how a bridge is supposed to be built, and whether this particular bridge was built in that manner, it will be difficult for the trier of fact to know whether the defendant is liable for building a bad bridge. For expert testimony (via an expert witness) to be allowed, it must be established to the court's satisfaction that this person (a) has specialized knowledge and skill, that (b) is relevant and necessary (reliable), and (c) helpful to the trier of fact. As such, the expert must be "qualified" before she can testify; often this involves a review of her training and expertise in the subject matter.

One might wonder why, if breastfeeding is a natural and biologic function that has been occurring for thousands of years, it would ever be necessary to have an "expert" testify on such a common, everyday occurrence. For the same reason that a cardiac surgeon might be required to testify on whether a common, everyday beating heart had proper surgery performed upon it. While mankind has invented nothing new about breastfeeding (or beating hearts) since the dawn of time, we have in the modern day found clever new ways to measure, study—and impact—those natural biologic functions. Someone who is a specialist in the underlying biology, who understands the results that will tend to occur when intervening factors occur (or fail to occur), can provide an expert opinion that will assist the court in figuring out how to decide the case.

Witnesses Are Not Advocates and Usually Don't Have Lawyers

The only advocates in the courtroom are the lawyers. Their job is to present a case most favorable to their client, and the process of advocacy started at the initial client–lawyer meeting when the attorney first got wind of the facts of the case. A thousand decisions, big and little, have occurred since then, all in the name of advocacy for the client: deciding which motions to file, which witnesses to call and experts to use (in the foreground or background); what offers at settlement to extend (or reject); which legal battles to cede in order to win on matters of greater import, and so on. Witnesses, whether offering facts or expert testimony, are *not* the advocates. To be plain: a lawyer is not going to use (and pay for) an expert witness that will offer unhelpful testimony. But it is up to the lawyer to ask the right questions, eliciting the best facts (from fact witnesses) and opinions (from expert witnesses) to meet the advocate's objectives in the case. Indeed, as we will see below, the credibility of a witness (whether fact or expert) can be impugned when they are seen to have strayed too far from the facts and too close to "siding" with one party. Such overt shows of favoritism cloud the objectivity of the rest of the witness's answers.

A witness does not need to have her *own* lawyer in order to be called to testify in a case. To be entirely accurate, there are situations were a party to the case (who will have a lawyer) may also take the stand to testify, in which case, that particular witness does indeed have a lawyer. But in the matter of an IBCLC being called to testify in a matter before the court, as either a fact witness or an expert witness, she will not have (nor be entitled to have) her own lawyer. If preparing the case responsibly, the lawyer calling the witness (plaintiff or defendant in a civil case; the prosecutor or defendant in a criminal case) should inform the witness about what to expect in the courtroom, what matters will be discussed, and even to practice offering testimony.

The attorney cannot tell the witness *what* to say: that is unethical for all attorneys everywhere, and is considered illegal in some jurisdictions. But it is perfectly ethical and legal for an attorney to learn from witnesses, ahead of the court date, the likely content of their testimony. Indeed, the entire "discovery" phase of litigation is designed to glean pertinent facts, through depositions (trial-like question-and-answer sessions, conducted in person, and recorded word for word), examination of documents that may be subpoenaed (compelled to be turned over) for that purpose, and the filing of written questions (interrogatories) that must be answered as if under oath (Winegar, 2009).

As the trial date approaches, lawyers may sit down and practice with (or "prepare") the witness for how the testimony will be elicited in the courtroom. The lawyer can offer stylistic suggestions ("Don't run on so long with the answer. Confine your answer to the specific question asked"). The lawyer must not coach on the substance ("It doesn't help us if you merely say it was dark out. I want you to tell the court you clearly saw the defendant with the smoking gun.").

By the same token, a witness can also choose not to be prepared by the attorneys in the case. Most welcome the opportunity: it can be nerve-racking to walk into a court-room, even as a nonparty witness, and be bombarded with all the mysterious practice and procedure with which everyone *else* seems so familiar. Experts, who are paid to pro-vide their testimony (a fee that is entirely ethical and legal; more on that below) would be foolhardy *not* to engage in as many preparation sessions as the lawyer will schedule. But a word of caution: no matter how sympathetic one is to the position espoused by one party in the case; no matter how friendly and helpful the lawyer who is doing the preparing, the lawyer's obligation is to the case, and his client, not the witness.

Pretrial Preparation

Once you have your contract in place, the next step is to do a little "due diligence" on your own. Do not rely on the lawyer alone to tell you the salient facts; he will be thinking in legal terms, and you will be thinking in lactation terms, and he may fail to mention elements that are critical to the IBCLC. Ask to review the files yourself, and to interview the mother or other important parties.

Discovery

Most litigation takes place before anyone gets near the courthouse. The discovery phase is critical to development of a case. Depositions have all the same procedural and evidentiary rules as testimony in a courtroom, except objections do *not* stop the flow of questions and answers. Many depositions are "fishing expeditions" (the lawyers are, after all, looking for any relevant information), but they also provide an invaluable sneak peak into what kind of a courtroom witness you'd be. Critically, a deposition supplies a *written, sworn* record, which can be used to impeach your testimony, months and even years later in trial. Depositions are often videotaped, and a word-for-word transcription is kept.

Privilege

The materials you assemble as part of pretrial preparation *may* be discoverable by the other side. Attorney "work product privilege" should keep confidential the information discussed between you and the attorney who is preparing the case, *once you are retained*. But written documents, drafts, email, and phone messages, voice mail, thumb drives, and cell phones could all be sought by opposing counsel if you do not have an official role vis-à-vis the mother's attorney. All the more reason to get that contract in writing and up front.

If you had prior dealings with a mother, perhaps as a patient/client of yours, you may be able to "claim a privilege" that these records are confidential and private. You may be required, nevertheless, to share that information, if it has been requested via a valid subpoena. The privacy and confidentiality requirements so familiar to us as IBCLCs (IBLCE, 2011b, CPC Principles 2.1, 2.4, 3.1, 3.2, 8.1, & 8.2; IBLCE, 2008, SOP para. 7, and ILCA, 2006, Standard 2) can be overridden by valid order of a court as part of legal proceedings (IBLCE, 2011b, CPC Definitions and Interpretations 5).

On the Witness Stand

The big day is at hand. You've prepared yourself by studying the information of the case and brushing up on your evidence-based lactation conclusions. It is perfectly understandable to be nervous when you take the stand and swear to tell the truth. As a witness (whether a fact witness or expert), you do not control the questions: the interrogator (the lawyer) does. And litigators are experts at *that*. The person(s) you need to impress is the trier of fact: the jury, or the judge. That is your audience, not the lawyer posing questions.

Conversely, the interrogator doesn't control the answers: you do. Remind yourself that lactation is *your* area of expertise, which is more important than familiarity with testifying in court. You will be forgiven a case of nerves if the quality of your answers is truthful and helpful. You are there because you are an expert on lactation, not an "expert on experting." Keep your preparation tips in mind: to answer only the question asked, to keep the answer simple, and to avoid rushing to fill the void of silence. Litigators know that silence is very unnerving, and the interrogator may intentionally have remained quiet after your answer to see if you might offer up something he can use to advantage.

Being Qualified as an Expert

If you are to be used to offer expert testimony, the first hurdle for the lawyer is to have you "qualified" as an expert in the area for which you will testify, and to convince the judge that your expert testimony will be reliable, relevant, and helpful. Sometimes this step is agreed to beforehand, when the lawyers stipulate (agree to) certain facts, including your qualifications as an expert. In any regard, your first step is to have a current and impressive curriculum vitae (CV) listing your training, experience, and accomplishments both in lactation and as an expert witness (Barsky & Gould, 2004). It is important to include everything, but do not inflate or overstate your experience or accomplishments. Your expertise (and CV) are subject to cross-examination. The CV should be on your own letterhead and include your:

1. Professional title
2. Contact information
3. Training and education
4. Degrees and professional licenses or certifications
5. Years of experience
6. Employment history
7. Supervisory experience
8. Special awards or citations
9. Provision of training (by you, to others)
10. Prior court experience (issues, representing which side, level of court, county and state where qualified as an expert)
11. Work under recognized experts
12. Memberships in professional organizations
13. Books or articles written
14. Positive book reviews or judicial comments on your work
15. Professional speaking experiences
16. Ongoing supervision or case consultation
17. Professional development and continuing education courses you have taken
18. Consultation work
19. Code(s) of ethics to which you prescribe (and other practice-guiding documents)

20. Methods of practice to which you prescribe
21. Professional development and continuing education courses you have taught
22. Your recognized specializations

Testimony as an Expert Witness

The trier of fact always decides the credibility of all the witnesses. Impeached credibility on one point means it is lost for *every* point, so the expert should avoid being caught in a mistake. How you testify is as important as what you say. Your demeanor says a lot about you, and may be far more influential to the trier of fact than the content of your expert testimony. Practice, practice, practice with the attorney who hired you, or the one who will depose or examine you.

The court is entitled to know the methodology used to reach your conclusions. This may not be so critical an element for the lactation expert as for the engineer or chemist who must explain complex formulae used in assessing evidence and drawing conclusions. But the IBCLC expert may well have to explain why there aren't "more studies" in a certain area (since the ethics of human research does not allow for whole populations—infants at that—to be assigned to a group that will be exposed to known health risks [Office of Research Integrity-Human Subject Research, University of Nevada, n.d.]).

Expert witnesses are unique in that they may be asked hypothetical questions by the lawyers or the judge ("If a mother is breastfeeding, and if she has a history of mastitis, and if she must be separated from her baby, and if she is unsuccessful in expressing milk using a breast pump, what lactation-related conditions could ensue?"). While no witness, not even the expert, can be asked the "ultimate issue" in the case (that is for the judge or jury to decide), hypothetical questions can come pretty darned close. The problem is that they are often very convoluted. If you are the expert, make sure you understand all the clauses and conditions of the question posed. It is perfectly okay to ask that the question be repeated, or read back by the stenographer.

Challenges to the Expert's Credibility

Cross-examination by opposing counsel is the most worrisome aspect of testifying, and with some justification. The expert can be challenged on her qualifications, her impartiality, the factual basis giving rise to the expert opinion, and the theoretical basis (i.e., reliance on various studies) giving rise to the expert opinion. Practice, practice, practice before the day of trial. Prepare by reading your own deposition, from the discovery phase, word for word. It will remind you of the issues covered then (probably many months ago), refresh you on the facts, remind you of opposing counsel's style (depositions are a 2-way sneak peek) and diminish the likelihood that you can be impeached for giving inconsistent answers on the stand from those offered at the deposition. Remind yourself that the cross-examiner's role is to make you feel dumb, stupid, untrained, immature, and out of control: anything to impeach your credibility. Repeat silently to yourself: "I know more about lactation than anyone else in this courtroom."

Be comforted knowing that there will be an opportunity on redirect to "rehabilita te" any damage to your testimony after cross-examination.

You may be challenged for having a "conflict of interest" because, as a lactation expert, you were called to testify by the lawyers for the breastfeeding mother. A quick review of the basics of conflict of interest will assure you that such a tactic is a red herring. You have a conflict of interest, as an expert, only if you have some *personal interest* in the outcome of the case. Your expertise as a breastfeeding proponent can certainly be offered objectively in a case involving a mother. That is the very reason you were called. It would hardly do the court any good to call an objective car mechanic to testify as an expert on breastfeeding issues.

You should also be prepared to be questioned about the fact that you got paid to be in the courtroom. Recall that it is perfectly acceptable and ethical to be hired as an expert in a court case. The jury is entitled to know that, and any litigator will be well practiced in explaining the utility of experts compensated for sharing their special knowledge. Remember, too, that if you have been hired by one side to serve as an expert, the other side will probably have one too, and she is fair game for the same sets of questions. So, hold your head high when your fee arrangements are discussed in open court. You are worth it; that is why you were hired.

Ten Rules of Testifying

1. Tell the truth, the whole truth and nothing but the truth. If you don't know or can't recall, say that!
2. Convey professionalism.
3. Respect the formalities of the tribunal.
4. Speak slowly, loudly, and without hesitation.
5. Provide clear and concise answers.
6. Let the attorney lead the questions.
7. Just the facts, ma'am (unless you are an expert; then, opinion is allowed).
8. Keep your composure.
9. Maintain eye contact.
10. Use notes to refresh your memory (if allowed by the judge) (Barsky & Gould, 2004).

Preparing a Written Report to the Court

In some situations, the court may request (or the lawyer may offer) that your testimony be offered by way of a written report to the court. This permits your information to be absorbed in a slower manner than on the witness stand, and because experts are often called to explain complex issues, many judges prefer this system. A report that lays out all of the circumstances, the evidence (or materials) considered, and how you came to your conclusions, is effective and persuasive. In many ways it is to be formatted like a legal brief. Your report should be on your own letterhead, and include:

1. Title of the proceedings
2. Submitted by (your information; attach a CV)
3. Purpose of report
4. Identifying information (individuals involved)
5. Materials reviewed
6. Positions of the parties
7. Primer (explaining your area of expertise)
8. Sources of information (data used to inform your report)
9. Relevant history
10. Present circumstances
11. Interpretation of data
12. Integration of data
13. Your expert opinion
14. Qualification of opinion
15. Conclusions and recommendations
16. Evaluative summary
17. Date and your signature
18. Appendices (CV, studies, etc.) (Barsky & Gould, 2004).

The IBCLC as a Party in a Lawsuit

The fateful day has arrived. You head to work to help mothers and babies happily breastfeed, and instead you are greeted by a smiling process server who hands you paperwork informing you that you have been named, as a defendant, in a lawsuit. Your stomach sinks, your heart races, your face flushes. What next?

While reported lawsuits (meaning the case went to trial and a judge wrote a decision) against IBCLCs are quite rare, getting sued (especially in the United States) is not. And when you have been named in a lawsuit, even a specious lawsuit, filed by an unstable party, that is laughable on its face, it must be answered. Customarily a lawsuit will be filed naming anyone and everyone who might have been culpable: it is easier to remove a defendant later in the proceedings than to add one. Being sued doesn't mean you have done anything wrong; it just means you have been sued. It also rather "shakes things up" when several employees of an institution are simultaneously served with process, and some attorneys feel this works to their advantage. While it may feel like it at the moment, this lawsuit is not the end of the world. Here are the steps the IBCLC should consider if she finds herself on the wrong end of a subpoena.

Professional Liability Insurance

This is why you have professional liability (medical malpractice) insurance. It is there to pay for a lawyer to represent you from start to finish, and to pay for any settlement or judgment that may result. Contact your insurer immediately. Not only are they very good at taking your teary-eyed call, and making you feel better about the whole mess, your rights are often triggered by your notice. If you sit on that subpoena too long, the insurer may come back with the unpleasant news that you voided the policy through your procrastination.

We suggested above, when you have been subpoenaed as a witness, to run it by the professional liability insurers even though most policies are intended to provide coverage and legal representation only in those cases where you are called as a party. To do so can't hurt, and you may find some little nugget of help or insight you didn't realize was there. But now you are a named defendant. As a person who is smart enough to have insurance, and unlucky enough to have to use it, the IBCLC should be cognizant of the many little loopholes in that policy that may leave her without counsel. How does that work?

Many of us wear several hats as an IBCLC and breastfeeding advocate. We work as an IBCLC at the hospital; volunteer as a La Leche League Leader; have a small business teaching childbirth and breastfeeding classes; work per diem to fill in at the local breastfeeding clinic when their regular IBCLCs are on vacation. Insurance companies are allowed to avoid coverage if they can. There is nothing illegal or unethical about that. One of their best options is the "exclusions" and "exceptions" portion of the professional liability policy. Exclusions are those occurrences the policy won't ever cover. Professional liability insurance for allied healthcare providers is designed to cover mistakes (negligence) by the practitioner, but it will not cover intentional acts of harm. Exceptions are used to deny coverage for occurrences that are normally covered, but are being denied here because of some extenuating circumstance. An example is the IBCLC who has professional liability insurance as a benefit of her employment at the hospital. But she also wears another hat when she runs a small private practice on the side. If she is sued by one of her private practice clients on a claim of negligence (an act covered by the professional liability policy), the IBCLC's insurer will *deny* coverage because she was not working as a hospital employee (Allied Healthcare Professionals Insurance Center, 2010).

There are other legitimate means by which an insurer may be able to restrict or deny coverage. The insurance you purchase will define the time period it covers. A "claims-made policy" (also called "prior acts coverage") will cover you for incidents that happened even before you got your insurance, so long as the lawsuit is filed when you do have the insurance. "Occurrence policy" (also called "extended reporting period") coverage will apply to claims that occurred while the policy was in effect, even if you no longer carry that insurance (Allied Healthcare Professionals Insurance Center, 2010). If you have retired from lactation consultancy, and no longer have professional liability insurance, and you get served with papers for an incident that happened back in your working days, you had better hope your old insurance was an occurrence policy rather than a claims-made policy.

The fine print of your insurance policy may reveal that it covers you for lawsuits that have been filed, but not an administrative or disciplinary proceeding (which can be just as expensive in terms of legal representation). Another pothole: your employer's liability insurance, which does cover you while at work, may not cover you when you need it most. They may claim that certain acts of negligence by you are your fault alone, not the employer's, and deny you coverage altogether.

The time to learn about all of this, of course, is now, not after the lawsuit papers have been served on you. Do not assume that an insurance policy handed to you by an agent will serve your best interests, and do not assume you are stuck with whatever they offer. An insurance policy is simply a contract: you agree to pay premiums to insure against the risks associated with a certain event (the lawsuit). Any contract can be negotiated. The good news is that professional liability insurance for an allied healthcare provider (like an IBCLC) is surprisingly affordable. Obtaining "rider" or "tail coverage" policies that fill in some of the coverage gaps described above is also easy and affordable (Allied Healthcare Professionals Insurance Center, 2010).

Resist the Urge to Patch Things Up

It feels awful when a mother whom you saw professionally is so disenchanted with that contact that she has filed a lawsuit. Resist, however, the urge to give her a call to try to make things right again. The time for extending olive branches is over (at least from her standpoint, right now) and any efforts toward that end will not likely be appreciated. Remember, too, it may backfire with medical malpractice insurer, who is always looking for ways to legitimately get out of the contract. One of them might be your interference with their appropriate defense of the case, defined as you picking up the phone to call mom without the lawyer's knowledge or permission.

Resist the urge to go back and make sure your files accurately reflect your sessions with the mother, your suggestions to her in the formation of a care plan, and her verbal or visible demonstrations of commitment to that plan. If you didn't write it down then, it is too late, and any efforts to fix the files will probably void your insurance coverage *and* leave you culpable on offenses far more serious than negligence. Recall IBLCE CPC Definitions and Interpretations 5 and 6, and Principles 2.4, 6.1, 7.2, & 8.2, speaking to the IBCLC's duties of honesty, accuracy, and fairness. Tampering with the lactation chart is not honest, accurate, fair—or likely even legal. Whereas you started out merely embarrassed because your files don't accurately reflect the good job you did, attempts to fix them with later-jotted notes will void your insurance, require you to pay out of pocket for your legal defense, and put your certification at risk if you are found liable.

Resist, too, the urge to immediately pull your friends and colleagues into a supportive circle, where you can vent and rage at the unfairness of it all. Don't send emails, don't have long phone calls or leave voicemails, don't meet for coffee (or a drink), don't post on your Facebook page, and don't type a text or tweet into your cell phone. *All* of those communications will be discoverable during the litigation; *all* of your friends can be subpoenaed to describe what you said; *all* of that provides opportunities for your inconsistencies to be exploited by the people suing you.

Movement Away from Blame and Toward Apology

But take heart. All is not cynical in the world. In recent years, there has been a movement away from the notion of blame-finding (as with negligence-based medical malpractice suits) and toward apology, explanation, and mitigation. The traditional posture has been for lawyers to tell their clients to remain mute about the incident: communicate with no one except the legal team. You read that advice just a few paragraphs above. Reaching out and apologizing was seen as (and argued in court to mean) an admission of guilt (Perfect Apology, 2012). However, many families who are traumatized over their medical care don't really want money damages (their only available remedy). They want to ensure that no other family goes through similar agony. They want to know that their caregivers really were trying their best, and were not cold, uncaring (or worse, arrogant) robots. They want to hear that their pain and heartbreak was heard and understood by the healthcare provider and the institution, that the healthcare provider is truly sorry, and that tangible measures have been taken to assure this mistake doesn't happen again (Cohen, 1999; Vitez, 2010).

This is something to raise with your lawyers, at the start of the case, and while you are (probably) under their orders to discuss nothing about the matter. It is an option they may well explore, but you will protect your own interests best if you collaborate with the attorneys' strategy to go the route of remediation, rather than to initiate it on your own.

When You Sue

An IBCLC may find herself in a situation where all avenues of informal redress have been exhausted, and now she must initiate legal proceedings on her own. Perhaps a mother is past due on her pump rental account. The IBCLC you subcontracted with to cover you while on vacation has taken all of your copyright-protected handouts and is using them word for word as her own. The contractor who was working to remodel your office damaged your computer when he triggered the automatic sprinklers, and he has yet to make good on his promise to replace it. The conference host that hired you to give a lecture last year still has not reimbursed your travel expenses. And on and on the nightmares go. IBCLCs are not immune to life's problems, and sometimes those problems need to be addressed formally.

As a litigant, your status as an IBCLC is largely irrelevant. Yes, the problem arose as part of your work, but in the situations described above, the causes of action are in: debt collection, intellectual property law, negligence causing property damage, and contract. They have nothing to do with breastfeeding or lactation. It is not surprising that this lawyer would suggest that the best starting point for any IBCLC who thinks she may have to sue to protect her rights is to hire excellent legal counsel.

Summary

An IBCLC may find herself involved in a legal case, as a witness to the occurrence, as an expert on breastfeeding and human lactation, or as a party herself. Laws can be created by the legislature (parliament), judicial decision (opinion), or administrative agencies (ministries) writing regulations. Actions involving lactation will tend to be grounded in tort (primarily the negligence of medical malpractice), family law, employment (labor) law, and civil rights. An IBCLC may provide support in an informal role (as an advocate for the mother, or a legal advisor to the attorney) or a formal role (as an expert witness). An IBCLC who is sued should turn first to her professional liability insurer to advise her on how to defend. An IBCLC who must sue someone else should find a good lawyer.

REFERENCES

Administrative law. (1979/1891). In H. Black (Ed.), *Black's law dictionary* (5th ed., p. 43). St. Paul, MN: West.

Alewell, D., & Pull, K. (2005, October). An international comparison and assessment of maternity leave legislation. *Comparative labor law and policy journal, 22*(2), 297–326. Retrieved from http://www.law.uiuc.edu/publications/cll%26pj/archive/vol_22/issue_2/PullArticle22-2-3.pdf

Allied Healthcare Professionals Insurance Center. (2010). *Understanding allied healthcare professional liability insurance.* Retrieved from http://ahc.lockton-ins.com/pl/understandingPLI.html

Americans with Disabilities Act, as amended, 42 U.S.C. § 12101 et seq. (1990), http://www.ada.gov/pubs/adastatute08.htm.

Barsky, A. E., & Gould, J. W. (2004). *Clinicians in court: A guide to subpoenas, depositions, testifying, and everything else you need to know.* New York, NY: Guildford Press.

Battery. (2010). In L. Duhaime (Ed.), *Duhaime legal dictionary* (para. 1). Retrieved from http://www.duhaime.org/LegalDictionary/B/Battery.aspx

Bornmann, P. G. (2008). A legal primer for lactation consultants. In R. Mannel, P. Martens, & M. Walker (Eds.), *Core curriculum for lactation consultant practice* (2nd ed., pp. 159–190). Sudbury, MA: Jones & Bartlett.

Breastfeeding at the Philadelphia Museum of Art [Web log post]. (2006, December 3). Retrieved from http://thewidetent.blogspot.com/2006/12/breastfeeding-at-philadelphia-museum-of.html

California Employment Development Department. (2010). *FAQ—Relation of the paid family insurance program to the family and medical leave act (FMLA) and the California family rights act (CFRA)* [Frequently asked questions]. Retrieved from http://www.edd.ca.gov/disability/FAQs_for_Paid_Family_Leave.htm

Canada Ministry of Labour. (2012, February 15). *Labour standards maternity-related reassignment and leave, maternity leave and parental leave.* Retrieved from http://www.hrsdc.gc.ca/eng/labour/employment_standards/publications/maternity/page00.shtml

Case law. (1979/1891). In H. Black (Ed.), *Black's law dictionary* (5th ed., p. 196). St. Paul, MN: West.

Christrup, S. (2001). Breastfeeding in the American workplace. *Journal of Gender, Social Policy & the Law, 9*(3), 471–503. Retrieved from http://www.iiav.nl/ezines/web/AmericanUniversityJournal/1999-2003/american/9-3christrup.pdf

Civil law. (1979/1891). In H. Black (Ed.), *Black's law dictionary* (5th ed., p. 223). St. Paul, MN: West.

Cohen, J. (1999). Advising clients to apologize. *Southern California Law Review, 72,* 1009–1069. Retrieved from http://www-bcf.usc.edu/~usclrev/pdf/072402.pdf

Common law. (1979/1891). In H. Black (Ed.), *Black's law dictionary* (5th ed., pp. 250–251). St. Paul, MN: West.

Cornell University Law School. (2010a). *Divorce laws.* Retrieved from http://topics.law.cornell.edu/wex/table_divorce

Cornell University Law School. (2010b). *Family law: State statutes.* Retrieved from http://topics.law.cornell.edu/wex/table_family

Cornell University Law School. (2010c, August 19). *Marriage.* Retrieved from http://topics.law.cornell.edu/wex/marriage

Cowling, M., & Sinclair, A. (2007, February). *Danger! UK at work!* (Monograph No. WP10). Retrieved from http://www.employment-studies.co.uk/pdflibrary/wp10.pdf

Criminal law. (2010). In L. Duhaime (Ed.), *Duhaime legal dictionary* (para. 1). Retrieved from http://www.duhaime.org/LegalDictionary/C/CriminalLaw.aspx

Dettwyler, K. A. (1995). A time to wean: The hominid blueprint for the natural age of weaning in modern human populations. In P. Stuart-Macadam & K. A. Dettwyler, *Breastfeeding: Biocultural perspectives* (pp. 39–74). New York, NY: Aldine De Gruyter.

Fair Packaging and Labeling Act, 15 U.S.C. § 1451–1461 (1966), http://www.ftc.gov/os/statutes/fpla/fplact.html.

Fair Packaging and Labeling Act, 16 C.F.R. § 500 (2000), http://www.ftc.gov/os/statutes/fpla/part500.shtm.

Family and Medical Leave Act, 29 U.S.C. § 2601 et seq. (1993), http://codes.lp.findlaw.com/uscode/29/28/2601.

Family Law Courts of Australia. (n.d.). *Family dispute resolution: Alternatives to going to court.* Retrieved from http://www.familylawcourts.gov.au/wps/wcm/connect/FLC/Home/About+Going+to+Court/Family+dispute+resolution/

Fine, T. (2008). *How the U.S. court system works.* Retrieved from http://www.lawyerintl.com/law-articles/2233-How%20the%20U.S.%20Court%20System%20Works

General information about expert witnesses and consultants. (2012). Retrieved from http://expertpages.com/news/new1.ht

Hall, J. K. (2002). *Law & ethics for clinicians.* Vega, TX: Jackhall Books.

In re Bisphenol-A (BPA) polycarbonate plastic products liability litigation, 687 F. Supp. 2d 897 (U. S. Dist. Ct., W. D. MO 2009), https://apps.fastcase.com/Research/Pages/Document.aspx?LTID=rHProKhQulgH5ydjd1ECASZgFu7dlW1ImzCmWjvsf7qkhIplkNMgKOfKy7GxFEnGdL2NLV3l22s3jpFVCUXiT8aVop%2bYh%2f7mRnryEnlVW6b%2f64EsQ8rHnFhdyexDAsvh.

International Board of Lactation Consultant Examiners. (2008, March 8). *Scope of practice for international board certified lactation consultants.* Retrieved from http://www.iblce.org/upload/downloads/ScopeOfPractice.pdf

International Board of Lactation Consultant Examiners. (2011a, September 24). *Disciplinary procedures for the code of professional conduct for IBCLCs for the international board of lactation consultant examiners (IBLCE).* Retrieved from http://www.iblce.org/upload/downloads/IBLCEDisciplinaryProcedures.pdf

International Board of Lactation Consultant Examiners. (2011b, November 1). *Code of professional conduct for IBCLCs.* Retrieved from http://iblce.org/upload/downloads/CodeOfProfessionalConduct.pdf

International Lactation Consultant Association. (2006). *Standards of practice for international board certified lactation consultants.* Retrieved from http://www.ilca.org/files/resources/Standards-of-Practice-web.pdf

International law. (1979/1891). In H. Black (Ed.), *Black's law dictionary* (5th ed., p. 733). St. Paul, MN: West.

Malfeasance. (1979/1891). In H. Black (Ed.), *Black's law dictionary* (5th ed., p. 862). St. Paul, MN: West.

Marcus, J. A. (2007, July/August). Lactation and the law. *Mothering, 143.* Retrieved from http://mothering .com/breastfeeding/lactation-and-the-law

Marcus, J. A. (2011, August 11). *Lactation and the law revisited.* Retrieved from http://mothering.com /breastfeeding/lactation-and-law-revisited

Martial law. (2010). In L. Duhaime (Ed.), *Duhaime legal dictionary* (para. 1). Retrieved from http://www .duhaime.org/LegalDictionary/M/MartialLaw.aspx

Military law. (1979/1891). In H. Black (Ed.), *Black's law dictionary* (5th ed., p. 896). St. Paul, MN: West.

Miller, R. (2006). *Problems in health care law* (9th ed.). Sudbury, MA: Jones & Bartlett.

Mittleman, D. (2009, October 11). *Woman sues Delta Airlines after being kicked off plane for breastfeeding daughter* [Web log post]. Retrieved from http://lansing.injuryboard.com/miscellaneous/woman -sues-delta-airlines-after-being-kicked-off-plane-for-breastfeeding-daughter.aspx?googleid=272364

National Conference of State Legislatures. (2011, May). *Breastfeeding state laws.* Retrieved from http://www .ncsl.org/default.aspx?tabid=14389

Office of Research Integrity-Human Subjects Research, Univ. of Nevada. (n.d.). *History of research ethics.* Retrieved from http://research.unlv.edu/ORI-HSR/history-ethics.htm#top

Orozco, N. K. (2010). Pumping at work: Protection from lactation discrimination in the workplace. *Ohio State Law Journal, 71*(6), 1281–1316. Retrieved from http://moritzlaw.osu.edu/students/groups/oslj /current-issue/archive-2/volume-71-number-6

Patient Protection and Affordable Care Act [Health Care Reform] amending the Fair Labor Standards Act, 29 U.S.C. § 207 (2010), http://www.usbreastfeeding.org/Portals/0/Workplace/HR3590-Sec4207 -Nursing-Mothers.pdf.

Perfect Apology. (2012). *Perfect medical apologies: Is honesty always the best policy?* Retrieved from http://www .perfectapology.com/medical-apologies.html

Pozgar, G. D. (2005). *Legal and ethical issues for health professionals.* Sudbury, MA: Jones & Bartlett.

Precedent. (2010). In L. Duhaime (Ed.), *Duhaime legal dictionary* (para. 1). Retrieved from http://www .duhaime.org/LegalDictionary/P/Precedent.aspx

Pro se. (2010). In L. Duhaime (Ed.), *Duhaime legal dictionary* (para. 1). Retrieved from http://www.duhaime .org/LegalDictionary/P/ProSe.aspx

Rathke, L. (2012, March 16). Emily Gillette, breastfeeding passenger settles airline lawsuit. *Huffington Post.* Retrieved from http://www.huffingtonpost.com/2012/03/16/emily-gillette-delta_n_1354582.html

Red herring. (2010). In L. Duhaime (Ed.), *Duhaime legal dictionary* (para. 1). Retrieved from http://www .duhaime.org/LegalDictionary/R/RedHerring.aspx

Rochman, B. (2011, December 27). The nurse-in: Why breast-feeding mothers are mad at Target. *Time.* Retrieved from http://healthland.time.com/2011/12/27/the-nurse-in-why-breast-feeding-moms-are-mad-at-target

Rule of law. (1979/1891). In H. Black (Ed.), *Black's law dictionary* (5th ed., p. 1196). St. Paul, MN: West.

Rule of law. (2010). In L. Duhaime (Ed.), *Duhaime legal dictionary* (para. 1). Retrieved from http://www .duhaime.org/LegalDictionary/R/RuleofLaw.aspx

Silver, K. (2009, November 6). Woman called indecent for breastfeeding in public. *Parents.* Retrieved from http://shine.yahoo.com/channel/parenting/woman-called-indecent-for-breastfeeding-in-public-542784

Stare decisis. (1979/1891). In H. Black (Ed.), *Black's law dictionary* (5th ed., p. 1261). St. Paul, MN: West.

Tort. (1979/1891). In H. Black (Ed.), *Black's law dictionary* (5th ed., p. 1335). St. Paul, MN: West.

U.S. Breastfeeding Committee. (2010). *Workplace accommodations to support and protect breastfeeding.* Retrieved from http://www.usbreastfeeding.org/Portals/0/Publications/Workplace-Background-2010-USBC.pdf

U.S. Breastfeeding Committee. (2011a). *Breastfeeding Promotion Act of 2011.* Retrieved from http://www.usbreastfeeding.org/LegislationPolicy/BreastfeedingAdvocacyHQ/BreastfeedingPromotionAct/tabid/115/Default.aspx

U.S. Breastfeeding Committee. (2011b). *FAQs: Break time for nursing mothers.* Retrieved from http://www.usbreastfeeding.org/Default.aspx?TabId=188

U.S. Breastfeeding Committee. (2011c). *Workplace support in federal law.* Retrieved from http://www.usbreastfeeding.org/Employment/WorkplaceSupport/WorkplaceSupportinFederalLaw/tabid/175/Default.aspx

U.S. Dept. of Labor Wage and Hour Division. (2010, December). *Fact sheet #73: Break time for nursing mothers under the FLSA.* Retrieved from http://www.dol.gov/whd/regs/compliance/whdfs73.pdf

U.S. Equal Employment Opportunity Commission. (n.d.). *Sexual harassment.* Retrieved from http://www.eeoc.gov/laws/types/sexual_harassment.cfm

Vitez, M. (2010, March 8). One hospital's simple measure to defeat infections. *Philadelphia Inquirer.* Retrieved from http://www.amh.org/aboutus/inquirer-series/handwashing-story.aspx

Walker, M. (2011). *Breastfeeding management for the clinician: Using the evidence* (2nd ed.). Sudbury, MA: Jones & Bartlett.

Winegar, T. (2009, July). *The ultimate trial notebook.* Philadelphia, PA: Philadelphia Bar Institute.

Chapter 7

The IBCLC as Advocate

If you've just plowed through the chapter about International Board Certified Lactation Consultants (IBCLCs) in the courtroom, you may be relieved to be reminded that the IBCLC can serve as an advocate in more places than the courtroom. Breastfeeding women and children need a good solid "shout out" every now and again. So does the IBCLC profession. Your advocacy can be offered for generic and positive reasons, but any efforts in the arenas of politics and policy making may have farther reach and overall impact than your work on behalf of one mother at a time. Do not underestimate your power. While your motivations may be altruistic, they are well-grounded in your practice-guiding documents:

1. The International Board of Lactation Consultant Examiners Scope of Practice (IBLCE SOP), a document describing professional behaviors we *must* engage in, tells us IBCLCs have a "duty to protect, promote, and support breastfeeding by educating women families, health professionals, and the community about breastfeeding and human lactation; facilitating the development of policies which protect, promote, and support breastfeeding; acting as an advocate for breastfeeding as the child-feeding norm" (IBLCE, 2008, SOP para. 4).

2. The International Lactation Consultant Association Standards of Practice (ILCA Standards), a document describing professional behaviors we *should* engage in, urges the IBCLC to "act as an advocate for breastfeeding women, infants, and children" (ILCA, 2006, Standard 1.4).

3. The *International Code of Marketing of Breast-milk Substitutes* (World Health Organization [WHO] Code, or International Code), is a document describing health worker behaviors that IBCLCs *should* follow, unless they *must* follow them. When *must* an IBCLC support the International Code? If laws or regulations enacting the International Code have been passed in her geopolitical region (legislation to restrict predatory marketing practices for products that inhibit breastfeeding), or if she works in a facility that is seeking or maintaining Baby-Friendly designation (Baby-Friendly USA, 2010a; UNICEF, 2012; WHO, 1981). The IBLCE Code of Professional Conduct (IBLCE CPC) states "a crucial part of an IBCLC's duty to protect mothers and children

is adherence to the principles and aim of the [WHO Code]" and subsequent relevant World Health Assembly resolutions (IBLCE, 2011, CPC Introduction at para. 3; International Baby Food Action Network [IBFAN], n.d.). Relevant sections of the WHO Code regarding health worker advocacy include:

a. Health authorities are urged to take appropriate measures to "encourage and protect breastfeeding and promote the principles of this Code" (WHO, 1981, Article 6.1).

b. Health workers (who include IBCLCs) "should encourage and protect breastfeeding" (WHO, 1981, Article 7.1).

c. "Governments should take action to give effect to the principles and aim of this Code . . . including the adoption of national legislation, regulations, or other suitable measures" (WHO, 1981, Article 11.1).

d. Monitoring of the Code, while a function of government, is to be aided in this regard by the manufacturers of products, and "appropriate nongovernmental organisations, professional groups, and consumer organisations" (WHO, 1981, Article 11.2).

e. "Nongovernmental organisations, professional groups, institutions, *and individuals* concerned should have the responsibility of drawing the attention of manufacturers or distributors to activities which are incompatible with the principles and aim of this Code, so that appropriate action can be taken" (WHO, 1981, Article 11.4) (emphasis added).

Let's examine how the IBCLC can advocate for the needs of breastfeeding families.

A Word About Language: Breastfeeding Has No Benefits

Many IBCLCs are familiar with the concept that "there are no benefits to breastfeeding." As the biologic norm for infant feeding since humans appeared on Earth, breastfeeding is just, well, normal. It doesn't imbue babies with "extra" super disease-fighting or brain-promoting powers. Thus, breastfed babies aren't "healthier;" rather, their formula-fed counterparts are less healthy. But the majority of literature (and advertising messages) presented to Millennial Mom will discuss the "advantages" of providing "the best/optimal/ideal/perfect food for your baby:" breastmilk. These messages are delivered not only by breastfeeding advocates, but by the manufacturers of formula itself (Wiessinger, 1996). Ironically, the one provision of the WHO Code that marketers universally seem to follow, even in countries where the International Code is not legislated and enforced, reads:

> Manufacturers and distributors of infant formula should ensure that each container has a clear, conspicuous and easily readable and understandable message printed on it . . . which includes . . . a statement of the superiority of breastfeeding. (WHO, 1981, Article 9.2 [b])

The inescapable result of messaging that breastmilk and breastfeeding is superior to formula and bottle-feeding is that:

> When we (and the artificial milk manufacturers) say that breastfeeding is the best possible way to feed babies because it provides their ideal food, perfectly balanced for optimal infant nutrition, the logical response is "So what?" Our own experience tells us that optimal is not necessary. Normal is fine, and implied in this language is the absolute normalcy—and thus safety and adequacy—of artificial feeding. The truth is, breastfeeding is nothing more than normal. Artificial feeding, which is neither the same nor superior, is therefore deficient, incomplete, and inferior. Those are difficult words, but they have an appropriate place in our vocabulary. (Wiessinger, 1996, p. 1)

This has ramifications in the way that research is conducted and reported, and as practitioners who are bound to use evidence-based practice in our work and advocacy (IBLCE, 2011, CPC Principles 1.2 & 1.3; IBLCE, 2008, SOP paras. 4, 5, & 8; ILCA, 2006, Standards 1.8 & 4.5) this is a concept worthy of full appreciation. The vast majority of people *outside* the field of lactation and human breastfeeding will find the notion of discussing the "risks of formula feeding" scary, threatening, and even a little crazy. Formula use is far too pervasive in modern day cultures to be seen and accepted as a population-wide threat requiring eradication, the way smoking has been (Akre, 2006). And yet, this is exactly how the information should be framed (ILCA, Spatz, & Lessen, 2011).

Most of the reported research on lactation still uses language that measures the "benefit" of breastfeeding or human milk. However: if breastfeeding is the *norm* for human infant feeding, then it should be considered (or used as) the *control* group in any research study. Use of formula or a different feeding method should then be the *intervention* whose introduction is being measured and assessed. Research results should be reported as either a risk or benefit of using this *intervention* (ILCA, Spatz, & Lessen, 2011; Smith, Dunstone, & Elliott-Rudder, 2009).

But most researchers do not use this parlance, and that makes a measurable difference in what the numbers (results) of the studies reveal. One analysis looked at many studies that compared exclusive breastfeeding and several infant illnesses. The researchers reconstructed the findings using exclusive breastfeeding as the standard. The recalculated odds ratios thus showed the risks of any formula use in the incidence of the infant illness.

> Overall, the results revealed that "any formula use" is associated with increased incidence of otitis media, asthma, type 1 diabetes, type 2 diabetes, atopic dermatitis, and hospitalization secondary to lower respiratory tract infections in infants in multiple studies. [E]xpression of the "risks of formula use" rather than only the "benefits of breastfeeding" could modify general perception, inform and reform clinical counseling, and lead to normalization of optimal infant feeding, that is, exclusive breastfeeding. (McNiel, Labbok, & Abrahams, 2010, p. 54)

To compound matters, the definition of "exclusive breastfeeding" remains highly variable from study to study (Aarts, Kylberg, Hornell, Hofvander, Gebre-Medhin, & Greiner, 2000; Labbok & Krasovec, 1990). The IBCLC advocate who is discussing lactation research and its implications with members of the healthcare and policy-making communities may find this concept of "no benefits of breastfeeding" initially difficult for others to swallow. And few of us could (or should) try to recalculate the study results to present the "real" results. Rather, we should be prepared to raise consciousness with others when discussing research, and know that the language used by others is borne of the familiarity of the "old" way of discussing breastfeeding. IBCLCs often find it difficult to stop pontificating about the transcendent effects of breastfeeding, and instead to focus on (merely) supporting the mother as she seeks to fit this normal, and sometimes even annoying, activity into everyday life. Cast in other terms: eating is something all humans do. It is sometimes a rich and luxuriant experience to sit down to a gloriously prepared meal, but other times we grab a banana on our way out the door. Breastfeeding can be the same, and mothers and healthcare policy makers should be told no differently:

> All of us within the profession want breastfeeding to be our biological reference point. We want it to be the cultural norm; we want human milk to be made available to all human babies, regardless of other circumstances. A vital first step toward achieving those goals is within immediate reach of every one of us. All we have to do is . . . watch our language. (Wiessinger, 1996, p. 4)

The IBCLC's Expertise Crosses Many Health Disciplines

The IBCLC is the premier allied healthcare provider (HCP) in breastfeeding and human lactation. Breastfeeding itself has been around since the dawn of humankind, but research in the past few decades has only begun to scratch the surface of examining how the simple process of breastfeeding reaps complex health and social "benefits" (reread the paragraphs above) lasting decades after weaning. While it is obvious that her expertise will be valuable and recognized in the fields of neonatology, pediatrics, midwifery, and obstetrics, the IBCLC's role, experience, and impact can also be used in other areas of health care and public health (ILCA & Henderson, 2011).

Childbirth and Maternity Practices

Before the baby can breastfeed, she has to be born. There is a growing (and alarming) body of evidence demonstrating that seemingly innocuous labor and delivery interventions can adversely affect breastfeeding: from inductions, to epidurals, to use of forceps/vacuum, separation from mother immediately after birth, to newborn baths, to injections and eye drops before the baby has even been placed in his mother's arms, to wholesale separation of mother and baby as part of postpartum care (Smith & Kroeger, 2010). As IBCLCs we usually see these problems "downstream," with babies who are sleepy, mucousy, and unresponsive (in large part because they are stressed), which leads to more interventions that adversely impact breastfeeding, such as the use of formula supplements, more separation of mother and baby (for various tests or procedures), and a tremendous amount of inappropriate and terrifying pressure placed on Millennial Mom to "feed the baby!"

The worldwide Baby-Friendly Hospital Initiative (BFHI), commenced by the World Health Organization (WHO) and United Nations Children's Fund (UNICEF) in 1991, is based on the simple premise that any place where a mother delivers a baby ought to be supportive of breastfeeding. Hospitals must meet certain criteria to be designated BFHI, including a rigorous review by external experts to be certain all elements are being met. A BFHI facility will meet each of the "Ten Steps to Successful Breastfeeding":

Every facility providing maternity services and care for newborn infants should:

1. Have a written breastfeeding policy that is routinely communicated to all healthcare staff.
2. Train all healthcare staff in skills necessary to implement this policy.
3. Inform all pregnant women about the benefits and management of breastfeeding.
4. Help mothers initiate breastfeeding within a half-hour of birth [one hour in the USA].
5. Show mothers how to breastfeed, and how to maintain lactation even if they should be separated from their infants.
6. Give newborn infants no food or drink other than breastmilk, unless *medically* indicated [emphasis in original].
7. Practice rooming in—allow mothers and infants to remain together—24 hours a day.
8. Encourage breastfeeding on demand.
9. Give no artificial teats or pacifiers (also called dummies or soothers) to breastfeeding infants.
10. Foster the establishment of breastfeeding support groups and refer mothers to them on discharge from the hospital or clinic. (Baby-Friendly USA, 2010b; WHO, 1998, p. 5)

In 2012, there were 15,000 facilities in 134 countries that had been awarded Baby-Friendly status (UNICEF, 2012). In the United States in 2007, there were roughly 3200 maternity hospitals and birth centers (DiGirolamo, Manninen, et al., 2008); 129 had been designated BFHI by March 2012 (Baby-Friendly USA, 2012). Clearly, this is a program that could use more advocacy "in the trenches" in the United States. Some facilities find it difficult to think about complying with requirements that no pacifiers/dummies be offered to babies, and that no low-cost or free infant formula be accepted (BFHI requiring that it be purchased, just as every other type of medicine or equipment must be purchased by healthcare facilities). A tremendous body of research backs up each of these 10 simple steps, compiled in a useful booklet that is "a tool for both advocacy and education" (WHO, 1998, p. 1). Implementation of even some of the 10 steps increases breastfeeding initiation, exclusivity, and duration (Bartick, Stuebe, Shealy, Walker, & Grummer-Strawn, 2009; DiGirolamo, Gummer-Strawn, & Fein, 2008).

Materials to assist the IBCLC advocate to discuss the Baby-Friendly Hospital Initiative abound. The U.S. Centers for Disease Control and Prevention (CDC) announced in October 2011 a major initiative to promote the Baby-Friendly Hospital Initiative in the United States, as a means of improving the public health (CDC, 2011). Peruse the UNICEF (www.unicef.org) and Baby-Friendly-USA (www.babyfriendlyusa.org) sites to learn more. BFHI was the focus of World Breastfeeding Week (WBW) in 2010, an annual policy and advocacy initiative sponsored by the World Alliance for Breast-feeding Advocacy (WABA) (World Alliance for Breastfeeding Action, 2010). The International Lactation Consultant Association (ILCA; www.ilca.org) also made the Ten Steps the focus of their 2010 WBW activities; both groups have materials for sale or free download from their websites.

The IBCLC advocate may also find it prudent to monitor infant formula recalls. They happen with disconcerting frequency in the United States. Searching for formula products already under recall may be conducted by brand name, lot number, or packaging size (U.S. Food and Drug Administration [FDA], 2009a). The FDA issues alerts when products are newly recalled (by FDA order, or voluntarily by the manufacturer) (FDA, 2010c). If facilities are giving out free samples of formula to patients, they have a duty to note the lot numbers for every single such sample distributed, and to whom, to allow for appropriate notice of any subsequent recall (Robbins & Beker, 2004). Recall the discussion on negligence: a duty of care, that is breached, that causes injury. It isn't hard to "connect the dots" if a healthcare institution has given a product to patients for their use, and it ends up making them sick. Avoiding such negligence is highly desired by large institutions (just ask those risk management officers). The headaches involved in tracking patient names and lot numbers may be a persuasive argument against formula samples being handed out by a healthcare facility in the first place.

As IBCLCs, we know that "it takes a village" to support a breastfeeding mother. A recent public health initiative from the U.S. Surgeon General recognizes that there are opportunities for healthcare providers, healthcare facilities, communities, governments, researchers, employers and family members *all* to assist mothers who wish to breastfeed. *The Call to Action to Support Breastfeeding* is an evidence-based advocacy piece that every IBCLC, including those outside the United States, can point to as credible support for the important role of IBCLCs and others in the public health imperative that breastfeeding represents (U.S. Dept. of Health and Human Services, Office of the Surgeon General, 2011b).

Mothers and Babies in Other Departments

If lactating women are everywhere in the world, then they (and their breastfeeding children) are coming to the emergency room after an accident, or having an appendix removed, or having an x-ray or MRI done, or recovering from some malady. The hospital where IBCLCs are happily and competently and ethically serving mothers in the postpartum wing may be the same facility whose other patients are getting incorrect and harmful lactation advice from the HCPs in charge of their care. It is probably because many HCPs just do not realize that lactation is an all day, every day process, that it is important (and actually easy) to protect, and that dire consequences may ensue if they do not (edema, plugged ducts, mastitis, abscess, premature weaning) (Riordan & Wambach, 2010). The risk management and quality assurance administrators in the hospital may be especially interested to know about that "dire consequences" part. Being admitted to the hospital as an ill or injured patient is fraught with worry. Many families find they must fight senseless battles to protect lactation and breastfeeding when they should be concentrating on the health issues that brought the loved one to the facility.

The IBCLC advocate can make a profound impact on the health and happiness of families at her institution by the simple act of offering to do an in-service training for care providers in other departments. Lactating women and breastfeeding children can show up in *every* department. That patient who just arrived for his appointment with the geriatrist was driven by his granddaughter, who has now asked the desk clerk where she might find a clean, private place to breastfeed her baby or use her breast pump while she waits. How will the clerk answer?

It is easy to protect breastfeeding.

1. Call or page the IBCLC for a consult! This simple step is often overlooked.
2. Keep the mother and baby together, wherever possible, and allow unfettered breastfeeding. This may require having a family member on site to tend to the baby when he or she is not actually breastfeeding, or providing a bed for the mother who is with her hospitalized breastfeeding child.
3. "Move the Milk," or perhaps "Move and Save the Milk." If breastfeeding cannot occur (for whatever *legitimate* reason; the IBCLC advocate can help describe what those might be), then regularly emptying the women's lactating breasts will preserve supply and ease discomfort.

Other HCPs may be aware of the importance of avoiding milk stasis (Amir et al., 2008), but may needlessly instruct the mother to "pump and dump" her breastmilk. It is better to pump, label, and *save* the milk until more research can be done in this particular clinical situation. If the milk truly cannot be used (ask the IBCLC) it can be discarded later. The initial instruction to discard the milk is often unfounded, and sends a very conflicting message about the value of breastmilk. The mother can also simply ask to take pumped milk home with her, and the IBCLC can back her up on this request.

Departments that will benefit greatly from evidence-based education by the IBCLC advocate include infection control, medical imaging, pediatrics, emergency department, postoperative care, and intensive care.

Infection Control

Customarily the handling of bodily fluids in a hospital is under strict guidelines, and for very good reason. Breastmilk, however, is not in and of itself an infectious by-product; it is packed with antiviral, antibacterial, and antiprotozoan factors (Lawrence & Lawrence, 2011). Contact with human milk by the HCP (spills or splashes) does not constitute an occupational exposure; indeed, the greater risk is that the milk will become contaminated when handled by those with unclean hands (Wight, Morton, & Kim, 2008).

Medical Imaging

X-rays, mammograms, MRIs, CT scans, contrast-media X-rays, even studies with radioactive nucleotides can nearly *all* occur without the need to cease breastfeeding (for any time period), nor to pump and dump ("Administration of Contrast Medium to Breastfeeding Mothers," 2001; Bonyata, 2011; Hale, 2010; Hoover, 2011).

Pediatrics

Children who are still breastfeeding sometimes need to go to the hospital. They may be ill, or require surgery. Families may be told that breastfeeding cannot occur for many hours prior to a procedure, the nerve-racking, even painful period when the comfort of breastfeeding is most needed. The IBCLC advocate can show evidence-based research to the pediatric surgeons and anesthesiologists that "mothers should limit the amount of breastfeeding after 4 hours [prior to surgery] and permit feeding on a pre-pumped breast, predominantly for comfort, to 2 hours before surgery" (Hale, 2010; Lawrence & Lawrence, 2011, p. 507).

Emergency Department

Not only will lactating women have emergencies, but lactating women will have lactation emergencies. Many mothers, unaware of the physiology of lactogenesis stage II (Lawrence & Lawrence, 2011), will visit the emergency room when their breasts become engorged and their temperatures rise. While advising the mother in this predicament is something the IBCLC can do with her eyes closed, it may be news to the emergency room (ER) physician that she should (a) call the IBCLC for a consult, (b) keep mother and baby together, and (c) move the milk. Similarly, when the ER physician is treating the woman for a more "conventional" emergency, it will be helpful to know that diagnostic tests can proceed without concern for lactation; that almost all medications are compatible with breastfeeding, or that pharmaceutical options exist that are breastfeeding-friendly; that regularly removing the milk (using the baby or a pump) will keep the mother's breasts comfortable and healthy when other parts of her are not.

Postoperative Care/Intensive Care

Lactating mothers who are recovering from surgery or other invasive procedures must regularly have their breasts emptied, to preserve supply and maintain comfort. A breast pump can be used even on a recumbent, anesthetized patient. While a nurse or IBCLC can certainly do this, it is the sort of task easily accomplished by a loving family member, who will not be as pressed for time to accomplish other clinical or administrative tasks. Another option is simply to bring the baby to breastfeed; again, a family member, "carer," or HCP can help "hold" the baby on mother's chest, and be sure that any postoperative tubes or bandages are not disturbed. The IBCLC advocate can help HCPs on the medical-surgery floors understand that as long as there is another competent adult to care for the baby the easiest means to protect the mother's lactation is recuperating with the baby. The anxiety and stress of mother–child separation will be greatly reduced in such circumstances, which can have a salubrious effect on recovery (Riordan & Wambach, 2010).

Public Health: Not Just Maternal and Child Health

Let's review the basics: breastfeeding has health impacts for mothers and babies. But it also has health impacts on the public at large because the mothers at some point wean, and their babies grow up to be men and women.

While noting that the following "language" springs from the original researchers, we have solid research showing that breastfeeding has short- and long-term health effects for both mothers and children. Meta-analyses evaluating data from around the world (Horta, Bahl, Martines, & Victora, 2007) and in developed countries (Ip et al., 2007) bears this out. What is remarkable is the broad range of health effects realized, and the dose-dependent nature of the benefit (meaning the more breastfeeding, the better the health result). Worldwide, subjects who were breastfed had lower blood pressure, lower serum cholesterol, less overweight/obesity, less type 2 diabetes, and higher intelligence test scores (Horta et al., 2007; ILCA, Spatz, & Lessen, 2011). In developed countries, breastfed infants had fewer cases of acute otitis media, less atopic dermatitis, fewer incidents of gastrointestinal infection, fewer hospitalizations for lower respiratory tract disease, less asthma, less obesity, less type 2 diabetes, reduced risk of leukemia, and less sudden infant death syndrome and overall infant mortality (Ip et al., 2007). These well-conducted meta-analyses can silence many doubters who think formula is "just as good" as breastfeeding, and the executive summaries of these reports will be handy for the IBCLC advocate to have at her fingertips.

An important document in support of breastfeeding as a public health imperative is from WHO and UNICEF: the Global Strategy for Infant and Young Child Feeding (GSIYCF) (WHO, 2003). It is *the* definitive policy document, grounded on "the best available scientific and epidemiological evidence" and building on important prior achievements in nutrition and child health reflected in the 1991 Baby-Friendly Initiative, the 1981 *International Code of Marketing of Breast-milk Substitutes* and the 1990 Innocenti Declaration (UNICEF, 1990, 2012; WHO, 1981, 2003, p. 2). The GSIYCF is an "integrated comprehensive approach" with a "degree of urgency" that recognizes the simple but profound concept: inappropriate feeding practices (that reduce optimal child growth and development) are obstacles to socioeconomic development growth (WHO, 2003, p. 4). Breastfeeding support and appropriate introduction of complementary foods play a large part in implementation of the GSIYCF.

Back-to-Sleep, Co-Sleeping and SIDS Awareness Campaigns

Early, strong messages from the Academy of Pediatrics (AAP), accompanied by public service campaigns initiated by public health departments about sudden infant death syndrome (SIDS), were very successful in selling the notion of placing babies on their backs during sleep, and not to allow the baby to sleep—at all—in bed with the parents (American Academy of Pediatrics Task Force on Sudden Infant Death Syndrome, 2005; Milwaukee Dept. of Health, n.d.). However, the research underlying these pronouncements does not support the conclusion that placing babies on their backs to sleep, and avoiding all co-sleeping with mothers and babies, will prevent the tragedy of SIDS (McKenna & McDade, 2005). Some policy statements have recently been revised to focus on education about safe sleep environments (American Academy of Pediatrics, 2011). Because we know that mothers *are* co-sleeping with their babies: 44% sleep with their babies at night. Often, babies start sleeping in one location, and end up in another. It is much riskier for a parent to fall asleep with the infant while in a chair, a recliner, or the sofa. Yet, that is just where many are going, in sleep-deprived droves in the middle of the night, because they have been told that co-sleeping in the parents' bed is the villain (Kendall-Tackett, Cong, & Hale, 2010; McKenna, Ball, & Gettler, 2007). Human infants are, in fact, much better off sleeping near or with their mothers, *in a safe sleep environment*:

> The AAP . . . is expanding its recommendations from focusing only on SIDS to focusing on a safe sleep environment that can reduce the risk of all sleep-related infant deaths, including SIDS. The recommendations . . . include supine positioning, use of a firm sleep surface, *breastfeeding*, room-sharing without bed-sharing, routine immunizations, consideration of using a pacifier[1], and avoidance of soft bedding, overheating, and exposure to tobacco smoke, alcohol, and illicit drugs. (American Academy of Pediatrics, 2011, p. 1030, emphasis added)

Demonizing one form or location for slumber does not consider the many variables that constitute "healthy, safe, and satisfying infant-child sleep" (McKenna & McDade, 2005, p. 150). Breastfeeding babies need to have access to their mothers at night; anything that hinders the dyad puts breastfeeding at risk. The IBCLC advocate will find that this is an area in which her calm, reasoned explanation of what the evidence better demonstrates may be sorely needed to prevent unsafe sleeping practices and diminished breastfeeding.

---

[1] "Delay pacifier introduction until breastfeeding has been firmly established, usually by 3 to 4 weeks of age," p. 1034.

Think Beyond Mothers and Babies

To those outside the field of lactation, and even to many within, it is easy to think of breastfeeding as something that concerns only mothers and newborns. That is, of course, essentially true, but as the research tells us (in whatever language is used) health effects are long term, even lifelong, for breastfeeding dyads (ILCA, Spatz, & Lessen, 2011). For those seeking to reduce or eradicate disease, it may come as a revelation that breastfeeding reduces the risk of certain conditions and diseases (or formula feeding increases their risk), and this is an angle in their public awareness and prevention campaigns that had never been considered.

Other areas of health care can benefit from advocacy by an IBCLC, with her access to evidence-based research about breastfeeding, to explain how lactation or breastmilk affects these subject areas:

- Brain, nerve and social development in children: The components of breastmilk and their manner of skin-to-skin delivery are ideally suited to the growing human infant's needs (Lawrence & Lawrence, 2011; Riordan & Wambach, 2010). Anti-infective properties of breastmilk are fairly well understood, even outside of maternal-child health, but it is not just about the breastmilk. It is the breastfeeding that provides a connection (literally) that helps the child's brain and social skills fully mature and to become a trusting adult (Bergman, Linley, & Fawcus, 2004; Guibert, 2010).
- Cancer: Breast cancer (Helewa et al., 2002), ovarian cancer (Danforth et al., 2007), endometrial cancer (Okamura et al., 2006), childhood leukemia and lymphoma (Bener, Hoffmann, Afify, Rasul, & Tewfik, 2008)
- Cancer treatment: Tumor cell death (Hallgren et al., 2008)
- Family planning (Labbok et al., 1997)
- Immune system (inflammatory response) development (Field, 2005)
- Motor (Dewey, Cohen, Brown, & Rivera, 2001) and cognitive (Kramer et al., 2008) development in children
- Mental health and depression (Kendall-Tackett, 2007)
- Obesity and diabetes, both of which are at epidemic proportions in some countries (U.S. Centers for Disease Control, 2007; U.S. Dept. of Health and Human Services, Indian Health Service, n.d.).

Breastfeeding Advocacy Beyond Health Care

The IBCLC profession, only 26 years old, can make great strides in cementing its credibility and in solidifying the need for IBCLCs in policy as well as clinical discussions by looking beyond the fairly insular world of pregnancy, childbirth, and the postpartum period. It has been said before: lactating women are everywhere, not just the maternity ward. That means their needs, and those of their children, can crop up anywhere. Some examples are discussed in the following sections.

Emergency Preparedness

The tsunami at Banda Aceh, Indonesia, in 2004; Hurricane Katrina in the southern United States in 2005; the devastating earthquakes in Haiti in 2010 and New Zealand and Japan in 2011: we all have vivid memories of these natural disasters just in recent years. Emergencies can be man-made, too: war, terrorist attacks, and industrial accidents can affect hundreds of thousands of people at a time. Besides the trauma and injury associated with the initial event, there can be weeks and months of privation for displaced and refugee families—including breastfeeding women and their children.

The Emergency Nutrition Network (ENN) "was set up in 1996 by an international group of humanitarian agencies to accelerate learning and strengthen institutional memory in the emergency food and nutrition sector" (Emergency Food Network, 2012, para. 1). They seek to assist in the immediate emergency, and take those lessons forward to better serve affected populations when the next disaster or emergency strikes.

For breastfeeding mothers and children, the goals are fairly simple: any relief activities are to be conducted in compliance with the *International Code of Marketing of Breastmilk Substitutes*, no small feat when well-meaning but misguided donors from around the world try to rush powdered or ready-made infant formula donations to the site, in a language that cannot be read by the population, and where clean water, electricity, and fuel for heating and cooking are unavailable. Emergency relief workers on the ground are to be trained in how to provide optimal feeding after the onset of the emergency, including support for and protection of breastfeeding. They assess the affected population (how many mothers, young children, pregnant women?) and their nutritional needs; support is to be offered to "maintain, enhance or reestablish breastfeeding using relactation. [I]f breastfeeding by the natural mother is impossible, make appropriate choices from among alternatives (wet-nursing, breastmilk from milk bank, unbranded [generic] infant formula, locally purchased commercial infant formula)" (Infant and Young Child Feeding in Emergencies [IFE], 2007, Part 5.2 at p. 11). Other features of the guidelines include providing a safe, private space for breastfeeding women and children to stay together. Something as simple as a blanket draped over a clothesline can offer "privacy" in a temporary shelter. Breastfeeding support activities should be kept separate from any relief efforts involving formula (where such families are also to be given 1:1 assistance). Evidence-based resources specific to the needs of infants detail the care to be used in supporting all families: those with breastfeeding children, and those who must safely prepare formula in emergency conditions (Gribble & Berry, 2011).

These guidelines can be applied anywhere in any emergency, no matter how big or small. An apartment complex fire affecting 20 families is every bit as uprooting and traumatizing to those people as a flood affecting thousands. IBCLC advocates can provide a great service by training "first-responders" (police, fire, and emergency medical team personnel) *before* the fact, even if the IBCLC is not in a position to assist mothers on the ground when the actual disaster strikes. Many relief agencies are involved in ongoing education and training efforts (American Red Cross 2010), and the IBCLC advocate may find her teaching niche there.

Breastfeeding Support as a Smart Business and Economic Decision

Women of child-bearing age make up a huge proportion of the workforce around the world. Many mothers must work outside of the home after their children are born. Readily accessible materials exist to allow the IBCLC advocate to show an employer how breastfeeding or lactation support programs are very cheap and easy to initiate. They reap bottom-line returns on the investment through reduced employee absenteeism (by mothers *and* fathers), reduced healthcare costs for the employer (of payments for the insurance benefit), and enhanced employee satisfaction/retention (U.S. Dept. of Health and Human Services, Office on Women's Health, 2010).

Globally, the right to paid maternity leave and the right to paid break time (to breastfeed or express milk) upon the return to work outside the home was affirmed during the International Labour Organization's (ILO) 2000 Convention on Maternity Protection (International Labour Organization, 2000).[2] The convention protects the health of both mother and child, assures maternity leave rights to 14 weeks, and prohibits discrimination/job loss based on pregnancy, maternity leave, or use of guaranteed break-time to breastfeed. These affirmative rights can be a powerful tool in advocating for women.

Getting the Message to Decision Makers

If you have the itch to advocate, how can you do it? Several tactics can be pursued.

Seek to Be "At the Table"

At your place of work, volunteer to be on the committee that reviews policies at your institution and suggests changes. There may be existing obstetrics, midwifery, pediatric, NICU, and nursing committees, or interdisciplinary groups containing representatives of these groups. The IBCLC should be there as well. If your facility does not already have a Breastfeeding Committee or Lactation Program, seek to set one up, ideally composed of members from many disciplines and job sectors (any reason why dietary and housekeeping would *not* be able to contribute ideas of how to better serve breastfeeding patients?) (Riordan & Wambach, 2010). Part of your effectiveness in making change is being seen as a competent professional: someone who attends meetings, makes meaningful contributions, is willing to listen to other viewpoints, comes back with results after receiving an assignment (Gastil, 1993).

Join breastfeeding coalitions or consortiums in your country or state. A cross-discipline model is effective when crafting public policy initiatives. HCPs, such as

---

[2] The International Labour Organization "is the only 'tripartite' United Nations agency that brings together representatives of governments, employers and workers to jointly shape policies and programmes promoting Decent Work for all. This unique arrangement gives the ILO an edge in incorporating 'real world' knowledge about employment and work" (International Labour Organization, 2012, para. 1).

physicians and IBCLCs, are appropriate, as are childbirth educators, early child development specialists, midwives, mother-to-mother breastfeeding counselors, government administrators, and private-sector leaders (e.g., human resources managers from companies). A blueprint for action was drafted for use in Europe, "based on a careful analysis of the situation, on a thorough review of effective interventions, on reports of successful national and local experiences, and on the consensus of hundreds of individual and groups committed to protecting, promoting, and supporting breastfeeding" (European Commission, Directorate Public Health and Risk Assessment, 2008, p. 1). This evidence-based roadmap provides suggestions for affecting change at local, national, and multinational levels, and its concepts are universal.

Whether the healthcare delivery system in your country is centralized or decentralized, there is always a governmental agency or ministry that is charged with protecting public health and safety. Most will provide some opportunity for the public to weigh in with their comments on proposed (or enacted) policy changes. Your ability to influence final decision making may depend on the procedures that have been devised: in the United States, at the federal level, a call for public comments is made on proposed regulations; after comments are solicited, their consideration must be accounted for in the report accompanying final regulations; comments can be submitted electronically (Office of the Federal Register, National Archives and Records Administration, n.d.). Sometimes calls for public comment are made, during hearings to be held on various matters, including those affecting the health of women and children (U.S. Dept of Health and Human Services, Healthy People 2020, 2011a). Such contributions may have to be kept to three minutes or less; it is an ideal opportunity for the IBCLC advocate to see if she can fashion her argument to promote and protect breastfeeding within this particular debate into "an elevator speech" (something that can be adequately explained in the time it takes to ride an elevator).

Empower Mothers to Advocate for Themselves

Much of our work as IBCLCs is to empower mothers to feel confident that their bodies and babies can do this fine work of breastfeeding. The IBCLC builds rapport with mothers by listening to their concerns and addressing their needs one mother at a time (even if it is the 15th time today the IBCLC has assured a new mother that she has "enough" milk). Often this rapport makes mothers see the IBCLC as a safe haven to whom they can complain about their (or their babies') treatment by or interactions with other HCPs.

If a colleague has given a mother incorrect lactation advice, or has not followed policy or procedure, it may give rise to an ethical or legal difficulty that the IBCLC will assess. Sometimes the issues raised by the mother are less obviously "problems," but go more to lousy bedside manner. Or, perhaps the mother feels as disturbed by a required hospital policy as you may be in your professional role (such as separation of mother and baby after birth, or routine use of pacifiers). Without telling the mother *what* to say, and while using demeanor that indicates you are a good listener (translation: do not telescope your own views on this topic), you can suggest that the mother be certain to fill out her hospital survey with these comments, or to write a letter to the administrators with her concerns. Sometimes one letter from a dissatisfied patient will do more to instigate change than months of committee meetings initiated by the IBCLC. It is empowering (and cathartic) for the mother to "take charge" of the dissatisfying situation by putting her thoughts into words, and sharing them with those who need to know.

When a mother has used a product that isn't doing the job—or worse, injured or sickened her or her child—encourage her (as the consumer) to file a complaint with the appropriate authorities or return the offending product.

As IBCLCs, we often work with mothers who are offering mixed feeds (breastfeeding and formula). Sometimes this is the situation we walk into during a consult: we have no idea why formula is in the picture. Sometimes the parents started using it on their own initiative. Sometimes it was medically indicated, and ordered by the pediatrician. Sometimes formula was suggested instead of offering appropriate breastfeeding assistance. Regardless, some babies have very bad reactions to infant formula. In the United States, infant formula is a product regulated as a food by the FDA. It is "generally recognized as safe (GRAS)" and does not have to undergo the stringent and ongoing quality controls required of mass-marketed drugs (FDA, 2011). Because formula is GRAS, the FDA has to be *told* when a problem occurs. They are not proactively seeking out and removing problems; they react when informed (FDA, 2009a, 2010a).[3] A mother should be encouraged to make her concerns known to the FDA. She doesn't have to "prove" anything. She just needs to make a simple report: "My baby drank 6 ounces of Brand *X* formula, had projectile vomiting within 30 minutes, and explosive, green mucousy stools for the next 24 hours."

Similarly, there are an increasing number of supplements, devices, gadgets, and machines out there, claiming to assist in all manner of breastfeeding issues. Whether it is a breast pump or a salve or a special bra or a nipple everter, the product is subject to all the same consumer protection regulations as any other product.

The Uniform Commercial Code in the United States recognizes implied "warranties of merchantability" and "fitness for a particular purpose," meaning the product was sold with the intent that it would perform as advertised. If the mother bought it, and it isn't doing what was promised, it can be returned, just as anything that is broken when it was purchased can be returned (Legal Information Institute, Cornell University Law School, n.d.).

---

[3] Healthcare providers also have a reporting site and phone line available for them to use, to alert FDA of "a serious adverse event, product quality problem or product use error that you suspect is associated with the use of an FDA-regulated" product (FDA, 2009c, para. 1). The IBCLC may use this secure and confidential site, as can the baby's HCP.

The FDA regulates breast pumps in the United States as a medical device; pumps that have been approved for use may be searched on their website (FDA, 2012), and a general information page about what type of breast pump to purchase or rent is offered (FDA, 2010b). Injuries caused by the device are to be reported by the mother/consumer to the FDA (FDA, 2009b), though complaints about the operation of the machine should be directed to the manufacturer (FDA, 2009b).

The Consumer Product Safety Commission does *not* have jurisdiction over foods, medicines, and medical devices (thus not infant formula or breast pumps), nor infant car seats, but they do oversee the safety of many products purchased by breastfeeding mothers, such as baby carriers/slings, cribs/bassinettes, toys, and so on. Consumers and HCPs alike may file complaints of "an illness, injury, or death, or the risk of illness, injury, or death related to use of the product" (U.S. Consumer Product Safety Commission, n.d., para. 1).

Informal Opportunities

Being an advocate means pleading for a cause, pushing an idea, arguing for a concept, and speaking up. But it doesn't have to be formal, it doesn't have to be hard, and it doesn't have to be boring. Little bits of evidence-based information may do more to enlighten your colleagues than a 30-minute in-service education session. Here are some suggestions:

- Put interesting journal articles on the staff bulletin board, highlighting the pertinent conclusions. Have you ever failed to read highlighted sentences in an article you've seen posted?
- Ask for 3 minutes (really) at the obstetrics or pediatric meeting; highlight one research-based fact about breastfeeding.
- Present a case study (anonymous or hypothetical) about treatment and care of a breastfeeding patient, and solicit discussion about how it was handled, and how it should have been handled.
- Praise what is working well. Thank colleagues who call to your attention mothers who need special help. Acknowledge when staff offers excellent breastfeeding support. Laud the family members who are providing a breastfeeding-supportive environment for the mother.
- Hang a wall calendar using "nonconventional" breastfeeding pictures: mothers with multiples; mothers with nursing toddlers, mothers who are tandem nursing; teen mothers; mothers out and about in public spaces.
- Post a lactation-related quiz question near the fax machine (or some other place where colleagues must stop for a minute or two) on Day 1; post the answer and a new quiz question on Day 2. Leave space for answers if you'd like; award a token prize.

- Practice "watching your language" when conversing with other HCPs about breastfeeding and human lactation.
- Smile, smile, smile when a colleague tries to "get your goat" by making inflammatory remarks about breastfeeding or lactation support. Sometimes we are so startled by the verbal zing that we can't immediately pull up an appropriate response (though it will, of course, occur to us during the commute home). Use the active listening tools you mastered as an IBCLC, in a nonthreatening way. Saying it with a smile, of course, try responding simply with "Tell me more." It usually throws your detractor off if you appear to be willing to engage in an honest discussion.
- Do a scavenger hunt of your workplace and count how many pictures, ads, or messages you see that promote breastfeeding, or formula/bottle use, or a pediatric medicine. Offer the information (lightly and nonjudgmentally) at the next staff meeting, to raise consciousness about good health messaging versus product messaging.
- Volunteer to do a bulletin board display for your facility during World Breast-feeding Week; or, when other health campaigns are being promoted, ask to include breastfeeding messages (e.g., breastfeeding reduces the risk of cancer, heart disease in women, and diabetes). If your colleagues balk that their target demographic isn't breastfeeding anymore, remind them that their patients may have daughters and granddaughters who could be inspired to breastfeed to improve their own odds against getting grandma's disease or condition.

Advocate for IBCLCs and Their Profession

Think of how long and hard you worked to be certified IBCLC. Don't be reluctant to toot your own horn or that of your profession. Many of the difficult ethical and legal situations described in this book would be eased if the clinical role of the IBCLC were better understood and respected. This isn't a surprising state of affairs. It makes sense that a group of allied healthcare providers, who specialize in breastfeeding and human lactation, and didn't even exist before 1985, would need to do a little marketing to secure their place at the table. Especially since breastfeeding straddles the medical world (where the need for HCPs is understandable) and the parenting world (where the HCP is *not* a required element). This doesn't have to be hard; a position paper from the international professional association puts it all into two free-to-download pages (ILCA & Henderson, 2011; www.ilca.org).

Introduce yourself as the "I-B-C-L-C" rather than the "lactation consultant." Yes, surely you will at some point use that more familiar and common term in describing your work, but let it come during the explanatory phase of the conversation, not the introductory phase ("Hi! I am your I-B-C-L-C [or] International Board Certified Lactation Consultant. I am here to talk to you about breastfeeding.")

Use your credentials on your letterhead, your business cards, your brochures, your website, and your social media pages. Describe how IBCLC differs from any other category of breastfeeding helper. Use your credentials on every single thing you write: on your charting notes; in your reports to HCPs, and in your marketing outreach for your private practice.

Wear a lapel pin from IBLCE, and from your professional association too, whenever you are out and about in your professional capacity. It's like "suiting up": whether you wear scrubs, suits or "casual professional" clothing, when you put on the insignia of your profession, it helps to mentally and emotionally prepare you for your day.

Take advantage of the many free downloads and ideas from the International Lactation Consultant Association (www.ilca.org), which celebrates IBCLC Day in March of every year (with a new theme each year).

Promote yourself with press releases to your local or neighborhood newspaper describing your work in the community.

Honor others. Mentors who have helped you get to where you are will appreciate a note of thanks.

Spread the word. The HCPs and nonmedical staff in your facility will see that your work is as worthy of praise and recognition as other professions.

Market your practice. Use IBCLC Day as an excuse to prepare a bulletin board at your birthing center describing the important role of IBCLCs on staff. Deliver your brochure and business cards to your referral sources, complete with a copy of your press release highlighting your accomplishments. Tell your facility's public relations department: this is an easy opportunity for them to trumpet the services IBCLCs provide to the hospital.

Your own excellence in everyday practice will advertise to the world the competence of IBCLCs.

Summary

IBCLCs have expertise that crosses many disciplines, providing opportunities to advocate for breastfeeding mothers and children in venues beyond traditional maternity and child health circles. We can help educate our HCP colleagues, and others working in aid of mothers and children, to know that "there are no benefits of breastfeeding": that this normal, biologic function is designed to provide optimal functioning of our children's minds and bodies. Advocacy can be accomplished formally (joining a committee, submitting comments to a legislative committee) or informally (factoids offered each day in our work setting). As a young profession, we need to be willing to advertise and promote ourselves, and our role, so the public at large can understand (and demand) our expertise.

REFERENCES

Aarts, C., Kylberg, E., Hornell, A., Hofvander, Y., Gebre-Medhin, M., & Greiner, T. (2000, December). How exclusive is exclusive breastfeeding? A comparison of data since birth with current status data. *International Journal of Epidemiology, 29*(6), 1041–1046. Retrieved from http://ije.oxfordjournals.org/content /29/6/1041.full

Administration of contrast medium to breastfeeding mothers. (2001, October). *ACR Bulletin, 57*(10), 12–13. Retrieved from http://www.urmc.rochester.edu/smd/Rad/CSIfaq/Breastfeeding.pdf

Akre, J. (2006). *The problem with breastfeeding: A personal reflection.* Amarillo, TX: Hale Publishing.

American Academy of Pediatrics. (2011, November). American Academy of Pediatrics policy statement on SIDS and other sleep-related infant deaths: Expansion of recommendations for a safe infant sleeping environment. *Pediatrics, 128*(5), 1030–1039. Retrieved from http://pediatrics.aappublications.org/content /early/2011/10/12/peds.2011-2284.full.pdf+html

American Academy of Pediatrics Task Force on Sudden Infant Death Syndrome. (2005, November 5). The changing concept of sudden infant death syndrome: Diagnostic coding shifts, controversies regarding the sleeping environment, and new variables to consider in reducing risk. *Pediatrics, 116*, 1245–1255. doi:10.1542/peds.2005-1499

American Red Cross. (2010, January 28). *American Red Cross looks ahead in Haiti.* Retrieved from http:// www.redcross.org/portal/site/en/menuitem.1a019a978f421296e81ec89e43181aa0/?vgnextoid=906bf4aa 95476210VgnVCM10000089f0870aRCRD

Amir, L., Chantry, C., Howard, C., Lawrence, R., Marinelli, K., & Powers, N. (2008, May). *Mastitis-Revision May 2008* (ABM Clinical Protocol No. 4). Retrieved from http://www.bfmed.org/Media/Files /Protocols/protocol_4mastitis.pdf

Baby-Friendly USA. (2010a). *Info for breastfeeding advocates/health care professionals* [Frequently Asked Questions]. Retrieved from http://www.babyfriendlyusa.org/eng/06.html

Baby-Friendly USA. (2010b). *The ten steps to successful breastfeeding.* Retrieved from http://www .babyfriendlyusa.org/eng/10steps.html

Baby-Friendly USA. (2012, March 6). *Baby-Friendly hospitals and birth centers.* Retrieved from http://www .babyfriendlyusa.org/eng/03.html

Bartick, M., Stuebe, A., Shealy, K., Walker, M., & Grummer-Strawn, L. (2009, October). Closing the quality gap: Promoting evidence-based breastfeeding care in the hospital. *Pediatrics, 124*(4), e793–e802. Retrieved from http://pediatrics.aappublications.org/cgi/reprint/124/4/e793

Bener, A., Hoffmann, G., Afify, Z., Rasul, K., & Tewfik, I. (2008). Does prolonged breastfeeding reduce the risk for childhood leukemia and lymphomas? [Abstract] *Minerva Pediatrica, 60*(2), 155–161. Retrieved from http://cat.inist.fr/?aModele=afficheN&cpsidt=20436295

Bergman, N., Linley, L., & Fawcus, S. R. (2004). Randomized controlled trial of skin-to-skin contact from birth versus conventional incubator for physiological stabilization in 1200 to 2199 gram newborns. *Acta Paediatrica, 93*, 779–785. doi:10.1080/08035250410028534

Bonyata, K. (2011, August 1). *Use of radioisotopes (and other imaging agents) during lactation.* Retrieved from http://kellymom.com/bf/can-i-breastfeed/meds/radioisotopes/

Danforth, K., Tworoger, S., Hecht, J., Rosner, B., Colditz, G., & Hankinson, S. (2007). Breastfeeding and risk of ovarian cancer in two prospective cohorts. *Cancer Causes Control, 18*, 517–523. Retrieved from http://www.springerlink.com/content/g86w9247j2282507/fulltext.pdf

Dewey, K., Cohen, R., Brown, K., & Rivera, L. L. (2001). Effects of exclusive breastfeeding for four versus six months on maternal nutritional status and infant motor development: Results of two randomized trials in Honduras. *The Journal of Nutrition, 131*, 262–267. Retrieved from http://jn.nutrition.org/content/131/2/262.full.pdf+html

DiGirolamo, A., Grummer-Strawn, L., & Fein, S. (2008, October). Effect of maternity-case practices on breastfeeding. *Pediatrics, 122*(Supplement 2), S43–S49. Retrieved from http://pediatrics.aappublications.org/cgi/reprint/122/Supplement_2/S43

DiGirolamo, A. M., Manninen, D. L., Cohen, J. H., Shealy, K. R., Murphy, P. E., MacGowan, C. A., . . . Scanlon, K. S. (2008, June 13). Breastfeeding-related maternity practices at hospitals and birth centers- United States, 2007. *Morbidity & Mortality Weekly Report [CDC], 57*(23), 621–625. Retrieved from http://www.cdc.gov/mmwr/preview/mmwrhtml/mm5723a1.htm

Emergency Nutrition Network. (2012). *About the ENN*. Retrieved from http://www.ennonline.net/about

European Commission, Directorate Public Health and Risk Assessment. (2008). *Protection, promotion and support of breastfeeding in Europe: A blueprint for action (revised 2008)* (N. SPC No. 2004326). Luxembourg: European Commission, Directorate Public Health and Risk Assessment.

Field, C. (2005, January). The immunological components of human milk and their effect on immune development in infants. *Journal of Nutrition, 135*, 1–4. Retrieved from http://jn.nutrition.org/content/135/1/1.full

Gastil, J. (1993). Small group democracy. In J. Gastil (Ed.), *Democracy in small groups* (pp. 15–47). Philadelphia, PA: New Society Publishers.

Gribble, K., & Berry, N. (2011, November). Emergency preparedness for those who care for infants in developed country contexts. *International Breastfeeding Journal, 6*(16). Retrieved from http://www.internationalbreastfeedingjournal.com/content/6/1/16

Guibert, S. (2010, September 17). *Research shows child rearing practices of distant ancestors foster morality, compassion in kids* [article on unpublished research by Darcia Narvaez]. Retrieved from://newsinfo.nd.edu/news/16829-research-shows-child-rearing-practices-of-distant-ancestors-foster-morality-compassion-in-kids

Hale, T. (2010). *Medications and mothers' milk* (14th ed.). Amarillo, TX: Hale Publishing.

Hallgren, O., Alts, S., Brest, P., Gustafsson, L., Mossberg, A.-K., Wullt, B., & Svanborg, C. (2008). Apoptosis and tumor cell death in response to HAMLET (human α-lactalbumin made lethal to tumor cells). *Advances in Experimental Medicine and Biology, 606*(2), 217–240. doi:10.1007/978-0-387-74087-4_8

Helewa, M., Levesque, P., Provencher, D., Lea, R., Rosolowich, V., & Shapiro, H. (2002, February). Breast cancer, pregnancy and breastfeeding [Abstract]. *Journal of Obstetricians and Gynaecologists of Canada, 24*(2), 164–180. Retrieved from http://www.ncbi.nlm.nih.gov/pubmed/12196882?ordinalpos=1&itool=PPMCLayout.PPMCAppController.PPMCArticlePage.PPMCPubmedRA&linkpos=3

Hoover, K. (2011, June). Breastfeeding and the use of contrast dyes for maternal tests. *Clinical Lactation, 2*(2), 31–32.

Horta, B., Bahl, R., Martines, J., & Victora, C. (2007). *Evidence on the long-term effects of breastfeeding: Systematic reviews and meta-analyses*. Retrieved from http://whqlibdoc.who.int/publications/2007/9789241595230_eng.pdf

Infant and Young Child Feeding in Emergencies (IFE) Core Group (Ed.). (2007, February). *Operational guidance for emergency relief staff and programme managers* (Version No. 2.1). Retrieved from http://www.who.int/nutrition/publications/emergencies/operational_guidance/en/index.html

International Baby Food Action Network (IBFAN). (n.d.). *The full code and subsequent WHA resolutions*. Retrieved from http://www.ibfan.org/issue-international_code-full.html

International Board of Lactation Consultant Examiners. (2008, March 8). *Scope of practice for international board certified lactation consultants*. Retrieved from http://www.iblce.org/upload/downloads/ScopeOfPractice.pdf

International Board of Lactation Consultant Examiners. (2011, November 1). *Code of professional conduct for IBCLCs.* Retrieved from http://iblce.org/upload/downloads/CodeOfProfessionalConduct.pdf

International Labour Organization. (2000, June 15). *International Labour Conference adopts new convention and recommendation on maternity protection* [Press release]. Retrieved from http://www.ilo.org/global /about-the-ilo/press-and-media-centre/press-releases/WCMS_007900/lang--en/index.htm

International Labour Organization. (2012). *About the ILO.* Retrieved from http://www.ilo.org/global/about -the-ilo/lang--en/index.htm

International Lactation Consultant Association. (2006). *Standards of practice for international board certified lactation consultants.* Retrieved from http://www.ilca.org/files/resources/Standards-of-Practice-web.pdf

International Lactation Consultant Association, & Henderson, S. (2011, June). *Position paper on the role and impact of the IBCLC* (Monograph). Retrieved from http://www.ilca.org/files/resources/ilca _publications/Role%20%20Impact%20of%20the%20IBCLC-webFINAL_08-15-11.pdf

International Lactation Consultant Association, Spatz, D., & Lessen, R. (2011). *Risks of not breastfeeding* (Monograph). Morrisville, NC: International Lactation Consultant Association.

Ip, S., Chung, M., Raman, G., Chew, P., Magula, N., DeVine, D., . . . Lau, J. (2007, April). *Breastfeeding and maternal and infant health outcomes in developed countries* (Rep. No. 153). Rockville, MD: U.S. Agency for Healthcare Research and Quality.

Kendall-Tackett, K. (2007, March 30). A new paradigm for depression in mothers: The central role of inflammation and how breastfeeding and anti-inflammatory treatments protect maternal mental health. *International Breastfeeding Journal, 2*(6). Retrieved from http://www.internationalbreastfeedingjournal .com/content/2/1/6

Kendall-Tackett, K., Cong, Z., & Hale, T. (2010, Fall). Mother-infant sleep locations and nighttime feeding behavior: U.S. data from the survey of mothers' sleep and fatigue. *Clinical Lactation, 1*(1), 27–31.

Kramer, M., Aboud, F., Mironova, E., Vanilovich, I., Platt, R., Matush, L., . . . Fombonne, E. (2008, May). Breastfeeding and child cognitive development. *Archives of General Psychiatry, 65*(5), 578–584. Retrieved from http://archpsyc.ama-assn.org/cgi/reprint/65/5/578

Labbok, M., Hight-Laukaran, V., Peterson, A., Fletcher, V., von Hertzen, H., & Van Look, P. (1997, June). Multicenter study of the lactational amenorrhea method (LAM): I. Efficacy, duration, and implications for clinical application [Abstract]. *Contraception, 55*(6), 327–336. Retrieved from http:// www.contraceptionjournal.org/article/S0010-7824(97)00040-1/abstract

Labbok, M., & Krasovec, K. (1990, July/August). Toward consistency in breastfeeding definitions [Abstract]. *Studies in Family Planning, 21*(4), 226–230. Retrieved from http://www.ncbi.nlm.nih.gov /pubmed/2219227

Lawrence, R., & Lawrence, R. (2011). *Breastfeeding: A guide for the medical profession* (7th ed.). Maryland Heights, MO: Elsevier Mosby.

Legal Information Institute, Cornell University Law School. (n.d.). *Uniform commercial code—Article 2—Sales* [Model legislative language for uniform commercial code]. Retrieved from http://www.law.cornell.edu /ucc/2/overview.html

McKenna, J., Ball, H., & Gettler, L. (2007). Mother–infant cosleeping, breastfeeding and sudden infant death syndrome: What biological anthropology has discovered about normal infant sleep and pediatric sleep medicine [Abstract]. *American Journal of Physical Anthropology, 134*(Suppl. 45), 133–161. Retrieved from http://onlinelibrary.wiley.com/doi/10.1002/ajpa.20736/abstract

McKenna, J., & McDade, T. (2005). Why babies should never sleep alone: A review of the co-sleeping controversy in relation to SIDS, bedsharing and breast feeding. *Paediatric Respiratory Reviews, 6*, 134–152. Retrieved from http://www.naturalchild.org/james_mckenna/cosleeping.pdf

McNiel, M., Labbok, M., & Abrahams, S. (2010, March). What are the risks associated with formula feeding? A re-analysis and review. *Birth, 37*(1), 50–58. Retrieved from http://onlinelibrary.wiley.com /doi/10.1111/j.1523-536X.2009.00378.x/pdf

Milwaukee Dept of Health. (n.d.). *City of Milwaukee health department's safe sleep awareness campaign.* Retrieved from http://city.milwaukee.gov/SafeSleep

Office of the Federal Register, National Archives and Records Administration. (n.d.). *About federal register.* Retrieved from http://www.gpo.gov/help/index.html#about_federal_register.htm

Okamura, C., Tsubono, Y., Ito, K., Niikura, H., Takano, T., Nagase, S., & Yoshinaga, K. (2006). Lactation and risk of endometrial cancer in Japan: A case-control study [Abstract]. *Tohoku Journal of Experimental Medicine, 208*(2), 109–115. Retrieved from http://www.jstage.jst.go.jp/article/tjem/208/2/208_109/_article

Riordan, J., & Wambach, K. (2010). *Breastfeeding and human lactation* (4th ed.). Sudbury, MA: Jones & Bartlett.

Robbins, S., & Beker, L. (2004). *Infant feedings: Guidelines for preparation of formula and breastmilk in health care facilities.* Retrieved from http://books.google.com/books?id=k8dNAyG2_DgC&printsec=front cover&dq=Robbins+Beker+Infant+Feedings&source=bl&ots=5vvoHEZaIy&sig=EMKU_iA7GHyMfnV -dOegPHLIwhY&hl=en&ei=LJz-TK_bCcK78gaXp9CXBw&sa=X&oi=book_result&ct=result& resnum=1&ved=0CBoQ6AEwAA#v=onepage&q&

Smith, J., Dunstone, M., & Elliott-Rudder, M. (2009). Health professional knowledge of breastfeeding: Are the health risks of infant formula feeding accurately conveyed by the titles and abstracts of journal articles? *Journal of Human Lactation, 25*(3), 350–358. Retrieved from http://jhl.sagepub.com/content/25/3/350

Smith, L. J., & Kroeger, M. (2010). *Impact of birthing practices on breastfeeding* (2nd ed.). Sudbury, MA: Jones & Bartlett.

UNICEF. (1990). *Innocenti declaration on the protection, promotion and support of breastfeeding* [Adopted by WHO policymakers 1990]. Retrieved from http://www.unicef.org/programme/breastfeeding/innocenti.htm

UNICEF. (2012, March 21). *The baby-friendly hospital initiative.* Retrieved from http://www.unicef.org /programme/breastfeeding/baby.htm

U.S. Centers for Disease Control and Prevention. (2011, October 13). *CDC announces new effort to boost number of baby-friendly hospitals.* Retrieved from http://www.cdc.gov/media/releases/2011/p1013 _babyfriendly_hospitals.html

U.S. Centers for Disease Control, National Center for Chronic Disease Prevention and Health Promotion (Ed.). (2007, July). *Does breastfeeding reduce the risk of pediatric overweight?* (Rep. No. 4). Retrieved from http://www.cdc.gov/nccdphp/dnpa/nutrition/pdf/breastfeeding_r2p.pdf

U.S. Consumer Product Safety Commission. (n.d.). *File a report.* Retrieved from https://www.saferproducts .gov/CPSRMSPublic/Incidents/ReportIncident.aspx

U.S. Dept. of Health and Human Services, Healthy People 2020. (2011a, April 4). *Public comment.* Retrieved from http://healthypeople.gov/2020/about/publicComment.aspx

U.S. Dept. of Health and Human Services, Indian Health Service. (n.d.). *Diabetes prevention and breastfeeding.* Retrieved from http://www.ihs.gov/MedicalPrograms/MCH/M/bfdiabetes.cfm

U.S. Dept. of Health and Human Services, Office of the Surgeon General. (2011b, January). *The surgeon general's call to action to support breastfeeding.* Washington, DC: U.S. Dept. of Health and Human Services, Office of the Surgeon General.

U.S. Dept. of Health and Human Services, Office on Women's Health. (2010, August 1). *The business case for breastfeeding.* Retrieved from http://www.womenshealth.gov/breastfeeding/government-programs /business-case-for-breastfeeding/index.cfm

U.S. Food and Drug Administration. (2009a, April 30). *Report a problem.* Retrieved from http://www.fda .gov/Safety/ReportaProblem/default.htm

U.S. Food and Drug Administration. (2009b, May 20). *Infection and injury.* Retrieved from http://www.fda
.gov/MedicalDevices/ProductsandMedicalProcedures/HomeHealthandConsumer/ConsumerProducts
/BreastPumps/ucm061964.htm

U.S. Food and Drug Administration. (2009c, October 23). *Report by health professionals.* Retrieved from
http://www.fda.gov/Safety/MedWatch/HowToReport/ucm085568.htm

U.S. Food and Drug Administration. (2010a, February 2). *How do I report a problem or illness caused by
an infant formula?* Retrieved from http://www.fda.gov/Food/FoodSafety/Product-SpecificInformation
/InfantFormula/ConsumerInformationAboutInfantFormula/ucm109056.htm

U.S. Food and Drug Administration. (2010b, September 8). *Choosing a breast pump.* Retrieved from
http://www.fda.gov/MedicalDevices/ProductsandMedicalProcedures/HomeHealthandConsumer
/ConsumerProducts/BreastPumps/ucm061939.htm

U.S. Food and Drug Administration. (2010c, September 23). *Infant formula products list.* Retrieved from
http://www.accessdata.fda.gov/scripts/infantformula/index.cfm

U.S. Food and Drug Administration. (2011, December 12). *Infant formula.* Retrieved from http://www.fda
.gov/Food/FoodSafety/Product-SpecificInformation/InfantFormula/default.htm

U.S. Food and Drug Administration. (2012, March 5). *Devices@FDA.* Retrieved from http://www
.accessdata.fda.gov/scripts/cdrh/devicesatfda/index.cfm?st=HGX%20or%20HGY

Wiessinger, D. (1996). Watch your language! *Journal of Human Lactation, 12*(1), 1–4. Retrieved from http://
jhl.sagepub.com/content/12/1/1.full.pdf+html

Wight, N. E., Morton, J. A., & Kim, J. H. (2008). *Best medicine: Human milk in the NICU.* Amarillo, TX:
Hale.

World Alliance for Breastfeeding Action. (2010). *World breastfeeding week 2010.* Retrieved from http://
worldbreastfeedingweek.org

World Health Organization. (1981). *International code of marketing of breast-milk substitutes.* Retrieved from
http://www.who.int/nutrition/publications/code_english.pdf

World Health Organization. (1998). *Evidence for the ten steps to successful breastfeeding (revised).* Geneva,
Switzerland: Author.

World Health Organization. (2003). *Global strategy for infant and young child feeding* [Monograph]. Geneva,
Switzerland: Author.

Chapter 8

The International Code of Marketing of Breast-milk Substitutes

It is formally named *The International Code of Marketing of Breast-milk Substitutes* (International Code, though often also called WHO Code) (International Code Documentation Centre [ICDC], 2007). It is a model policy coming out of the renowned World Health Organization. Governments around the world are to demonstrate their support for this public health policy by turning it into the law in their land. It is a statement that declares marketing of certain commercial products (infant formula and breastmilk substitutes, bottles, and teats/nipples) should not prevail over marketing of good health. It recognizes a simple truth: breastfeeding is the biologic imperative for humans; governments, healthcare providers (HCPs), and manufacturers alike should support and protect breastfeeding, free from inappropriate commercial influences.

Yet many International Board Certified Lactation Consultants (IBCLCs) around the world find the International Code nearly impossible to understand and support in their daily professional lives. They wonder what HCPs and IBCLCs must do, and what happens if they fail to act "the right way." Passions and accusations seem to run high with this subject matter, which further clouds understanding and makes practitioners skittish. According to a 2009 survey of IBCLCs, support for the International Code was identified as the third most difficult tenet under the then-prevailing code of ethics for IBCLCs "to understand" and the most difficult "to abide by" (Noel-Weiss, 2009). Add to this the notion that most IBCLCs toss and turn over ethics problems involving their colleagues (rather than themselves) (Noel-Weiss, 2009), and you have a real quagmire: IBCLCs don't understand the International Code, find it difficult to support, and are troubled by their colleagues whom they think have got it all wrong, too.

The International Code is a *should* that may be turned into a *must* for the IBCLC. This is discussed in detail previously, but the synopsis goes like this: If the International Code has been legislated into law in the geopolitical region where an IBCLC works or lives, then—as a matter of law—the IBCLC will be fully expected to comply with the legislation and/or regulations. Any provisions to enforce the International Code will be a function of the law that was enacted, and the enforcement and sanctions provisions that were included.

The implementation of the International Code is very important for the protection and promotion of breast-feeding and the healthy growth and development of infants. Therefore, any implementation has to be done in a suitable legal instrument, be it a statute, regulations, a decree and so on, within the relevant national context. The implementation of the Code should be done in a reasonable, pragmatic and flexible manner, providing legal bases, in the instrument itself, to meet future changes and developments. Unfortunately, thirty years after the adoption of the Code by the WHA, very few Member States have implemented is as envisaged by the Assembly. (Shubber, 2011, pp. 221–222)

Some countries have taken this responsibility quite seriously: India's law (the Infant Milk Substitutes, Feeding Bottles, and Infant Foods Act of 1992 [amended 2003]) "provides sanctions including fines and imprisonment for violations" (Sokol, 2005, p. 262). In Yemen, sanctions include fines, confiscation, and destruction of products that are either prohibited or not in compliance with standards; sanctions double for repeat offenders and the courts can even order that *any* activity "related to food, infant food or products for children" be halted temporarily or permanently (Sokol, 2005, p. 296).

Another way support for the International Code becomes mandatory is when the IBCLC works at a facility that is seeking or maintaining designation under the Baby-Friendly Hospital Initiative, as such facilities will be expected to support the aims of the International Code (Baby-Friendly USA, 2010; Shubber, 2011; UNICEF, 2012a; World Health Assembly, 1996). Thus, support for the International Code becomes a condition of employment for the IBCLC.

Under the now-replaced International Board of Lactation Consultant Examiners Code of Ethics (IBLCE COE), the IBCLC was required to "adhere to those provisions of the [International Code] which pertain to health workers" (IBLCE, 2003, COE p. 2). The IBLCE Code of Professional Conduct (IBLCE CPC), which replaced the IBLCE COE on November 1, 2011, states that "a crucial part of an IBCLC's duty to protect mothers and children is adherence to the principles and aim of the [International Code]" (IBLCE, 2011a, CPC Introduction at para. 3). However, that language comes in the Introduction, *before* the enumeration of 8 principles (broken down further into 26 subparts) which every IBCLC is "required" to follow (IBLCE, 2011a, CPC Principles Overview, p. 2). The IBLCE Scope of Practice (IBLCE SOP), a *must* document for IBCLCs, states "IBCLCs have the duty to protect, promote and support breastfeeding by complying with the [International Code]" (IBLCE, 2008, SOP para. 4). Similarly, the International Lactation Consultant Association Standards of Practice (ILCA Standards), which describes professional best practice an IBCLC *should* engage in, states "the IBCLC has a responsibility to maintain professional conduct and to practice in an ethical manner [within] the scope of the [International Code]" (ILCA, 2006, Standard 1.2 at p. 1).

Fortunately, the International Code also ranks as the number two subject matter about which IBCLCs are willing to learn more (Noel-Weiss, 2009). And the good news is that the International Code is really *not* all that complicated or difficult to support. This chapter will endeavor to put the International Code, and the expectations for IBCLCs, into plain language.

Who Is WHO, What Is WHA, and When Did It Happen?

Some brief explanation will help put this topic into context. The World Health Organization (WHO), an intergovernmental agency related to the United Nations (UN), is the premiere international health organization. It is multilateral, meaning it gets its funds from many government and nongovernmental sources. It is a separate, autonomous body that works with the UN, and by agreement, with other organizations and countries. Its 1948 constitution states that WHO's main goal is "the attainment by all peoples of the highest possible level of health" (World Health Organization [WHO], 1948, Article 1, p. 2). The governing body of WHO is the World Health Assembly (WHA), which meets annually to set international health policy; the 190+ member nations send delegations to this deliberative body. The Secretariat (with a staff of 4500 around the world) carries on the day-to-day operations of WHO; the executive board (made up of health experts designated by WHA) acts as the liaison between WHA and the Secretariat (International Medical Volunteers Association, n.d., para. 7).

In May 1981, after much advocacy by health experts, governments and nongovernmental organizations (NGOs), intense lobbying on the part of infant formula manufacturers, and politicking between the member delegations (Sokol, 2005), the member states of the World Health Organization adopted, at the annual World Health Assembly deliberations on health policy, the *International Code of Marketing of Breastmilk Substitutes*, by a vote of 118 member states in favor, 1 against (the United States), with 3 abstentions.[1]

They were joined in support of this document by the United Nations Children's Fund (which still goes by the acronym UNICEF, even though the original name of "United Nations International Children's Emergency Fund" was abandoned in 1953) (UNICEF, 2012b). Procedurally, the document passed as an "annex to WHA Resolution 34.22," which urges member states to adopt legislation or regulations within their boundaries to give the International Code effect (ICDC, 2007). As a "recommendation" (versus the more powerful, but hard-to-pass, WHA "convention" or "regulation" [Sokol, 2005]), the statement is a *minimum model policy* outlining the general public health objectives of promoting and protecting breastfeeding against the inappropriate commercial influence of heavily marketed breastmilk substitutes. It must be implemented country by country, but was considered a ground-breaking piece of policy: "perhaps the most significant international consumer protection standard of modern time" (Baumslag & Michels, 1995, p. 164).

But the document isn't contained in a 1981 time capsule. It was recognized at passage that the policy objectives would need to be revisited over time.

---

[1] "In 1994 the United States voted for the first time in favor of a World Health Assembly resolution on infant and young child feeding (Resolution 47.5). The resolution reaffirmed support for the International Code and the subsequent relevant resolutions, meaning that the United States finally joined in supporting the Code and resolutions that endorse it" (Armstrong & Sokol, 2001, p. 6).

The Director General of WHO was charged with producing a report in even years on the state of implementation, and to give suggestions for further action. Accordingly resolutions have been adopted *clarifying and amplifying* the International Code. These subsequent, relevant resolutions enjoy the same status as the International Code itself. (International Baby Food Action Network [IBFAN], n.d.f., para. 6, emphasis added)

Thus, while updating and modernizing the International Code is allowed, resolutions cannot be used as a backdoor means to substantively alter the original policy document. Resolutions can be used to offer the clarity or amplification that countries seeking to implement (or advocates seeking to support) the International Code may need.

And so, approximately every two years, WHA has adopted resolutions that clarify the International Code. Resolutions carry the same legal weight and status as the original document that they seek to clarify. Thus, the International Code, to be fully understood, must be read together with all the subsequent relevant WHA resolutions that have been passed since 1981. For this reason, the document is most correctly cited as *"The International Code of Marketing of Breast-milk Substitutes* and all subsequent relevant World Health Assembly Resolutions."* By far the easiest means to view these materials is on the International Baby Food Action Network (IBFAN) website, which has the full text of the International Code and all the WHA resolutions (IBFAN, n.d.c.) (www.ibfan.org/issue-international_code-code.html).

Spellings and Shorthand

The original document used the spelling *breast-milk*, as was prevalent in the day. Since then, *breastmilk* has been adopted as the preferred spelling by most practitioners, research journals, and major health organizations, including UNICEF, IBFAN, and the International Code Documentation Centre (ICDC), which is charged with tracking International Code compliance by companies and governments (Sokol, 2005). These august organizations use the spelling *breastmilk* and *breastfeeding* even when citing the original policy document itself.

The International Code of Marketing of Breast-milk Substitutes has been shortened into several phrases: *International Code, WHO Code, WHO/UNICEF Code,* or simply *the Code.* While perhaps *International Code* is the more appropriate shorthand term given the original title, the phrase *WHO Code* is commonly used by IBCLCs. So, for this chapter, as throughout this book, shorthand reference to the document in discussion will be *WHO Code* or *International Code,* and IBCLCs may be similarly correct in either usage.

Here we are, thus far, in our plain language explanation for IBCLCs of the WHO Code:

- The WHO Code is a minimum model policy that seeks to support and promote breastfeeding and to limit improper marketing of certain products.

- It says governments should restrict inappropriate marketing of breastmilk substitutes.
- Anyone may choose to support WHO Code objectives, but it must be enacted into law to have enforcement power.

The WHO Code in a Nutshell

The Preamble and Article 1 of the WHO Code are very clear and synopsize what IBCLCs know, overall, about human lactation: breastfeeding is unequalled food for the healthy growth and development of infants. Inappropriate feeding practices lead to infant malnutrition, morbidity, and mortality. Protection and promotion of breast-feeding is an important part of health care offered by HCPs and their institutions, and supported by governments. Further, while there is a legitimate market (as in, commerce) for infant formula (meaning: it can be sold and purchased), such products should not be *marketed* (as in, advertised) in a way that disrupts breastfeeding (ICDC, 2007). Thus, the title gives you a major clue about WHO Code: it concerns *marketing* and *breastmilk substitutes.*

Article 2 tells us the scope of the WHO Code: it applies to the *marketing* of four product types:

1. Infant formula
2. Feeding bottles
3. Teats [nipples]
4. Breastmilk substitutes: other foods or liquids meant to replace breastmilk, in whole or part. Examples of this hard-to-summarize category: cereals meant to be dissolved in breastmilk or formula and fed by bottle; follow-up formula/ milks meant to replace breastfeeding; sugary or fruit drinks given by bottle/ teat before 6 months of age; baby foods pushed on babies before 6 months of age,[2] the age to which they should be exclusively breastfed according to the Global Strategy for Infant and Young Child Feeding (GSIYCF) (WHO, 2003, p. 7). Basically, "breastmilk substitutes" are anything that is suggested to be given to a child in lieu of breastfeeding at breast.

---

[2] It didn't take the formula makers long to try to find a loophole. They figured, maybe if we call our product something other than infant formula, we won't have to comply with the International Code. So a flurry of "add-on" and "toddler" and "specialty" formulas was quickly packaged and marketed (Walker, 2001). WHA Resolution 39.28, passed in 1986, clarifies that these "follow-up milks" are not needed for the baby's health, to emphasize that the WHO Code proscriptions should be extended to cover marketing practices for them (ICDC, 2007, p. 29). In 1996, WHA Resolution 49.15 also emphasized that marketing of complementary foods in ways that undermine exclusive breastfeeding up to 6 months, and sustained breastfeeding from months 6–24, is inappropriate.

Article 3 provides definitions of important words and phrases in the WHO Code.

Article 4 gives governments (whose motivation is the public health of their citizens), rather than marketers of commercial products (whose motivation is profit) the job of ensuring families receive objective and consistent information about child feeding. The superiority of breastfeeding and the risk of artificial feeding must be emphasized.

Article 5 states no marketing directly to the public, which means mothers. No samples, no coupons, no ads in magazines, no website specials, no mothers' clubs, no incentives—nothing. And marketers or sales people should not have direct contact with mothers.

Article 6 warns healthcare systems against being a conduit for commercial messages about infant feeding. Do not promote products covered by the International Code, do not have displays or posters about them, and do not freely give out samples.

Article 7 covers "health workers," which includes IBCLCs. Our requirements under WHO Code Article 7 are:

a. Encourage and protect breastfeeding.
b. Do not *accept* financial or material inducements from the marketers of products covered by the International Code: No freebies, no gifts, no mugs, no bags, no mouse pads, no books, no vacations, no stethoscopes, no stethoscope clip-ons, no ID badge holders, no meals, no pens, no calendars, no posters, and so on.
c. Report to your employer if you accept any funds or grants from the makers of such products.

As for the manufacturers and marketers, their responsibilities under Article 7 are:

a. Provide only scientific and factual information about the products to health workers (offer the research results, not a four-color brochure, brand-and-logo covered, touting the product's virtues, as written by the sales promotions department).
b. Do not *offer* financial or material inducements to health workers: No freebies, no gifts, no mugs, no bags, no mouse pads, no books, no vacations, no stethoscopes, no stethoscope clip-ons, no ID badge holders, no meals, no pens, no calendars, no posters, and so on.
c. Provide samples of products only if they are to be used for research at the institutional level.
d. Report to institutions any contributions given to their health workers in the form of funds or grants.

Article 8 covers persons employed by the manufacturers and distributors of products covered by the International Code. Their salary is not to be tied to sales volumes; sales persons should not be conducting any education of mothers.

Article 9 defines the rules for labels that must appear on any of the products covered by the WHO Code. The superiority of breastfeeding must be stated, with a warning that substitutes should be used only under advice of a health worker. Pictures and language may not idealize the use of breastmilk substitutes. Proper ingredient, preparation, and storage instructions must be shown.

Article 10 requires that any product covered by the WHO Code must meet international food quality and safety standards.

Article 11 covers implementation and monitoring: governments should enact legislation or regulations to make the International Code the law of their land; they should monitor marketing activities and report infractions. Manufacturers should take it upon themselves to comply. Governments should be aided in monitoring and enforcement by manufacturers, NGOs, professional groups, consumer groups, and individuals. Periodic reports will be made to WHO on the progress of international implementation of the WHO Code.

The WHO Code in a Nutshell for the IBCLC: What Is Allowed

Any IBCLC may talk to any mother, one-on-one, about any product, in a clinical setting. This bears repeating, because nearly every concern a conscientious IBCLC has about complying with the International Code is based on a misimpression that she has some sort of gag order on discussing the proper use or sale of the products covered by the WHO Code. *Any IBCLC may talk to any mother, one-on-one, about any product, in a clinical setting.*

You can talk about the proper use (and cleaning) of bottles and teats, along with the use of the many other options for getting expressed breastmilk or a breastmilk substitute into a baby (e.g., dropper, cup, syringe, and tube feeder). You can talk about the use of formula. It may have been ordered by the pediatrician or neonatologist; the IBCLC will discuss how to properly prepare it (World Health Organization & Food and Agriculture Organization of the United Nations, 2007), and offer it to baby (along with appropriate suggestions about increasing mother's milk supply or assisting the baby to better transfer what milk is there). You can talk about breast pumps (not covered by the WHO Code) even if the pump manufacturer has failed to meet its obligations under the International Code for its marketing of bottles and teats. When there is an IBCLC and a mother in a consultation about lactation, and in development of a care plan, the IBCLC may offer evidence-based information and support on any aspect, whatsoever, of lactation care. This notion is also supported by the IBLCE SOP (at paragraph 4).

Some IBCLCs are under the further misimpression that they have special (or extra-onerous) responsibilities and duties under the International Code. Not so. We fall under the WHO Code definition at Article 3 for "health worker" in a "healthcare system" just like any other healthcare provider or volunteer breastfeeding supporter who works with mothers and babies:

Health care system means governmental, nongovernmental, or private institutions or organisations engaged, directly or indirectly, in health care for mothers, infants, and pregnant women; and nurseries or child-care institutions. It also includes health workers in private practice. For the purposes of this Code, the healthcare system does not include pharmacies or other established sales outlets.

Health worker means a person working in a component of such a healthcare system, whether professional or nonprofessional, including voluntary, unpaid workers. (Article 3 Definitions, in ICDC, 2007, p. 4)

If she does not have a retail component to her practice, it will be especially easy for the IBCLC to support the WHO Code, particularly when she is already following the IBLCE CPC, IBLCE SOP, and ILCA Standards of Practice cautioning against conflicts of interest when using or discussing any commercial products. What the WHO Code requires is really pretty simple:

- Promote and protect breastfeeding (WHO Code Article 7.1).
- Do not accept any "material or financial inducements" (gifts or money) from those who market the products falling under the WHO Code (WHO Code Article 7.3).
- Do not accept free samples of products covered by the WHO Code, unless you are doing legitimate scientific research (WHO Code Article 7.4).
- Do not give free samples to families of products covered by the WHO Code, period (WHO Code Article 7.4).
- If you do accept any money or gifts from a marketer covered by the WHO Code, disclose it (WHO Code Article 7.5).

If the IBCLC does have a retail component to her practice, or she is in a position at her facility to negotiate contracts, she may have to meet with manufacturers of the products falling under the International Code. This is perfectly acceptable. The whole notion of the WHO Code is to remove unnecessary and unfair commercial marketing practices from the discussion and conduct of breastfeeding support. To have formula, bottles, nipples/teats, and breastmilk substitutes *purchased* (for subsequent resale or use with patients), under a fair contract negotiated at arm's length and in accord with prevailing market standards, is exactly what should be occurring. Have the meeting and conduct it with the same professionalism and seriousness as any other business- or practice-related meeting. This is required under Baby-Friendly Hospital Initiative (BFHI) objectives as well: formula should be purchased by hospitals (UNICEF, 2012a), just as they purchase foods to feed patients and medical supplies to treat them.

The WHO Code in a Nutshell for the IBCLC: What Is Not Allowed

What the IBCLC cannot do is market anything to a mother, overtly or subtly, while acting in the position of consultant to a mother or patient. If you walk in looking like a billboard, using the formula company pen to write on the bottle company clipboard, using the "add-on formula" brochure (complete with brand and logo) to discuss introduction of solids, while wearing an ID lanyard from the teat company, you are inappropriately marketing products covered by the International Code. This is frowned upon by the WHO Code itself at Articles 4.2, 4.3, 5.1, 6.2, 6.3, 7.2, and 7.3 (ICDC, 2007). Not just WHO Code tensions but any direct or implied conflicts of interest are problematic, under *all* of your practice-guiding documents: the IBLCE CPC at the Introduction and Principles 1.4, 5.1, 5.2, and 6.1; the IBLCE SOP at paragraphs 4 and 8; and the ILCA Standards of Practice at Standards 1.2 and 1.3.

If you have a retail side to your practice, you will have to be especially cognizant of the many hats you wear, and not cross the line into International Code violation or conflicts of interest territory. Bear in mind that the WHO Code does *not* prohibit you, in your retail capacity, from *selling* products covered by the International Code. And mothers may come in and buy them.

> The Code Preamble specifies that there is a legitimate market for infant formula. Article 1 elaborates the aim, one part of which is "ensuring the proper use of breastmilk substitutes, when these are necessary, on the basis of adequate information and through appropriate marketing and distribution." The Code clearly intends to correct *un*necessary use of breastmilk substitutes, *in*adequate information, and *in*appropriate marketing and distribution. (Armstrong & Sokol, 2001, pp. 6–7, emphasis in original)

What Products Are Not Covered by the WHO Code?

Many products we come across in our IBCLC practice are not covered by the WHO Code at all. We may use the products or devices as part of our clinical practice; mothers will often ask us about these items. A non-exhaustive list includes:

- Breast pumps (whether manual or electric)
- Milk collection containers (a.k.a. bottles) that get attached to a breast pump for use, and then sealed with a flat cap (not a teat/nipple)
- Nipple shields and breast shells
- Feeding tube devices for use at breast or by finger
- Nursing bras, or bustiers for hands-free pump use
- Nipple creams and salves
- Teas, tinctures, vitamins, homeopathic or herbal remedies intended to affect milk supply
- Slings, baby seats, baby carriers, "coverings" for breastfeeding in public
- Stools, nursing pillows, books, maternity clothing, rockers, cribs/bassinettes, side-car sleepers, infant car seats
- Specialty feeders for use by babies with congenital conditions precluding effective feeds at breast
- Medicines (prescription, over-the-counter, and street drugs)

- Paladais, syringes, cups, or spoons to offer supplements to an infant
- Pacifiers (dummies)

Pacifiers and dummies deserve a bit of discussion, because many believe this product is covered by the International Code. The text accompanying a model statute, drafted by ICDC to be used by countries seeking to pass WHO Code legislation, recognizes that while the original International Code did not cover pacifiers/dummies, the WHO Code is a *minimum* model of support for breastfeeding, and countries may expand upon definitions in enacting their own laws:

> *Pacifiers (also known as dummies), are not included in the scope of the International Code*, but there is compelling evidence that they can also inhibit breastfeeding and can be harmful to a baby's health and development [citing to BFHI]. Other devices that can interfere with breastfeeding, such as nipple shields are also included in certain countries. Some countries use a catchall phrase to include other implements. (Sokol, 2005, p. 61) (emphasis added)

There are some countries that have done just that, when enacting legislation in their borders to give force and effect to the WHO Code. Pakistan did so in 2002, going beyond the model WHO Code language (as encouraged by ICDC), to include pacifiers/dummies (and even valves for feeding bottles, and nipple shields) in the definition of products whose inappropriate marketing would be restricted:

> This legislation adopts all provisions of the International Code and subsequent WHO resolutions. It prohibits promotion of any milk produced as partial or total replacement for mother's milk or represented as a complement to mother's milk to meet the growing nutritional needs of an infant. Promotions of feeding bottles, teats, *valves for feeding bottles, pacifiers or nipple shields are also forbidden.* Health workers are not permitted to receive any offers including gifts, free samples, and sponsorship from these companies. (Salasibew, Kiani, Faragher, & Garner, 2008, para. 10, emphasis added)

The confusion about pacifiers/dummies is certainly understandable, since the BFHI walks hand in hand with the WHO Code as an international policy promoting breastfeeding support as a best practice for infant feeding and health. BFHI, launched in 1991 as a joint WHO/UNICEF effort, recognizes birthing and maternity centers that support breastfeeding by implementing the Ten Steps to Successful Breastfeeding (UNICEF, 2012a). And, right there in the Ten Steps is No. 9: "Give no artificial teats or pacifiers (also called dummies or soothers) to breastfeeding infants" (WHO, 1998, p. 5). Combined with the BFHI requirement that birthing facilities provide *no* free or below-cost samples of infant formula (similar to the WHO Code's prohibition; see Articles 5.2, 5.3, 5.4, 6.6, 6.7, and 7.4), it is no wonder that some IBCLCs have a difficult time keeping track of which products are subject to marketing prohibitions, and which are not.

Where are we now, in our plain language explanation for IBCLCs of the WHO Code? To repeat and build upon what we have learned thus far:

- The WHO Code is a minimum model policy that seeks to support and promote breastfeeding and to limit improper marketing of certain products.
- It says governments should restrict inappropriate marketing of breastmilk substitutes.
- Anyone may choose to support WHO Code objectives, but it must be enacted into law to have enforcement power.
- It covers four product-types: infant formula, bottles, teats, and breastmilk substitutes meant to replace breastfeeding.
- IBCLCs are health workers who must support the WHO Code, by promoting and protecting breastfeeding and by refusing gifts or money from marketers of products covered by the WHO Code.
- The WHO Code allows the covered products to be sold and purchased; it prohibits them from being inappropriately marketed.
- Any IBCLC may talk to any mother, one-on-one, about any product, in a clinical setting.

Who Is Who in WHO Code Monitoring and Enforcement?

Many IBCLCs will freely admit that keeping track of the hierarchy of decision makers and enforcers for this international policy document, as important as it is to the field of human lactation, is hard to understand. Here's the plain language version.

There Is No "WHO Code Court"

There is *no* "WHO Code Court." There is no single, penultimate arbiter of all matters involving the International Code whose decisions carry the weight of law. But what about WHO and WHA? Recall the following concepts: the "rule of law," "precedence" (the importance of respect for the prior rulings on the same subject matter), and a hierarchy in the legal system to define who shall decide questions of law or controversies of fact. The International Code is a model document. It is not a law unto itself; "as an international recommendation the Code is to be put into effect at the national level" (Sokol, 2005, p. vii). To be sure, having WHO, the premiere international body supporting public health, encourage nations to enact this legislation carries significant weight and panache. But WHO can't force a country to enact the law; that is up to leaders of the individual nations. "This process continues to be very slow. [It] was not a matter of disinterest; it was rather that governments found it complicated to transform global recommendations into national legislation or other measures that could be implemented and monitored" (Sokol, 2005, p. ii).

As such the WHO Code has enforcement teeth *only* in those countries that have turned it into law, and their law only extends as far as their own borders. Without legislative action to back up the International Code, support is voluntary (as is the case in the United States). As expansive as is the 2002 legislation passed in Pakistan (described a few paragraphs above), it is the law of the land *only* in Pakistan. A listing of the countries that have enacted all or part of the WHO Code is issued every 3 years by the ICDC; newer reports are available for purchase, and older ones may be downloaded (www.ibfan.org) (IBFAN, 2011).

WHO Code Experts and Monitors

There are several organizations that exist to provide education about and monitoring of the WHO Code. IBFAN actually predates the WHO Code and was instrumental in organizing support for and original passage of the International Code:

> The International Baby Food Action Network, IBFAN, consists of public interest groups working around the world to reduce infant and young child morbidity and mortality. IBFAN aims to improve the health and well-being of babies and young children, their mothers, and their families through the protection, promotion, and support of breastfeeding and optimal infant feeding practices. IBFAN works for universal and full implementation of the International Code and Resolutions. IBFAN is one of the longest-surviving single-issue organisations. IBFAN was founded on October 12, 1979, after the joint meeting of WHO and UNICEF on Infant and Young Child Feeding (IBFAN, n.d.e, paras. 1–2).

IBFAN has an international office headquartered in Malaysia, with eight regional offices located through the world (IBFAN, n.d.a., n.d.e.). IBFAN is actually a dense network of organizations (large, small, volunteer, and paid) all over the world that support the goal of WHO Code implementation. The International Code Documentation Centre (ICDC) was created in 1985 to track WHO Code implementation efforts worldwide and to offer legal and legislative expertise toward such efforts (IBFAN, n.d.d.). IBFAN and ICDC are considered the preeminent experts on the history of the International Code, and are continuing efforts to implement it and monitor compliance worldwide. They both serve to push a political and policy agenda, but it happens to be one that lactation professionals can (and should) agree with.

The International Code at Article 11 calls for implementation *and monitoring*, and in keeping with the latter requirement, IBFAN and ICDC publish triennial monitoring reports of WHO Code compliance, broken out by countries (that have enacted WHO Code legislation) and companies (for whom WHO Code violations have been reported) (IBFAN, 2011). These reports are always entitled *Breaking the Rules; Stretching the Rules* and the changing year of publication will be included in the title. They are compiled from reports of WHO Code violations submitted to IBFAN (IBFAN, n.d.b.) or its member organizations. The National Alliance for Breastfeeding

Advocacy (in the United States) has published two reports of International Code violations in the United States (Walker, 2001, 2007), as part of their monitoring efforts (NABA, n.d.b.).

Anyone who supports the WHO Code can be a "monitor." The reported violations can come from anyone: a mother, a professional association, an IBCLC, or a public health minister. Nearly all of IBFAN's member organizations serve as monitors of the WHO Code by collecting reports of Code-violating activities in their region. Some groups are more visible than others in advocacy efforts, depending on their organization and funding; well-known groups in the lactation community are INFACT Canada (Infant Feeding Action Coalition [INFACT], n.d.), Baby Milk Action in the United Kingdom (Baby Milk Action, n.d.), and the Geneva Infant Feeding Association (GIFA), also acting as the European Regional Coordinating Office for IBFAN (Association Genevoise pour L'Alimentation Infantile, 2007).

WHO Code Advocacy

These WHO Code experts and monitors serve another important purpose for marketers who seek to comply with the WHO Code's objectives: they advise companies on how to change their practices to align with the WHO Code (National Alliance for Breastfeeding Advocacy, n.d.a.; Massachusetts Breastfeeding Coalition, 2007). They focus all day, every day, on the WHO Code, which is critically important in the swiftly evolving commercial and marketing world. When the International Code was first passed in 1981, no one had ever heard of the elements making up the core of Millennial Mom's modern day life: the Internet, home and laptop computers, cell phones, and social networks. The means of marketing WHO-Code-covered products directly to mothers has increased exponentially since 1981. Companies themselves are in constant flux; corporate buyouts and mergers result in changes in names, missions, and product lines at a dizzying pace. Having motivated, articulate, and politically savvy advocates looking out for the WHO Code and its purposes is tremendously important to mothers, babies, and public health worldwide. IBCLCs are well served to remind themselves, when reviewing materials from any source whatsoever, to ponder what might motivate the commentary. Advocates all have an agenda of one kind or another; that is the essence of advocacy. Being passionate about a cause (or agenda) is vital for true advocacy. Advocates must be careful not to overstep or misstate their lines of authority, or overall credibility (and the goal for the advocacy) suffers.

Compliance as Easy as 1-2-3

If the International Code still mystifies you, recall the following motto, which will serve the IBCLC well for both WHO Code, and general conflicts-of-interest purposes: *Don't take the freebies and gifts.* Not a one of them, from any company. Follow this motto in your professional clinical practice, and you will not have to keep track of which products fall under the WHO Code, or which companies are complying with it. And by removing the appearance of an implied (or real) conflict of interest with any commercial entity, the IBCLC meets her general professional requirement (much broader than that involving the International Code) against conflicts of interest (IBLCE, 2011a, CPC Principles 1.4, 5.1, 5.2, & 6.1; IBLCE, 2008, SOP para. 8; ILCA, 2006, Standards 1.3 & 3.3.6; ICDC, 2007, Preamble and Articles 4, 5, 6, & 7).

Some Quiz Questions

What happens when we apply our understanding of International Code support and compliance to real-life situations? What follows are a series of quiz questions, drawn from real situations IBCLCs have faced. The answers are the result of the author's analysis of the facts, in light of the requirements of the IBCLC's practice-guiding documents (including, of course, the WHO Code). Bear in mind that, as these answers are not provided by a national government that has enacted the International Code, they carry no weight of law. Similarly, recognized experts and monitors of the WHO Code may offer well-informed responses to inquiries about the WHO Code, but their opinions carry the weight of respect, without the weight of law.

WHO Code Problem? RN IBCLC in Hospital NICU

Question: RN IBCLC works in a hospital-based neonatal intensive care unit (NICU). The neonatologist has ordered formula for an infant/patient, to be given by bottle, after 20 minutes spent feeding at breast. RN IBCLC must talk to the mother about implementing this care plan. Is this an International Code problem?

Answer: Not at all. Any IBCLC may talk to any mother, one-on-one, about any product, in a clinical setting. She is working in collaboration with the neonatologist who is the infant's primary HCP, discussing with the mother the use of products that are pertinent to the care plan for this baby. The IBCLC may have a different clinical approach she'd like to suggest (e.g., offering the supplement via a non-bottle method); her ability to raise these aspects of care is subject to all the "ordinary" professional tensions of such a discussion. But there is no International Code violation here. The RN IBCLC is not marketing products covered by the WHO Code; she is discussing them in a clinical context.

WHO Code Problem? Private Practice Lactation Consultant (PPLC)

Question: IBCLC in private practice (PPLC) sees mothers in their homes, by appointment. Client called PPLC at her general practitioner's (GP) suggestion; baby is 2 weeks old, still below birth weight, and GP has ordered formula supplements. Baby transferred 0.2 ounces (5 mL) at breast at the lactation consultation; mother now needs to know how to feed the formula supplement to the baby. Is this an International Code problem?

Answer: Not at all. Any IBCLC may talk to any mother, one-on-one, about any product, in a clinical setting. Under these facts, we have a baby who is not gaining appropriately, and is not transferring milk at breast. There could be any number of reasons for this; that is why the IBCLC is on the scene. Rule No. 1 is Feed the Baby (Smith, 1997), and this baby not only needs a supplement, it has already been ordered by the baby's HCP. Indeed, it would be a violation of WHO Code Article 6.5 *not* to instruct this mother, as a health worker, on the proper preparation of and feeding of infant formula:

> 6.5 Feeding with infant formula, whether manufactured or home-prepared, should be demonstrated only by health workers, or other community workers if necessary; and only to the mothers or family members who need to use it; and the information given should include a clear explanation of the hazards of improper use. (ICDC, 2007, p. 7)

Of course, the IBCLC will also be working closely with the mother to protect and increase her milk supply, discussing techniques to improve baby's latch and suckling, and charting or sending reports to the HCP on the care plan devised. But this situation does not present an International Code problem.

WHO Code Problem? Hospital-Based IBCLC Part 1

Question: Hospital with a large maternity floor accepts free formula from the manufacturer, which is used for any patient babies. It is administered by the HCPs to the babies, or provided to the mothers to offer to their newborns. The facility also gives, to every discharging mother, a free gift bag (also called a "discharge bag") containing product samples of formula, brochures about baby care and breastfeeding showing the formula company's brand and logo, and coupons to purchase more of the product. IBCLC is asked to give the bags to the discharging mothers as part of her work. Is this an International Code problem?

Answer: Yes: this is the quintessential International Code problem. The facility is accepting free formula (rather than purchasing it, like any other supply in the hospital). It is asking HCPs to give out WHO-Code-covered product samples to mothers. This goes against WHO Code Articles 5.2 (manufacturers may not indirectly distribute samples [through HCPs]); 6.2 (healthcare facilities should not promote WHO-Code-covered products), 6.3 (healthcare facilities should not distribute promotional materials), 6.6 (donations of formula allowed under restrictive, not general purposes) and 7.4 (health workers should not distribute samples of WHO-Code-covered products) (ICDC, 2007). The scenario does provide an opening for the IBCLC to educate her colleagues and superiors about why distribution of such discharge bags presents a conflict of professional interest, in addition to violating the WHO Code (the IBLCE CPC at Introduction and Principles 1.4, 5.1, 5.2, & 6.1; the IBLCE SOP at paras. 4 & 8; and the ILCA Standards of Practice at Standards 1.2 & 1.3).

WHO Code Problem? Hospital-Based IBCLC Part 2

Question: Hospital with a large maternity floor accepts free formula from the manufacturer, which is used for any patient-babies. The facility also gives, to every discharging mother, a free gift bag (also called a "discharge bag"). IBCLC does not touch those discharge bags. She has been able to convince her supervisor that her professional practice-guiding documents, and her own ethics as an allied healthcare provider, require support for the WHO Code. Thus, she cannot distribute those formula samples. She does, however, get her paycheck from the hospital, and the hospital is violating the WHO Code by accepting the formula samples for other HCPs to distribute. Does this make the IBCLC a Code violator, too, by accepting her paycheck? Is this an International Code problem?

Answer: No. The International Code looks to regulate the marketing behaviors of manufacturers and marketers. The healthcare system in this example should *not*, under the International Code, be accepting free samples or handing them out (and unless the facility is in a country where the WHO Code has been legislated into law, there will be no sanctions that can be brought to bear). But the International Code does not go beyond this "first tier" of analysis. "Any practice related to any of the activities covered by the definition of marketing, would, in general be subject to the International Code, [as] long as it concerns a product covered by the Code" (Shubber, 2011, p. 68). This is pretty plain on its face: look to see if the product involved is covered by the WHO Code; next, see if inappropriate marketing is going on. The IBCLC in this scenario gets her paycheck from the hospital, *not* the formula manufacturer. Unless she gets paid directly by the formula manufacturer, she is not taking "financial or material inducements" from the WHO Code marketer (which violates Article 7.3 of the WHO Code). As a practical matter, if IBCLCs around the world could only work and by paid by WHO-Code-supporting or BFHI facilities, there would not be many IBCLCs hired to provide education and support to breastfeeding families and healthcare providers. So long as the IBCLC is receiving her compensation from the facility, she is secure in knowing that she may continue to work there, advocating for change to help breastfeeding mothers and supporting the WHO Code by eradicating undue commercial influences.

WHO Code Problem? Hospital Gift Shop

Question: Hospital has a retail gift store in the lobby, where it hopes to capture business from the families who delivered their children there, and the visitors who come to see them. Among other items, the gift store sells (a) pacifiers, (b) nursing bras and tops, (c) bottles and teats, and (d) breastfeeding and parenting how-to books. Is this an International Code problem?

Answer: No, *unless*. The only products that matter, for purposes of International Code analysis, are the bottles and teats; the other items do not fall under the WHO Code at all. The International Code does not prohibit the sale of bottles and teats, but it does seek to restrict inappropriate marketing. The *unless* part means it is not a WHO Code problem to sell the bottles/teats *unless* they are being *inappropriately marketed* by the gift store (which is run by the healthcare facility). The bottles may not have any special language on the packaging that idealizes their use or suggests they are just as good or a replacement for breastfeeding (WHO Code, Article 9). Consumers should not be induced to buy through coupons, special sales, and flashy shelf ads (WHO Code, Article 5.3). Simple descriptions of the bottles can be on the packaging (size, materials used in manufacturer, cleaning instructions, price), but not much more.

WHO Code Problem? Pediatric Office

Question: Sales representative for the formula company has visited the administrative office manager at a small pediatric practice. He left behind pens, mugs, and sticky note-pads emblazoned with the company's formula brand logo. The office administrator is thrilled, because her budget for office supplies is just about depleted, and this will save the practice lots of money. She doesn't see patients, she works in the office all day. Is this an International Code problem?

Answer: Yes. Even though the office administrator does not work directly with patients, she is part of an office that is engaged in the healthcare of infants (WHO Code, Article 3). These gifts and freebies are the kind of inducements to healthcare professionals prohibited by Article 7.3 of the WHO Code. That the sales represen-tative offered the gifts to the office staff rather than the clinicians is irrelevant: he is trying to curry favor, and a sense of reciprocity, which is just the sort of aggres-sive marketing the International Code is designed to prevent. It is marketing to the general public—not just mothers and infants, but everyone—that is prohibited by Article 5 of the WHO Code.

WHO Code Problem? Public Health Clinic

Question: The staff at a public health clinic (that primarily serves low-income women and children) wants to liven up the office a bit. The maker of baby foods, marketed to children 4–6 months of age, has some gorgeous color posters of mothers and chil-dren. Their logo and brand is on the bottom of the poster. The staff wants to use the posters, but they will cut off the part with the brand name and logo before they are put on the walls, so no one knows that a company made them. Is this an International Code problem?

Answer: Yes. Even if a clinic patron may not realize that the poster came from a company that violates the WHO Code, the health workers and the public health clinic know it. Such posters not only violate Article 6.3 of the International Code, but obtaining them from the company necessarily means the sales representative is in the office, chatting up the staff, and creating those friendly relationships that later can be exploited for commercial purposes.

WHO Code Problem? Lactation Conference

Question: Your small hospital wants to have a one-day breastfeeding conference, and invite speakers to offer education to hospital staff, local breastfeeding support group counselors, and others HCPs who work with families. To offset costs, they will allow exhibitors to set up booths to show and sell their wares. A formula company wants to set up a booth. Is this an International Code problem?

Answer: No . . . but be careful. Manufacturers may provide information about WHO-Code-covered products to health professionals as long as it is "scientific and factual" information (WHO Code, Article 7.2). Note that giving out trinkets with the brand and logo on it, or passing out brochures written by the marketing department, is not offering "scientific and factual" information. "Information relating to factual matters may cover the questions of the storage of the product, its correct preparation for use, and the quantities to be used and so on. Therefore, any information which goes outside this field, be it promotional, educational or public relations, would not be compatible with Article 7.2" (Shubber, 2011, pp. 159–160). At a professional educational conference, where HCP colleagues rub elbows, they are "on their toes" and thinking critically not only about the speakers and educational sessions, but about the products and services advertised in the exhibit hall. What better place to clarify or challenge the claims being made, than in a teaching/learning environment? This is an entirely different "audience" than the unsuspecting pregnant woman, who sits down in her obstetric office, and flips open a magazine, only to be inundated with ads for products she is told she "has to have" to make her baby smart, or non-fussy, or able to sleep all night.

Be aware that the trend, for educational offerings to any medical professionals, is to preclude the conflict of interest inherent in any commercial influences by pharmaceutical and medical device manufacturers (e.g., those making formula and breast pumps) (Lo & Field, 2009). The International Board of Lactation Consultant Examiners will deny Continuing Education Recognition Points (CERPs) for education sessions that cannot meet this standard (IBLCE, 2011b).

WHO Code Problem? Breast Pump Rental Station

Birthing doula and childbirth educator run a storefront operation with classes for pregnant/new mothers, and offer a range of products of interest to families with young children. The owners are supporters of the International Code, even though it is not legislated in their country. One of their active retail services is breast pump sales and rentals. One breast pump company begins to market bottles and teats in a manner that does not meet their obligations under the WHO Code. The owners wonder if they must now stop renting those pumps. Do they have an International Code problem?

Answer: No. Breast pumps are not covered under the International Code. Once the company moved into inappropriate marketing of bottles and teats, the company failed to meet its obligations under the WHO Code, and thus it "tainted" the whole company. The retailer who supports the International Code will take care not to be seen as *marketing* for the Code violator. Recall that the International Code does *not* prohibit the *sale* of covered products (infant formula, bottles, teats, and breastmilk substitutes meant to replace breastfeeding). Marketing of the breast pump company's products may now need to be curtailed at the storefront location, because of their changed status vis-à-vis the International Code, but the owners may continue their business relationship with breast pump company. Indeed, the WHO Code envisions that transactions with any companies should be done on an arms-length, business-only basis, and not be subject to coercive marketing tactics. If a customer comes in and asks about one of those pumps, the owners can discuss the pump and its various pros and cons, and even rent or sell one. But they should not, now, be marketing the product by having it prominently displayed in the window, or subject to discounts, and so on.

WHO Code Problem? NICU with Exclusive Breast Pump Contract

Question: A large hospital, part of a chain, has an exclusive contract with one breast pump company to supply pumps at all their facilities. The folks in the procurement office were able to negotiate very favorable terms, due to economies of scale. This hospital has a 25-bed Level III NICU for sick and premature babies, and thus has many mothers who are heavily reliant on breast pumps to establish and maintain breastmilk supply until their babies are able to feed well at breast. The breast pump company is now heavily marketing a bottle and teat as "most like mother." Thus, it is not meeting its obligations under the International Code. Does the exclusive breast pump contract now present an International Code problem?

Answer: No. The hospital procurement officers can, and should, engage in arms-length, business-only negotiations with any vendor. That the contract is with one company only is not an issue; this is a common business practice that brings benefits to both parties. We know that any IBCLC may talk to any mother, one-on-one, about any product, in a clinical setting. Having these pumps in the NICU as part of a care plan is not an issue. There may be repercussions in the future: when the contract is to be renegotiated, the IBCLCs may well suggest that the hospital procurement officers instead negotiate with a company that complies with the WHO Code, allowing the facility to "put its money where its mouth is."

WHO Code Problem? Conference Speaker

Question: IBCLC agrees to speak at a large dietitians' conference that will be held in 10 months' time. When she arrives at the venue, she is mortified to see that it has been heavily sponsored by a formula company: their logo is on the conference syllabus, on the tote-bags given to attendees, even on the podium where the speakers will stand to give their presentations. The speaker verifies with the planners that her honorarium will be paid from funds generated by attendee fees, not sponsor fees. She is solely responsible for the content of her presentation. She is expected to come to a dinner afterward for all the speakers, paid for by the formula sponsor. Is this an International Code problem?

Answer: No as to speaking; Yes as to dinner . . . but be careful. Even though the speaker knows her fees do not come from formula company, this set-up may not pass her personal smell test. It may give the appearance that the IBCLC "endorsed" the product, since she is listed on the syllabus with the formula company logo on it, and will stand (and be photographed) at the podium with the same logo on it. Offering the meal (by the formula company) and accepting it (by the IBCLC) are both prohibited by WHO Code Article 7.3. The speaker is between a rock and a hard place: she has been contracted to speak, and the attendees will expect to see her. She can certainly request that the logo be removed from the podium during her talk; she can declare at the start of her session that she is herself fully compliant with the International Code. The speaker will benefit from this hard-learned lesson by revising her speaking contract template to include her right to be informed of all sponsors, and to withdraw from the contract without penalty if she determines in her sole discretion that sponsors are violators of the International Code.

Summary

To repeat and build upon what we have learned thus far, this is how we end up, in our plain language explanation of the International Code:

- The WHO Code is a minimum model policy that seeks to support and promote breastfeeding and to limit improper marketing of certain products.
- It says governments should restrict inappropriate marketing of breastmilk substitutes.
- Anyone may choose to support WHO Code objectives, but it must be enacted into law to have enforcement power.
- It covers four product types: infant formula, bottles, teats, and breastmilk substitutes meant to replace breastfeeding.
- IBCLCs are health workers who must support the WHO Code, by promoting and protecting breastfeeding, and by refusing gifts or money from marketers of products covered by the WHO Code.
- The WHO Code allows the covered products to be sold and purchased; it prohibits them from being inappropriately marketed.
- Any IBCLC may talk to any mother, one-on-one, about any product, in a clinical setting.
- WHO Code experts and monitors track reports of violations of the WHO Code, and can advise companies seeking to be Code compliant or governments seeking to enact WHO Code legislation.

REFERENCES

Armstrong, H., & Sokol, E. (2001). *The international code of marketing of breastmilk substitutes: What it means for mothers and babies world-wide* [Monograph]. Raleigh, NC: International Lactation Consultant Association.

Association Genevoise pour L'Alimentation Infantile. (2007). *GIFA* [Home page]. Retrieved from http://www.gifa.org

Baby Friendly USA. (2010). *Info for breastfeeding advocates/health care professionals.* Retrieved from http://www.babyfriendlyusa.org/eng/06.html

Baby Milk Action. (n.d.). *About us* [Home page]. Retrieved from http://info.babymilkaction.org

Baumslag, N., & Michels, D. (1995). *Milk, money and madness: The culture and politics of breastfeeding.* Westport, CT: Bergin & Garvey.

Infant Feeding Action Coalition (INFACT) Canada. (n.d.). *What is INFACT?* Retrieved from http://www.infactcanada.ca/about.htm

International Baby Food Action Network. (n.d.a.). *Coordinating the networks activities.* Retrieved from http://www.ibfan.org/ibfan-regional_coordination.html

International Baby Food Action Network. (n.d.b.). *Forms for reporting violations: Monitoring the code.* Retrieved from http://www.ibfan.org/code_watch-form.html

International Baby Food Action Network. (n.d.c.). *The full code.* Retrieved from http://www.ibfan.org/issue-international_code.html

International Baby Food Action Network. (n.d.d.). *Our network: International code documentation centre.* Retrieved from http://www.ibfan.org/our_network-documentation.html

International Baby Food Action Network. (n.d.e.). *What is IBFAN?* Retrieved from http://www.ibfan.org/ibfan-ibfan.html

International Baby Food Action Network. (n.d.f.). *What is the international code?* Retrieved from http://www.ibfan.org/issue-international_code-code.html

International Baby Food Action Network. (2011, October). *ICDC Monitoring.* Retrieved from http://www.ibfan.org/our_network-documentation-monitoring.html

International Board of Lactation Consultant Examiners. (2003). *Code of ethics for international board certified lactation consultants.* Retrieved from http://www.iblce.org/upload/downloads/CodeOfEthics.pdf

International Board of Lactation Consultant Examiners. (2008, March 8). *Scope of practice for international board certified lactation consultants.* Retrieved from http://www.iblce.org/upload/downloads/ScopeOfPractice.pdf

International Board of Lactation Consultant Examiners. (2011a, November 1). *Code of professional conduct for IBCLCs.* Retrieved from http://www.iblce.org/upload/downloads/CodeOfProfessionalConduct.pdf

International Board of Lactation Consultant Examiners. (2011b, November 1). *Minimizing commercial influence on education policy.* Retrieved from http://www.iblce.org/upload/downloads/CommercialInfluenceOnEducation.pdf

International Code Documentation Centre (Ed.). (2007, May). *International code of marketing of breastmilk substitutes and relevant WHA resolutions (annotated)* (2nd updated edition). Penang, Malaysia: IBFAN Penang.

International Lactation Consultant Association. (2006). *Standards of practice for international board certified lactation consultants.* Retrieved from http://www.ilca.org/files/resources/Standards-of-Practice-web.pdf

International Medical Volunteers Association. (n.d.). *The major international health organisations.* Retrieved from http://www.imva.org/Pages/orgfrm.htm

Lo, B., & Field, M. (Eds.). (2009). *Conflict of interest in medical research, education, and practice.* Retrieved from http://www.ncbi.nlm.nih.gov/books/NBK22942/

Massachusetts Breastfeeding Coalition. (2007, October 25). *News item: Evenflo to become code-compliant* [Press release]. Retrieved from http://www.massbfc.org/news/#evenflo

National Alliance for Breastfeeding Advocacy. (n.d.a.). *Code help center.* Retrieved from http://www.naba -breastfeeding.org/nabareal.htm

National Alliance for Breastfeeding Advocacy. (n.d.b.). *Code monitoring.* Retrieved from http://www.naba -breastfeeding.org/nabareal.htm

Noel-Weiss, J. (2009, July 24). *Ethics and lactation consultants: A needs assessment.* Lecture presented at ILCA Annual Conference, Orlando, FL.

Salasibew, M., Kiani, A., Faragher, B., & Garner, P. (2008, October 17). Awareness and reported violations of the WHO international code and Pakistan's national breastfeeding legislation; a descriptive cross-sectional survey. *International Breastfeeding Journal, 3,* 24. Retrieved from http://www.international breastfeedingjournal.com/content/3/1/24

Shubber, S. (2011). *The WHO international code of marketing of breast-milk substitutes history and analysis* (2nd ed.). London, UK: Pinter & Martin.

Smith, L. (1997). *Coach Smith's rules for breastfeeding helpers.* Retrieved from http://www.bflrc.com/ljs /breastfeeding/rulbfhlp.htm

Sokol, E. (2005). *The code handbook: A guide to implementing the international code of marketing of breastmilk substitutes* (2nd ed.). Penang, Malaysia: International Code Documentation Centre and International Baby Food Action Network.

UNICEF. (2012a, March 21). *The baby-friendly hospital initiative.* Retrieved from http://www.unicef.org /programme/breastfeeding/baby.htm

UNICEF. (2012b). *What does UNICEF stand for?* Retrieved from http://www.unicefusa.org/about/faq/what -does-unicef-stand-for.html

Walker, M. (2001). *Selling out mothers and babies: Marketing of breast milk substitutes in the USA* [Monograph]. Weston, MA: NABA REAL.

Walker, M. (2007). *Still selling out mothers and babies: Marketing of breast milk substitutes in the USA.* Weston, MA: NABA REAL.

World Health Assembly. (1996, May 25). *WHA Resolution 49.15—1996.* Retrieved from http://www.ibfan.org /issue-international_code-full-4915.html

World Health Organization. (1948, April). *Constitution of the World Health Organization* [Monograph]. Retrieved from http://www.who.int/governance/eb/who_constitution_en.pdf

World Health Organization. (1981). *International code of marketing of breast-milk substitutes.* Retrieved from http://www.who.int/nutrition/publications/code_english.pdf

World Health Organization. (1998). *Evidence for the ten steps to successful breastfeeding (revised).* Geneva, Switzerland: Author.

World Health Organization. (2003). *Global strategy for infant and young child feeding* [Monograph]. Geneva, Switzerland: Author.

World Health Organization & Food and Agriculture Organization of the United Nations. (2007). *Safe preparation, storage and handling of powdered infant formula: Guidelines* [Monograph]. Retrieved from http://www.who.int/foodsafety/publications/micro/pif_guidelines.pdf

Chapter 9

Intellectual Property Law and the IBCLC

The International Board of Lactation Consultant Examiners Code of Professional Conduct (IBLCE CPC) retains a principle that had been added in 2004 to the predecessor document, the IBLCE Code of Ethics (IBLCE COE). Under the new IBLCE CPC, IBCLCs *must*:

Principle 2: Act with due diligence.

Principle 2.5: Every IBCLC shall [r]espect intellectual property rights. (IBLCE, 2011, CPC p. 2)

It seems unusual that, of all the laws on the books, respect for intellectual property (IP) law was singled out for attention by the organization that administers a certification exam for allied healthcare providers specializing in breastfeeding and human lactation. Why not single out required respect for public health law measures? Or laws upholding women's or children's rights? That seems more pertinent to the professional mission of International Board of Certified Lactation Consultants (IBCLCs). Surely IBCLCs ought to be law-abiding citizens wherever they live, respecting all the laws of their country or state. And yet, there IP law is, singled out as a requirement of the ethical code for our profession. This can be problematic: some IBCLCs have moral or philosophical opposition to such notions as the patenting of human milk components (McClain, 2007), or the use of trade pacts and trademark law to defeat legislation enacted to enforce the *International Code of Marketing of Breast-milk Substitutes* (Love, 1997). The IBLCE did not offer any legislative history when it changed the old IBLCE COE to add this principle, nor was explanation offered when it was retained in the IBLCE CPC. We are left to our imaginings as to why this principle was made a permanent part of the IBLCE CPC.

Intellectual property law is a legal concept that has been embraced for hundreds of years, all over the globe. It has long been used to protect rights over creative works such as books, art, and music. Today, the World Trade Organization (WTO) recognizes the important role in international trade of fair sharing of ideas and knowledge, which is at the root of all intellectual property law. The WTO Agreement of Trade-Related Aspects of Intellectual Property Rights (TRIPS) is an attempt to bring "order and predictability" to trade agreements and transactions between countries by recognizing and defining universal intellectual property concepts (World Trade Organization [WTO], 2012, para. 3). In short: Intellectual property sells.

Most IBCLCs are not negotiating international trade agreements, but every single day we benefit from the use of something that was created via processes that are protected under intellectual property law. The clothes we wear, the manner in which they were marketed to us, the "look" of the store at which they were sold, even the logo on the credit card we used to make the purchase—all have intellectual property rights attached to them, meaning rights (including money) are associated with their creation and use. This book was typed on a computer with a mechanical design under patent protection, using software programs under copyright and license agreements; it was published using machines and techniques that are patented. The content is copyright protected; the design and artwork and marketing for the published book were executed under protected means of trade and merchandising.

As an inescapable part of our lives, and a required element of our IBLCE CPC, intellectual property law is something about which an IBCLC should have a basic understanding. We will explore copyright law in greater detail, as the appropriate use and reproduction of written and Web-based materials is something that IBCLCs come up against nearly every day in their work. One would hope their goal would be to comply with copyright law for its own sake and not only as a function of an IBLCE CPC requirement.

Intellectual Property Law in a Nutshell

Intellectual property laws are similar around the world; IP definitions are fairly constant. In different countries one's means of remedy may be different. IP rights were considered so important that they were recognized in the U.S. Constitution:

> The Congress shall have the Power . . . To promote the Progress of Science and useful Arts, by securing for limited Times to Authors and Inventors the exclusive Right to their respective Writings and Discoveries. (U.S. Constitution, 1787, Article I, Section 8, Clause 8)

The theme underlying intellectual property law is that individuals who are creative and inquisitive and entrepreneurial, those people who are clever enough to invent machines, or create works of art, or write great literature, ought to be the "masters of their work." They should control, at least for a while, the distribution and use of that work, and have first rights to whatever monies might be earned for allowing their product or design to be seen or used by someone else. After a certain period of time, however, their material ought to be made fully and freely available to everyone;

it should be accessible in the "public domain." This will foster innovation (which will spur economic development) because, as more people are given access to the clever ideas of those who came before them, the more innovative and creative their own thinking and design can become. But the originators of the concept ought to be able to have a monopoly on the rights and earnings for that initial time period, to reward their considerable time and effort in coming up with the idea in the first place (Fields, 2004). To be sure: there are those who find this approach to the commoditization of ideas unsound; famously, Thomas Jefferson (Kelty, 2004). But this is now the prevailing legal theory used by governments that have intellectual property laws.

The following sections describe the major categories of intellectual property.

Patents

Patents are granted for physical objects (inventions of: machines, articles of manufacture, composition of matter) or methods of production. A patent may also be awarded for any improvements on any such items. Applications are filed in the national office each country has designated for this purpose; they are enforceable within that country. Under the Patent Cooperation Treaty (PCT), an inventor can file one application, in one language, using a simplified application process should he seek patent protection in several countries (U.S. Patent and Trademark Office, 2011c). But if he plans to have an international market for his product, he will need to seek individual patent protection in all the countries where he hopes to sell. In the United States, the governmental agency that will scrutinize the application (for originality and authenticity) is the U.S. Patent and Trademark Office (USPTO) (USPTO, 2011c). Earning a patent is an arduous and exacting process.

To be patentable, an invention must meet several criteria: (a) it is novel, (b) it is nonobvious (meaning it is more than a simple idea: using a breadknife to open an envelope is "obvious," whereas inventing a specially adapted slicer that cuts paper but not fingers is "nonobvious"), (c) it falls within the statutory definition of what may be patented (such as machines, or a specific manufacturing process), and (d) it meets disclosure requirements (meaning the inventor describes his product with enough detail that once his patent rights expire, others will be capable of accessing and using the information) (USPTO, 2011b).

Once a patent has been granted, several rights flow from it:

- A time-limited (usually 20-year) grant of a *negative* right "to *exclude others* from making, using, offering for sale, or selling the invention" (USPTO, 2011c, para. 2, emphasis added)
- Right to compensation
- Right to sell, assign, or license
- Right to prevent use/sale of goods made by infringing processes (those that copy the patent's process or design) (Fields, 2004)

In the United States, only the human beings who were the inventors may apply for and be granted a patent. Thus, corporations do not own patents; individual inventors do. To be sure: Through contractual arrangement and assignments of rights by the inventor, companies may reap the financial rewards of a good invention. Large corporations with research and development divisions, which employ scientists and inventors to work in their laboratories, will often have employment contract language that requires the inventor to sign over to the company any rights (e.g., royalties, or earnings) in patents that may be granted. This is a fair arrangement: customarily the scientists are paid handsomely, working in well-equipped labs, and are eligible for employee bonuses for their excellent work even if they are not earning direct royalties from the patent. And, the distinction and fame go to the inventor, not the company. Legend has it that the inventor of the hugely successful Post-it Note was paid one dollar in exchange for assigning the rights to the patent to his employer 3M (Fields, 2004). And yet, it was the Post-it Note inventor Arthur Fry who was a 2010 inductee into the National Inventors' Hall of Fame (Invent Now, 2010), not 3M.

Any rights associated with a patent are triggered by the granting of the patent. Unlike copyright (as we will see below) patent rights do not spring from the mere creation (invention) of the object, but rather from proactively completing the legal processes for obtaining a patent. If you invent a machine that turns straw into gold, you will not be able to stop someone else from selling a similar machine using your gold-producing process unless you are the first patent holder for the device.

Historically in the United States, patents were given to the "first to invent." This differs from the law used nearly everywhere else in the world, where patent protection was recognized for "the first inventor to file" (for a patent). However, by March 2013, the law in the United States will align with that used elsewhere (Leahy-Smith America Invents Act of 2011; Leppo, 2011). Under the soon-to-expire patent law in the United States, an inventor has a 1-year grace period after he has revealed his invention (through disclosure, use, or sale) to apply for a patent on the invention. In contrast, in most other countries (and again, by 2013 in the USA), the patent will go to the inventor who demonstrates "absolute novelty" of his invention, or (in some cases) that he was the "first to file." The disparity in legal requirements across the world was apparent if the inventor had "disclosed" his invention in the United States (relying on that 1-year grace period to actually complete his patent application in the USA). He would thus be shut out from patent protections elsewhere, in countries that require him to file his patent application first, *before* showing (or disclosing to) the world his clever device (Kilner, 1998). While there are several international treaties and trade agreements (such as the Patent Law Treaty) to allow patent holders to have their rights recognized and enforced in other countries (USPTO, 2011c), for the inventor it is critical to be recognized as the first person with the patentable idea.

For IBCLCs, a discomfiting aspect of their IBLCE CPC requirement to support all intellectual property law is that patents can (and are) being awarded in the 21st century for processes that manipulate elements found in nature: plants, plant chemicals, and human breastmilk and its various components. International trade agreements requiring respect for intellectual property law (WTO TRIPs) means mandated respect for biodiversity patents, and patents that parse out elements of human breastmilk:

> The debate on the relationship between intellectual property and biodiversity mainly evolves [sic] around the alleged contradiction between the recognition . . . of the states' sovereign rights over their generic resources (or biological material) and the possibility, under the TRIPs Agreement . . . to provide patents on inventions incorporating genetic resources. (European Trade Commission, 2005, para. 1)

This raises the penultimate question: does the legality of a process (i.e., the issuance of the patent) make the result ethically and morally correct? While the philosophers and ethicists debate the notion, tens of thousands of patents involving biological elements have been filed around the world (Lever, 2008).

Trademarks, Service Marks, Certification Marks, and More

Whereas patents are *granted* to demonstrate an enforceable intellectual property right, trademarks and other marks are *registered* to establish enforcement rights (USPTO, 2011a). Having a product bear a trademark (or other such mark) designates the origin of the product or service. This serves as a type of quality control for customers. Buyers are assured that if they buy something with the brand or trademark on it, they are getting what that symbol represents. Similarly, the maker of the product wants to protect that good image and reputation and avoid having his trademark "diluted" because poor-quality knock-offs have been sold with his brand and logo on them. A strong body of common law, in the United States and other countries, also protects the trade and commerce rights that are at issue (usually based on unfair competition or likelihood of confusion theories). Unlike patents, there is no time limit on this intellectual property right: as long as the marks continue to be used in commerce, the registrations may be renewed forever. The different types:

- Trademarks (® once issued; ™ in the registration phase) are used on goods and products, and are the most common form of intellectual property right in this group. They are brand names, and also cover symbols, logos, sounds, designs, even distinctive color configurations on packaging, to identify the source (or maker) of the goods. Trademarks for well-known products include Sharpie permanent markers, Kleenex facial tissues, Verizon telephones, Reebok shoes.
- Service marks (® once issued; SM when in the registration phase) also cover symbols, logos, sounds, and designs that distinguish services offered by one provider over another. Examples include Citibank banks and credit cards, Greyhound bus lines, Wal-Mart retail stores.

- Certification marks (®) are for symbols, logos, sounds, or designs that indicate services are provided by someone who is a member of a [certified] group, or for products that come from a specific location. The obvious example: IBCLC is a certification mark, registered by IBLCE. Another is the UL certification mark, registered by Underwriters Laboratories, to indicate a product meets UL safety requirements. Only potatoes grown in Idaho may be called "Idaho" or "Grown in Idaho."
- Collective marks (®) indicate the person providing the service is a member of a collective [union] (USPTO, 2012). Examples include AAA (American Automobile Association), which provides ratings for hotels and motels along with its roadside assistance, and ILGWU labels, indicating an item of clothing was produced by a member of the International Ladies' Garment Workers Union.
- Geographical indications show that goods originated in a certain place, where location provides an essential attribute (think Champagne, or Vidalia onions, or Scotch whiskey, or, the example used above: Idaho potatoes). Geographical indications have been registered as trademarks, certification marks, and collective marks (USPTO, 2010a).

These insignia for which registration is sought will be evaluated on a continuum, to determine how distinctive and unusual the intended use for the mark is. The more fanciful (Xerox, an invented name), arbitrary (Mercury for a car, not a Greek god), suggestive (Roach Motel, a catchy phrase describing only one product), and distinctively descriptive (Beer Nuts vs. nuts; they have acquired special meaning through use), the better. Owners of these marks (whether trademarks, service marks, certification marks, or collective marks) must be careful to protect their registration, using it as an adjective rather than a noun ("Kleenex-brand tissues"). Otherwise, their protection is lost through common usage (as occurred with *aspirin* and *escalator*, former trademark-protected terms) (Fields, 2004).

The initials I-B-C-L-C are registered as a certification mark. As you may recall, IBLCE registered as certification marks the acronym *IBCLC* and the phrase *Registered Lactation Consultant (RLC)* with the USPTO. Only those who have been designated as *IBCLC* by IBLCE are entitled to use those initials, as "the certification mark, as used by persons authorized [by IBLCE], certifies the quality of the services performed by those approved by the certifier" (IBLCE Certification Mark Reg. No. 2042667, 2007). Similarly, "Registered Lactation Consultant . . . as used by authorized persons, certifies that persons performing lactation consulting have met the standards, qualifications, and testing of the certifier" (IBLCE Certification Mark Reg. No. 2749041, 2003).

Here's an example that can put several intellectual property concepts, literally, onto a piece of paper. Imagine you are an IBCLC, and you want to have some business cards printed to describe your business. The sketches of your logo and company, that you redraw and recolor until you are satisfied, are all copyright protected. Once you have settled on a design, that logo along with your business name can be trademark or service mark protected. The section showing your IBCLC designation is an indication of a certification mark.

Trade Secrets

Patent applications must include very specific details about the invention to determine if the inventor is entitled to a patent because this invention is novel (USPTO, 2011a). There is nothing secret about the process; the designs are all revealed in the application. Similarly, trademarks and other registered marks are for goods and services whose very purpose is to be seen (and sold) in commerce.

Trade secrets are just the opposite: their commercial value derives from their secrecy, which gives the owner a distinct advantage over his competitors. Think of unrevealed recipes for food and drink products, or customer lists, or business plans. Trade secrets tend not to involve technology; as a practical matter, as soon as the physical object is purchased by a competitor, it can be "reverse engineered" to learn its mechanical secrets.

Trade secret protection is a function of state or common law, and generally operates only to protect a commercial enterprise from the unfair appropriation of whatever information it has taken steps to protect (Kelty, 2004). There is no federal law in the United States protecting this right (as with patents, trademarks, and copyrights), but state law provides trade secret protection, and the United States is a party to the WHO TRIPS agreement to give force and effect, in other countries, to trade secret protection (USPTO, 2010b). Like trademark and other marks, there is no time limit on the protection so long as a company can demonstrate continuous efforts to protect the trade secret.

Compare this to the separate concept of a trade *name*. Many jurisdictions will require businesses to register their trade names, along with the names of their (human) business leaders. This is for practical reasons: imagine an abandoned van marked "Acme Baking Co." on the side of the road. The police will use the trade name to determine who the owners are, so as to send them a ticket for the towing and recovery charges. Or, if someone wants to sue Acme Baking Co., they need to be able to find an actual person to whom the process (lawsuit papers) may be served.

Copyright Law

Copyright is the intellectual property right that IBCLCs are most likely to encounter in their professional lives. The concepts are fairly consistent throughout the world, as are the misconceptions. The mechanisms to enforce copyright may differ from country to country (a theme well visited by now in this book), but the basics will remain the same both in the description of the right and its protection. There is no "international copyright" to protect one's work against unauthorized use throughout the world, but treaties between countries have made it simpler to protect and enforce copyright (U.S. Copyright Office, 2011a). We will explore copyright in some detail.

If You Create It, It Is Automatically Copyrighted
Copyrights belong to "original works of authorship" including literary, dramatic, musical, artistic, and other intellectual works (U.S. Copyright Office, 2011a). This includes the research and journal articles that form a significant portion of the IBCLC's required evidence-base for practice (IBLCE, 2011, CPC Principles 1.2 & 1.3; IBLCE Scope of Practice for IBCLCs [IBLCE SOP], 2008, paragraphs 4 & 5; the International Lactation Consultant Association Standards of Practice for International Board Certified Lactation Consultants [ILCA Standards], 2006, Standards 1.8 & 4.5). Copyright is born right along with the creation of the work: "copyright protection subsists from the time the work is created in fixed form" (U.S. Copyright Office, 2011a, p. 2), meaning your child's artwork hanging on your refrigerator is copyrighted; your To Do List for this week is copyrighted; that song you made up and hummed in the shower this morning is copyrighted; that email you sent to your cousin is copyrighted.

Copyright lasts a long time under the law: in the United States, any work produced after January 1, 1978, has automatic copyright protection for "the author's life plus an additional 70 years after the author's death" (U.S. Copyright Office, 2011a, p. 5). Works made "for hire" (e.g., a writer contracted by a magazine to produce a column every month) have a copyright duration of 95 years from publication or 120 years from creation, whichever is shorter. Copyright may be transferred via written agreement, or after death, according to laws of succession (U.S. Copyright Office, 2011a).

Copyright Means Control Over What Happens to the Work
The owner of a copyright has several exclusive rights over which he or she has sole control. The copyright holder may choose to share, sell, transfer, or even ignore these rights, in whatever manner the copyright holder chooses. Copyright provides the *exclusive* right to:

- Reproduce the work (copies, recordings, tapes, etc.)
- Prepare derivative works (e.g., write an edited chapter, for a magazine, from your previously written book)
- Distribute copies to the public, by sale, rental, lease or lending
- Perform the work publicly (in the case of literary, musical, dramatic and choreographic works, pantomimes, movies, and audio-visual works)
- Display the work publicly, for all the works described above, including an individual image of a movie or other audio-visual work
- Perform a sound recording publicly by means of digital audio transmission (U.S. Copyright Office, 2011a)

Registration Is Nice but Not Required by the Law
In the United States, the U.S. Copyright Office of the U.S. Library of Congress is the agency with which one may register a copyrighted work. This is not necessary in order to establish copyright—remember, the copyright was born the minute the item

was created. Registration, however, allows for a convenient form of public notice, and a powerful means to enforce one's legal rights for violations of copyright (in that registration fixes in time when a work has been created, and many copyright disputes center on who-created-what-first) (U.S. Copyright Office, 2011a). It is quite simple and inexpensive to register a copyright, and may be done on-line (U.S. Copyright Office, 2011c) or via paper using forms also available online (U.S. Copyright Office, 2011a). One may also register the copyright for an online work (such as a webpage) (U.S. Copyright Office, 2009a).

Works Not Covered by Copyright, but Perhaps by Other Intellectual Property Law
Some works are not able to be covered by copyright, even though they were conjured in someone's mind, just the way an article, painting, or song is created. They include:

- Works not yet fixed in tangible form
- Titles, names, short phrases and slogans; symbols and designs; variations of typographic ornamentation, lettering or coloring; mere listings of ingredients. Note, however, that many of these elements may be given protection under trademark law: "Just do it" is not a copyrightable phrase, but you can be certain that Nike has trademark-protected that phrase for the distinct association it has with the marketing of their athletic shoes (Nike, 1994).
- Ideas, procedures, methods, systems, processes, concepts, principles, discoveries or devices. These (such as manufacturing processes) may enjoy patent law protection, but not copyright—until they are distilled into a tangible work or illustration. Albert Einstein would not have been able to copyright his scientific concept $E = mc^2$, but if he doodled the equation on a piece of paper, that rendering of the work would enjoy copyright protection.
- Works that consist entirely of information that is common property, and has no original authorship (such as standard calendars or height and weight charts) (U.S. Copyright Office, 2011a)
- Works of the U.S. federal government are not copyright protected, but they ought to be attributed (i.e., you can copy the report, but always show or credit where it came from) (U.S. Copyright Office, 2011b, p. 16 [section 105 of copyright law])

Want to Use It? Ask First
The basic premise underlying copyright law is that *you must seek permission of the copyright holder if you would like to reproduce, exhibit, perform or display the work*. Period. You may have to pay for the right to do so (a license), or the copyright holder may attach certain conditions (i.e., reproduce it without any changes or deletions), but your requirement, if you are supporting and upholding copyright law, is to ask the copyright holder for permission first. Researchers and writers work long and hard, and don't appreciate it when others waltz off and share those documents with others. Some infringers go

so far as to pretend they wrote the handout or PowerPoint, behavior which not only violates copyright law and Principle 2.5 of the IBLCE CPC, but ignores several other required elements of our practice-guiding documents (IBLCE CPC Principle 2.3 [be responsible and accountable for personal conduct and practice], Principle 2.4 [obey all laws including those regulating IBCLCs]; Principle 6.1 [behave honestly and fairly as a health professional], Principle 7.2 [provide only accurate information regarding lactation consultant services]; IBLCE SOP paragraph 3 [work within legal framework or setting]; ILCA Standard 2 [legal considerations]). But even those who distribute with proper attribution (though without prior permission) may be diminishing the author's ability to present her own materials, in the fashion she prefers. Seek permission first.

Limitations on the Exclusive Rights of Copyright Owners: The "Fair Use" Defense
We have seen there are some works that are not subject to copyright protection at all. For everything else, there is a requirement to seek permission from the copyright holder any time one seeks to reproduce, adapt, publish, perform, or display a work. Is there ever a situation where one may use someone else's work without first seeking permission? When the use may be excused, or is a valid defense to the charge of copyright infringement? The answer is yes, and some situations are readily understandable: news reporters can show and quote materials in their reports. Literary, drama, and movie critics can discuss and show the materials they are critiquing. Researchers and scholars may copy some sections of material as part of their work; correctly citing to such sources is part of any scholarly work. Educators and teachers are specifically allowed to make multiple copies of some works for classroom use (more on that below).

"Fair use" provides a *defense* against the improper use of copyrighted material. It is not a legitimate use of someone else's property; it is an explanation that may mitigate the damage for a wrong that admittedly occurred. "Fair use" is much misunderstood and abused, especially the notion that copies may be made liberally for classroom use. Those who think they have carte blanche to download and copy materials without limit, because they are learning or teaching or simply because it is easy to do, may be surprised to learn that U.S. copyright law is not quite so liberal.

The copyright law language, in the U.S. statute, describes fair use as follows:

107. Limitations on exclusive rights: Fair use

Notwithstanding the provisions of sections 106 and 106A [regarding a copyright owner's exclusive rights], the fair use of a copyrighted work, including such use by reproduction in copies or phonorecords or by any other means specified by that section, for purposes such as criticism, comment, news reporting, teaching (including multiple copies for classroom use), scholarship, or research, is not an infringement of copyright. In determining whether the use made of a work in any particular case is a fair use the factors to be considered shall include—

(1) the purpose and character of the use, including whether such use is of a commercial nature or is for nonprofit educational purposes;

(2) the nature of the copyrighted work;

(3) the amount and substantiality of the portion used in relation to the copyrighted work as a whole; and

(4) the effect of the use upon the potential market for or value of the copyrighted work.

The fact that a work is unpublished shall not itself bar a finding of fair use if such finding is made upon consideration of all the above factors. (U.S. Copyright Office, 2011b, p. 19 [section 107 of copyright law]).

There are no hard and fast rules—no "bright line tests"—about fair use. Everything is taken in context, and considered case by case. It is evaluated reviewing all four fair use elements along a continuum, something like a teeter-totter, to determine whether the reproduction, adaptation, publishing, performance, or display tips one onto the side where the use is excused from the requirements of permission, or the other side where such permission should have been sought. Where permission was needed and not received, it is considered a copyright infringement, subject to associated federal penalties and fines (U.S. Copyright Office, 2011b).

What do we look at on this teeter-totter?

- Nonprofit/educational vs. commercial use: If you intend to sell or profit from your use of someone else's work, without having first sought permission from the copyright owner, your use will be considered less "fair" than if you have a benevolent, educational, nonprofit purpose.
- Fact and published vs. imaginative and unpublished use: The "nature of the work" goes to its distinctiveness: if the piece is a one-of-a-kind rendering, your unsanctioned wholesale reproduction of hundreds of copies will diminish the rarity of the original, and thus be considered an unfair use.
- Small vs. large amount of copyrighted material used: If you copy a few paragraphs of a book, your use will be seen as more fair than if you copied the entire book.
- Whether your widespread use of the work affects the market of the original (e.g., sales for the copyright owner would diminish): If the unsanctioned use will impinge upon a small market for the material, that is considered unfair. Imagine a local professional association, which produces and sells a newsletter to generate income for the group. If one person copies that newsletter and hands it out to every other member, the organization will have lost its entire market, making that use unfair, indeed (Fields, 2004).

Teach Me About Teachers and Fair Use

Let's explore the phrase describing an allowed, fair use of copyrighted material: "teaching (including multiple copies for classroom use)." Many IBCLCs believe (or have been told) that when one is not selling the material, and when one "is learning something" from the materials, that it is a "fair use" to download or copy (indeed, make multiple copies of) breastfeeding and lactation-related journal articles, presentations, drawings, tables, or any other materials.

When revisions to copyright law were enacted in 1976, the fair use exemption described for teachers was the subject of much study, debate, lobbying, and (ultimately) compromise between the U.S. House, the U.S. Senate, and members of teachers' unions and librarian associations. The need for teachers to be able use materials in a timely manner (for purposes of educating students) was balanced against the well-established exclusive rights of copyright holders. The pertinent portions of the House and Senate reports, the Conference Report, and the floor debates, have been assembled in Circular 21 of the U.S. Copyright Office (which, ironically, means it may be freely downloaded and copied, as it is a federal government publication, so long as the source is shown and credited) (U.S. Copyright Office, 2009b).

But this loophole is not as large is it seems. The allowed ("fair") uses of copyrighted materials by teachers are subject to the following conditions:

- The fair use exemption is for photocopying from *books and periodicals only*, and does not apply to musical or audiovisual works (U.S. Copyright Office, 2009b).[1] An audiovisual work familiar to IBCLCs is a PowerPoint presentation. The fair use exemption by teachers/scholars does *not* extend to such a presentation; the author/copyright holder must first grant permission if any part of his or her presentation is to be reproduced, adapted, published, performed, or displayed.
- A teacher may, for scholarly research or use in teaching, make *single* copies of a chapter, or an article (from a journal or newspaper), or a short story/poem, or a chart/diagram/cartoon, but not an entire book, periodical, or newspaper (U.S. Copyright Office, 2009b).
- A teacher may make *multiple* copies (not to exceed the number of students in the class) of materials, provided that:
  (a) she is the teacher for the class
  (b) the copied material meets the tests of "brevity" and "spontaneity"
  (c) each copy includes a notice of copyright (the symbol ©, the word "Copyright," or the abbreviation "Copr." *and* the year of first publication of the work *and* the name of the rightful copyright holder (U.S. Copyright Office, 2009b, 2011a)

"Brevity" is specifically defined: poems of less than 250 words; prose of a complete article or essay if less than 2500 words, or an excerpt of 10% or less of a longer work; one "chart, graph, diagram, drawing, cartoon, or picture per book or per periodical

---

[1] The issue of fair use of copyrighted materials by educators was intensely debated by teachers, writers, publishers, and legislators before and during the 1975–1976 hearings for revision of U.S. copyright law. At the urging of Rep. Kastenmeier, Chair of the Judiciary Subcommittee hearing the matter, interested parties met separately to see if they could devise a compromise agreement on the use of copyrighted materials by scholars. They were able to do so, and the Ad Hoc Committee of Educational Institutions and Organizations on Copyright Law Revision, the Authors League of America and the Association of American Publishers produced an Agreement on Guidelines for Classroom Copying in Not-for-Profit Educational Institutions with Respect to Books and Periodicals, provisions of which were included in the House Committee Report (Agreement on Guidelines) (U.S. Copyright Office, 2009b).

issue" (U.S. Copyright Office, 2009b, p. 6). "Spontaneity" requires that the copying is at the "instance and inspiration" of the individual teacher, and the decision "to use the work, and the moment of its use for maximum teaching effectiveness are so close in time that it would be unreasonable to expect a timely reply to a request for permission" (U.S. Copyright Office, 2009b, p. 6).

- No teacher may make multiple copies under the fair use exception of more than one item per author, and on no more than nine occasions in a class term. Translation: One cannot copy an article by Jane Doe, and an essay by Jane Doe, and a different article by Jane Doe, all in the same semester/term. Pick the one item of Jane Doe's that you like best, because that is your limit until next semester (U.S. Copyright Office, 2009b). You can do this for a grand total of nine articles per semester, from nine different sources.
- Teachers may never copy a "consumable" such as a workbook, standardized test, or test booklet/answer sheet. These are items that were originally intended to be purchased/obtained by the individual students as part of their course of study (U.S. Copyright Office, 2009b).
- Teachers may not use their fair use copying exception to substitute for the purchase of books or periodicals, or to copy the same item from term to term. And, copying "shall not be directed by higher authority" (U.S. Copyright Office, 2009b, p. 7). In other words: Your boss can't make you copy it. If you decide on your own to make a copy, consider it a one-time deal.

For the IBCLC scholar/teacher, the implication is clear: Permission is the preferred and desired (and required, legal) avenue for use of any materials; fair use without permission is for a very limited number of materials in a few precise situations. There may be the rare circumstance where you are dealing with "late-breaking lactation news." Imagine you are a conference speaker presenting about increasing low milk supply, and two days before your session you learn of a newly published journal article discussing research of galactogogues. Certainly it is pertinent to your presentation; you want to distribute the abstract in a handout. While permission should immediately be sought to share this material, the authors may not get back to you in 48 hours. The fair use doctrine was intended for these rare and unforeseeable events. Otherwise, the requirement to seek permission to use previously published materials is reasonable, and ought to be honored. And in the case of the conference speaker, she should still initiate the permission-seeking process, even if she expects not to hear an answer in time for the live session.

It Was On the Internet. Can I Use It?

Not without permission first:

> Copyright protection subsists from the time the work is fixed in any tangible medium of expression from which it can be perceived, reproduced, or otherwise communicated, either directly or with the aid of a machine or device. (U.S. Copyright Office, 2009a, p. 1)

Just because you can easily find it, and effortlessly copy and paste it, does not mean you can use something you found on the Internet. You are still required to seek permission from the copyright holder to use the material. Indeed, scroll down and look at the bottom of just about any website: you'll see the copyright symbol. Look at their About Us or Home pages; you'll probably find a link to a page telling you the procedures needed to seek permission for reuse or republishing of content.

Copyright Law Compliance as Easy as 1-2-3

It should be pretty clear by now that there will be few instances where your use of a copyrighted work will be defensible without honoring the rights of the copyright holder. Fortunately, seeking permission is fairly easy to do.

Seek Permission from the Copyright Holder

If you found it on the Internet, you can probably get permission to use it via the Internet. There is no special format or letter or legal document to seek or demonstrate permission sought and received: Just ask! Call, write, email, or fax. Tell the person who you are, clearly identify the materials you are interested in, explain why you want to use their materials, and the context in which you seek to republish their materials. Keep a copy of your inquiry, and a copy of their response. In some cases you may need to seek permission from a publisher (i.e., journals will maintain copyright over research articles they publish).

Records in the Copyright Office
If the work does not clearly indicate who holds the copyright, the U.S. Copyright Office contains the records of all copyright holders who have registered their works. Remember that copyright is generated the minute the work takes tangible form, but not everyone will go to the extra step of registering his or her work with the U.S. Copyright Office. If the work is more than 30 years old, your search may require sifting through microfiche or paper records. For materials registered after January 1, 1978, you can use online searchable records (www.copyright.gov; U.S. Copyright Office, 2012). For a fee the Copyright Office staff will do the search for you (U.S. Copyright Office, 2010).

The Copyright Holder May Have Limitations on Use
Be aware that some copyright holders may have limitations on their own use of materials. A common situation for IBCLCs involves the use of photographs of mothers who have had a lactation consult. Prior written consent must be sought from a mother before she or her child may be photographed, recorded, or taped, for any purpose (IBLCE, 2011, CPC Principle 3.2; ILCA, 2006, Standard 2.3). However, the mother may only have agreed to allow her own IBCLC to use that photograph for teaching purposes. Perhaps the mother is comfortable knowing that her IBCLC will discuss and explain

her case, in a live teaching session, showing PowerPoint photographs of her damaged nipples. But she may not be keen on the idea that the photograph will be reproduced in a conference handout, or used by another speaker in her PowerPoint.

Add Photograph Permission to Your Consent Form
If your lactation consultancy is one where you may influence the wording on consent-to-be-seen forms (IBLCE, 2011, CPC Principles 3.2 & 4.1; IBLCE, 2008, SOP paragraph 6; ILCA, 2006, Standard 2.3), it may be a good idea to include language whereby the mother also consents to have photographs or other recordings taken of her and her baby. Under the language of IBLCE CPC Principle 3.2, such written consent is required if the photograph is to be used for *any* purpose, including photographs that will only be seen by you, and stored in your clinical file. Draw the mother's attention to the language when she reviews the papers prior to signing. It is a lot simpler for the mother to sign just one form up front, rather than scrambling to find a camera and the right consent form in the middle of the consult, all while you are trying to explain what you are doing, before the fleeting photographic moment ends. You can give the mother the option of having her face or identifying characteristics not be shown in any reuse of any photograph.

An IBCLC doesn't have to take clinical photographs, but having the consent language there may move her to use a camera when she is confronted with one of those strange and unusual cases. An IBCLC isn't restricted to using the photo in a classroom teaching situation: she can ask permission from the mother to take the photo, to share with a handful of colleagues, in an attempt to determine the cause of the problem. Dermatological conditions just cannot be described with words as readily as they can be shown in a photograph.

If the mother does not agree, simply cross off that language on her consent form. Both of you should initial the edit before the mother signs. Most mothers are more than happy to have their own unhappy situation used to train IBCLCs, to help future mothers avoid similar breastfeeding issues. On a similar note, your consent form can contain items to prove other signature-required elements. For example, in the United States, the Health Insurance Portability and Accountability Act (HIPAA) requires that an IBCLC demonstrate that she has given a mother the required Notice of Privacy Practices. The consent form for the visit, and photography, can also indicate that HIPAA documents have been provided (Health Insurance Portability and Accountability Act [HIPAA], 1996, codified at 45 CFR § 164.520(c)(2)(ii)).

Find Copyright-Free or Permission-Granted Materials
Big Brother is watching you: if you search the Internet for a nifty photograph to download and use in a PowerPoint you are creating, be aware that most commercial sites have software programs that allow them to capture Internet addresses of those who visit their site. If their photograph shows up in your materials, and you have not sought

permission or paid an appropriate royalty or licensing fee, they will have grounds to sue for infringement. If you use fancy computer software to remove the "watermark" that overlies a Web-based photograph (placed there by the copyright owner to diminish unauthorized use), that is infringement as well.

Handouts

Rather than trying to evade the law (or stretching the facts to convince yourself that your use is "fair") it is very easy to comply with the statute and use materials or images that are clearly intended for your use. There are many sources that make their information available to others, with a minimum of fuss, at no fee, and some are even lactation specific. If you visit just about any website catering to breastfeeding women, look on the Home page or About Us page (some even have a Permissions page) to determine what materials may be used and under what circumstances. For example, one well-known pediatrician and IBCLC makes his materials freely available as downloads from his site, with the following condition:

> All of our information sheets may be copied and distributed without further permission on the condition that it is not used in *ANY* context that violates the *WHO International Code on the Marketing of Breastmilk Substitutes* (1981) and subsequent World Health Assembly resolutions. If you don't know what this means, please email us to ask. (International Breastfeeding Centre, n.d., p. 1, emphasis in original).

One advantage to searching for materials from an Internet website is that nearly all have a means of contact (often called a Contact Us page) making it extremely easy should you need to seek for and ask permission of the copyright holder.

Photos or Illustrations

Go to your favorite Internet search engine, and enter *copyright free photo* or *royalty free photo*. You are likely to get more than 500,000 options. Visit a few sites, and learn how each operates. Some will offer a mere handful of freebies, with many others available for purchase. If the item is worth it, certainly do purchase the rights to use it. But it won't take long to find the sites that have a wide choice of materials available for your use, free of charge, and with permission. Some sites provide access to materials that are very old, and now in the public domain, and hence free to be reused. Other sites merely seek attribution: tell everyone where you got the nifty photo. Others permit use if certain conditions are met: do not sell or alter the work, for example.

One valuable resource for media of all kinds is Creative Commons (www.creative commons.org):

> The Creative Commons copyright licenses and tools forge a balance inside the traditional "all rights reserved" setting that copyright law creates. Our tools give everyone from individual creators to large companies and institutions a simple, standardized way to grant copyright permissions to their creative work. The combination of our tools and

our users is a vast and growing digital commons, a pool of content that can be copied, distributed, edited, remixed, and built upon, all within the boundaries of copyright law. (Creative Commons, n.d., para. 1)

Different kinds of licenses may be attached to works by their authors, indicating how they will permit their materials to be used by others. For example:

Attribution. This license lets others distribute, remix, tweak, and build upon your work, even commercially, as long as they credit you for the original creation. This is the most accommodating of licenses offered. Recommended for maximum dissemination and use of licensed materials. (Creative Commons, n.d., p. 1)

The Creative Commons website provides links to resources for images and materials, although they caution that one should verify that the work is actually under a Creative Commons license by following the link.

Another popular photo-sharing site is Flickr.com, which has an archive they call "the Commons" with images from such august institutions as the U.S. Library of Congress, the National Galleries of Scotland, the Australian National Maritime Museum, and Bibliotheque de Toulouse. One main objective: "To *increase access* to publicly held photography collections" (Flickr.com, 2012, p. 1).

Materials to Avoid (Even If They Are Free)
Anything produced by a company that is not meeting its obligations under the *International Code of Marketing of Breast-milk Substitutes* (WHO or International Code) should be considered off-limits for the IBCLC. The IBLCE CPC in its introduction says "a crucial part of an IBCLC's duty to protect mothers and children is adherence to the principles and aim of the [International Code]." This includes *not* distributing freebies (including printed materials or DVDs) offered by companies who improperly market bottles, teats, infant formula, and breastmilk substitutes (WHO, 1981). The companies are more than happy to have their materials freely distributed, and their handouts will no doubt grant such permission at the customary copyright line. Product branding is their paramount interest, not breastfeeding education. The IBCLC should be wary of using materials offered from any commercial source, regardless of their compliance with the WHO Code, because use of such materials puts the IBCLC at risk of a conflict of interest (IBLCE, 2011, CPC Principles 1.4, 5.1, & 5.2; IBLCE, 2008, SOP para. 8; ILCA, 2006, Standard 1.3; WHO, 1981, Preamble and Articles 4, 5, 6, & 7).

Establishing Your Own Copyright

You know by now that the minute you create the work, it enjoys copyright protection. But it is nice to "put the world on notice" that you are aware of your copyright, and intend to defend it. You may simply insert the copyright symbol (©) somewhere on your work: customarily it is on the very last page, but you may put it in a footer that appears on every page of your work. Include the date it was created, and your name. Example: "© 2008 Jane Doe" (U.S. Copyright Office, 2011a). This helps to make your materials look polished and professional. If you frequently revise and update your work, you can add a month as well as the year. This will be handy for cross-checking should you share or discuss revised materials. IBCLCs often see mothers years later, with subsequent children, and the evidence-based information one has to share now may supersede that which the mother received at prior visits. And while registering your copyrighted materials is not necessary, to do so is fairly easy, and provides better enforcement options should there be infringement by others.

Summary

IBCLCs are required by IBLCE CPC Principle 2.5 to "respect intellectual property rights." IP law covers patents (on machines and processes), trademarks and other marks (on materials and services sold in commerce), trade secrets (under business and commercial law), and copyright law (original works of authorship including literary and other intellectual works). For most IBCLCs, understanding the rights and responsibilities associated with copyright law will be important, as it covers works they use in everyday lactation consultancy: written materials, photographs, and audiovisual works such as PowerPoint presentations and instructional DVDs. Copyright attaches the minute the item is created, but it helps to provide public notice of copyright by including the copyright symbol, date, and author in the work. Registering the material with your national copyright enforcement office will facilitate enforcement, should someone infringe the copyright. Some exceptions to copyright law exist ("fair use") allowing materials to be reused by others without first seeking permission, but the exceptions are limited and precise. Seeking permission to use copyrighted materials is a fairly easy process, and IBCLCs should endeavor to do so unless they are using materials that are clearly designated as in the public domain or available for use of others.

REFERENCES

Creative Commons. (n.d.). *About the licenses*. Retrieved from http://creativecommons.org/licenses

European Trade Commission. (2005, August 1). *Biodiversity*. Retrieved from http://ec.europa.eu/trade/creating -opportunities/trade-topics/intellectual-property/biodiversity

Fields, S. (2004, November 15). *Intellectual property primer*. Lecture presented at Philadelphia Bar Institute, Philadelphia, PA.

Flickr.com. (2012). *Flickr—The commons*. Retrieved from http://www.flickr.com

Health Insurance Portability and Accountability Act [HIPAA] Administrative Simplification, 45 C.F.R. § Parts 160, 162 & 164 (1996), http://www.hhs.gov/ocr/privacy/hipaa/administrative/privacyrule /adminsimpregtext.pdf.

International Board of Lactation Consultant Examiners. (2003). *U.S. Patent No. Certification Mark 2749041 [Registered Lactation Consultant]*. Washington, DC: U.S. Patent and Trademark Office.

International Board of Lactation Consultant Examiners. (2007). *U.S. Patent No. Certification Mark 2042667 [IBCLC]*. Washington, DC: U.S. Patent and Trademark Office.

International Board of Lactation Consultant Examiners. (2008, March 8). *Scope of practice for international board certified lactation consultants*. Retrieved from http://www.iblce.org/upload/downloads/Scope OfPractice.pdf

International Board of Lactation Consultant Examiners. (2011, November 1). *Code of professional conduct for IBCLCs*. Retrieved from http://iblce.org/upload/downloads/CodeOfProfessionalConduct.pdf

International Breastfeeding Centre. (n.d.). *Information sheets—English*. Retrieved from http://www.nbci.ca/ index.php?option=com_content&view=category&layout=blog&id=5&Itemid=17

International Lactation Consultant Association. (2006). *Standards of practice for international board certified lactation consultants*. Retrieved from http://www.ilca.org/files/resources/Standards-of-Practice-web.pdf

Invent Now. (2010). *Invent now hall of fame inventor profile: Arthur Fry*. Retrieved from http://www.invent .org/hall_of_fame/412.html

Kelty, C. (2004, April 23). *A primer in modern intellectual property law*. Retrieved from http://cnx.org/content /m11795/latest

Kilner, C. (1998). *U.S. "novelty" vs. international "absolute novelty."* Retrieved from http://ram.timberlake publishing.com/files/usnoveltyvsinternationalabsolutenovelty.pdf

Leahy-Smith America Invents Act of 2011, 35 U.S.C. § 100 et seq. (2011), http://www.gpo.gov/fdsys/pkg /BILLS-112hr1249enr/pdf/BILLS-112hr1249enr.pdf.

Leppo, S. (2011, October 17). *The changing face of U.S. patent law*. Legal education seminar presented at Philadelphia Bar Institute, Philadelphia, PA.

Lever, A. (2008). Is it ethical to patent human genes? In A. Gosseries, A. Marciano, & A. Strowel (Eds.), *Theories of justice and intellectual property*. Retrieved from http://www.alever.net/DOCS/Is%20It%20 Ethical%20to%20Patent%20Human%20Genes.pdf

Love, J. (1997, May). *A free trade area for the America: A consumer perspective on proposals as they relate to rules regarding intellectual property; trademarks and infant formula marketing*. Hearing testimony presented at Working Group on Intellectual Property Rights, Third Trade Ministerial and Americas Business Forum, Belo Horizonte, Brazil. Retrieved from http://www.cptech.org/pharm/belopaper.html

McClain, V. (2007, October 31). *A slogan of illusion* [Web log post]. Retrieved from http://vwmcclain .blogspot.com/2007_10_01_archive.html

Nike, Inc. (1994; renewal 2004). *U.S. Patent No. Word Mark 1817919*. Washington, DC: U.S. Patent and Trademark Office.

U.S. Constitution. (1787, September 17). Retrieved from http://www.house.gov/house/Constitution /Constitution.html

U.S. Copyright Office. (2009a, May). *Circular 66: Copyright registration for online works*. Retrieved from http://www.copyright.gov/circs/circ66.pdf

U.S. Copyright Office. (2009b, November). *Circular 21: Reproduction of copyrighted works by educators and librarians*. Retrieved from http://www.copyright.gov/circs/circ21.pdf

U.S. Copyright Office. (2010, November). *Circular 22: How to investigate the copyright status of a work*. Retrieved from http://www.copyright.gov/circs/circ22.pdf

U.S. Copyright Office. (2011a, August). *Circular 1: Copyright basics*. Retrieved from http://www.copyright .gov/circs/circ01.pdf

U.S. Copyright Office. (2011b, December). *Circular 92: Copyright law of the United States and related laws contained in title 17 of the United States code*. Retrieved from http://www.copyright.gov/title17/circ92.pdf

U.S. Copyright Office. (2011c, December 1). *eCO online system*. Retrieved from http://www.copyright .gov/eco

U.S. Copyright Office. (2012, February 22). *Search copyright information*. Retrieved from http://www.copyright.gov/records

U.S. Patent and Trademark Office. (2010a, October 4). *Office of the administrator for policy and external affairs: Geographical indications (GIs) protection*. Retrieved http://www.uspto.gov/ip/global/geographical/protection/index.jsp

U.S. Patent and Trademark Office. (2010b, October 4). *Office of the administrator for policy and external affairs: Patent trade secrets*. Retrieved from http://www.uspto.gov/ip/global/patents/ir_pat_tradesecret.jsp

U.S. Patent and Trademark Office. (2011a, June 24). *Trademarks*. Retrieved from http://www.uspto.gov/inventors/trademarks.jsp#heading-2

U.S. Patent and Trademark Office. (2011b, November). *General information concerning patents*. Retrieved from http://www.uspto.gov/patents/resources/general_info_concerning_patents.jsp#heading-4

U.S. Patent and Trademark Office. (2011c, December 19). *Patents*. Retrieved from http://www.uspto.gov/inventors/patents.jsp

U.S. Patent and Trademark Office. (2012, March 9). *Trademark FAQs*. Retrieved from http://www.uspto.gov/faq/trademarks.jsp#DefineServiceMark

World Health Organization. (1981). *International code of marketing of breast-milk substitutes*. Retrieved from http://www.who.int/nutrition/publications/code_english.pdf

World Trade Organization. (2012). *Intellectual property: Protection and enforcement*. Retrieved from http://www.wto.org/english/thewto_e/whatis_e/tif_e/agrm7_e.htm

Chapter 10

The Law as It Affects Breastfeeding Women

IBCLCs are not trained to be lawyers, nor should they offer legal advice to breast-feeding mothers. True, they can play a role in court cases involving breastfeeding women. However, as trusted allied healthcare providers, International Board Certified Lactation Consultants (IBCLCs) can't help but encounter mothers who are struggling to maintain breastfeeding in unfriendly environments. As such, we may be witness to situations where we suspect the mothers' rights are being compromised. Perhaps the mother is seeking advice from the IBCLC about how to wean because she must return to work outside the home and her boss (erroneously) told her she cannot take breaks to express her milk or feed her baby. Perhaps the mother herself suspects her rights are being squeezed, and she has come directly to the IBCLC, seeking non-lactation-related help and support.

If we IBCLCs are doing our jobs well, we have earned trust from the mother with our empathic provision of evidence-based support and information. Mothers feel comfortable turning to us as allies in their plight. In other situations, the mother may be wholly unaware that her breastfeeding status entitles her to certain rights and privileges; there, the IBCLC can offer proactive support. In this chapter, we review those areas of law that commonly have a nexus with the breastfeeding mother, and some generalized suggestions of how the IBCLC may *support* the mother by steering her to information or resources she may need.

The Role of the IBCLC When the Mother's Rights Are Infringed

Some IBCLCs get very nervous when a mother, tearful and clearly under stress, comes to them describing a sad situation and beseeching the allied healthcare provider for help. The IBCLC may feel "out of her league" or fear that she will get entangled in a messy, lengthy proceeding of some kind or another if she offers even a little bit of assistance beyond pure lactation consultancy. Recall, however, the following: *The IBCLC's legal and ethical responsibility is to provide evidence-based information and support, so the mother can make an informed decision about lactation.* On breastfeeding matters, we ask the mother to make her own decisions, and we help craft a care plan she can implement given the totality of her circumstances, after hearing what evidence-based information and support we have to offer. Similarly, with a little flexibility, the IBCLC can suggest to the mother options to sort out the legal issues, without taking on the role of the mother's legal advocate, and even without having to reveal the IBCLC's position on the matter. The mother can be guided to resources that will allow her to make her own informed decision in a non-lactation context.

The conscientious IBCLC will become familiar with the kinds of legal and ethical issues that breastfeeding mothers (as a whole) face. As compared to the mother, the IBCLC is not (or, more accurately, should not be) emotionally entangled in the outcome. The IBCLC may be the one calm voice of reason and information that the mother needs to hear. No, the IBCLC is not expected to become a legal expert, but there are a handful of issues that will arise over and over again. Finding credible support or legal resources to whom you can refer the mother is as important as building your referral list for specialists treating mothers' or babies' clinical conditions. The IBCLC can assist the lawyers in finding other expert lactation advisors if she is not willing to take on such a role herself.

Several sections of our practice-guiding documents encourage us, as IBCLCs, to have at least passing familiarity with the mother's home and work situation in order to better craft a care plan to address lactation issues, and support the mother to achieve her breastfeeding goals. It is not too much of a stretch to interpret these practice-guiding documents to mean that an IBCLC should be able to identify matters for which a lactating mother will need nonlactation help. Recall these documents describe the professional behaviors in which the IBCLC *must* or *should* engage:

- Know when to refer to clinical or other support specialists: International Board of Lactation Consultant Examiners Code of Professional Conduct (IBLCE CPC) (2011) Principles 2.1, 2.2, and 4.2 (*musts*); International Board of Lactation Consultant Examiners Scope of Practice (IBLCE SOP) (2008) paragraphs 5, 6, and 8 (*musts*); International Lactation Consultant Association Standards of Practice (ILCA Standards) (2006) Standards 3.2.3, 3.3.5, 4.2, and 4.4 (*shoulds*).
- Know and respect the laws of the land (which would include those addressing the mothers' rights): IBLCE CPC Principles 2.4, 2.5, 6.1, 6.3, and 8.2 (*musts*); IBLCE SOP paragraph 3 (*must*); ILCA Standards at Preface and Standards 1 (Introduction), 2 (Introduction), 2.5, 3 (Introduction) (*shoulds*); *The International Code of Marketing of Breast-milk Substitutes* (WHO Code or International Code) at Preamble and Article 11 (*should that could be a must*[1]).

---

[1] The International Code is a model public health policy, endorsed by the World Health Organization, meant to curtail certain marketing practices that subvert breastfeeding. Member nations are encouraged to pass legislation enacting the International Code within their borders. If this has occurred in the geopolitical region where the IBCLC practices, then the WHO Code is a *must* (International Code Documentation Centre, 2007). Alternately, if the IBCLC works in a facility that is seeking or maintaining Baby-Friendly status under the worldwide WHO/UNICEF Baby-Friendly Hospital Initiative (BFHI), support for the International Code is a mandatory element (Baby-Friendly USA, 2010; UNICEF, 2012).

- Respect individual needs/values of the client/patient: IBLCE CPC Principles 1.2, and 1.5 (*musts*); IBLCE SOP paragraph 8 (*must*); ILCA Standards at Preface and Standards 3.2, 3.3.1, 3.3.2, and 4.2 (*shoulds*).
- Offer information without personal bias, recognizing legitimate differences of opinion: IBLCE CPC Principles 1.5 and 6.3 (*musts*); IBLCE SOP paragraphs 4, 5, 6, and 8 (*musts*); ILCA Standards 3 (Introduction), 3.2, and 3.3 (*shoulds*); WHO Code at Preamble and Articles 1 and 2 (*should that could be a must*).
- Provide support to the client/patient: IBLCE CPC Principles 1.1, 1.3, 1.4, and 6.3 (*musts*); IBLCE SOP paragraphs 4, 5, and 8 (*musts*); ILCA Standards 3.3.1, 3.3.2, 3.3.4, 4.3, and 4.4 (*shoulds*); WHO Code at Preamble (*should that could be a must*).

Where Lactation and the Law Meet

Breastfeeding is something of an anomaly in the law, where specific support for a breastfeeding mother's rights is not as clear as one might assume. We previously discussed an active advocacy role that an IBLCE might take, in or out of the courtroom, on a matter that involves lactation issues. Let us review here some areas of the law where the mother's right to breastfeed (or) to have access to her baby (or) to express and transport her breastmilk are described, regardless of whether there is a court action pending.

Family Law Actions

Marriage, divorce, separation, custody, visitation, alimony, child support, adoption, foster care, and so on may generally be described as "family law" or "domestic relations" matters. Family law customarily falls under local or state court jurisdiction because traditionally these matters are considered to reflect the common law of the locality. This is why marriage requirements can differ from state to state (Legal Information Institute, Cornell Univ. Law School, n.d.a). Similarly, the laws governing dissolution of a marriage, and the care and custody of children, will vary from jurisdiction to jurisdiction (Legal Information Institute, Cornell Univ. Law School, n.d.b). Some states in the United States, as well as the Family Law Courts of Australia, have voluntary arbitration, mediation, or alternative dispute resolution tracks for resolving family law matters (Family Law Courts of Australia, n.d.).

The classic situation involving breastfeeding tensions is when the non-lactating parent seeks extended periods of time with the still-breastfeeding child: overnights, or for several days in a row. Such visitation/custody periods are quite common in divorce arrangements, but they do not easily accommodate the round-the-clock physical proximity requirements of a breastfeeding dyad. The mother who is caught up in this situation will find several easy-to-understand and informative articles on the La Leche League website, geared to give her some legal background and some advice on looking beyond lactation to the entirety of the custody/visitation scenario (http://www.llli. org/Law/LawUS.html). This is the first resource to which the IBLCE may send a distraught mother, so she can read pragmatic suggestions about how to protect her (and her baby's) rights in a family law struggle (La Leche League International, 2011). The overall theme of attempting to find an amicable arrangement without resorting to court action will resonate for any mother, in any geopolitical location. Another excellent online resource about breastfeeding-related law in the United States is Breastfeedinglaw.com (http://wwww.breastfeedinglaw.com; Marcus, 2012).

What the mother needs most in this situation is a very good family law attorney who practices in the local jurisdiction. The profession may be called solicitor, barrister, or advocate depending on one's country, but the goal is the same: Find an excellent person, familiar with the law of the geopolitical region, to represent the mother. Many mothers, especially those who are at home, caring for children, and who have no independent source of income, are fretful about the cost of such representation. She can save money by doing a lot of homework herself (such as reading through the pages at the websites mentioned above). Then, when she does the hiring interview for a lawyer, she will know whether each candidate knows something, or nothing, about lactation and the law. The mother can survey friends or relatives who hired a good attorney to handle their own domestic law disputes; word of mouth is a reliable barometer for a good barrister. The IBCLC can also suggest that the mother call her local bar association (the professional association for lawyers), which are usually organized by geography (city, county, or state). Most have good websites and referral lines, and many have programs to assist low-income clients with free or low-cost legal counsel if the circumstances warrant.

Informal Assistance to the Mother in Trouble

Most mothers make outreach to the IBCLC in the very early stages of the domestic tensions. Maybe the mother doesn't have a lawyer yet, or doesn't think she needs one. IBCLCs, in addition to offering suggestions to the mother about how to find a good lawyer, can offer other means of support. Some ground rules:

- Refer the mother to resources to obtain the legal help she needs. She should understand you are *not* a substitute for a legal expert.
- Often, the mother just needs a sympathetic shoulder. Distraught mothers may take advantage of your kind heart. Lay boundaries clearly, and early. If the current atmosphere is friendly between mother and father, suggest that mother take the time and effort to get her custody, support, and visitation orders squared away *now*. Difficult topics are better discussed when tempers are calm and emotions are in check. Suggest that mother offer up plenty of parenting time to the father *now*. That is healthy for both the father and the child, and provides a much clearer picture of the stress and time involved in capable parenting. If things are starting to turn sour between the parents, especially if mother has concerns about her own or her child's safety, suggest she keep a simple notebook where she contemporaneously writes down the facts giving rise to her worries

(with date, time, and a list of others present). Just the act of writing can be very cathartic and empowering for a woman who feels increasingly powerless in a deteriorating situation. It can also be a very helpful tool, later on, as a good memory-jogging tool. The diary will not be accepted as "evidence" but it can be used (even at trial) to allow the mother to be reminded of an event, about which she can then testify in person.

- If you do offer "soft shoulder" support for the mother, you have removed yourself forever from being used as an expert or fact witness, because of your demonstrated partiality.

Domestic Violence

Nearly every city, county, province, state, or country has a program to provide immediate protection to women who fear for their own or their children's safety because of emotional or physical abuse. Victims do not easily reveal their terrifying situations to others, and IBCLCs are not trained domestic violence counselors, but IBCLCs do connect with mothers, and the victim may reach out and confide details of her situation. Every IBCLC should know, and carry with her, the local hotline numbers and/or website pages for the programs that operate in her territory. The National Domestic Violence Hotline in the United States is 1-800-799-SAFE (7233); of course, any situation that is an emergency will warrant a call to 9-1-1. At any hint of concern mentioned by the mother during the lactation consultation, the IBCLC should share the resource numbers. It can be done compassionately and nonjudgmentally: "You sound worried/scared. Here is the number for an office where you can have a private, safe conversation with someone who will help you sort out your options. Will you be able to find some private time to make that call or look at this website?"

The IBCLC in the United States can learn more about the topic of violence against women, generally, from the National Coalition Against Domestic Violence, a private–public partnership designed to provide support for victims of domestic violence (National Coalition Against Domestic Violence, 2011a). The website (www.ncadv.org) has materials the mother herself may find helpful (a "Protect Yourself" page). There are also links to international organizations that non-USA IBCLCs may find helpful, for services/programs serving other countries or regions (National Coalition Against Domestic Violence, 2011b).

Employment or Labor Law Actions

Alternate phrases may be used by different countries to describe this general area of law, but it covers all areas of the employer-employee relationship. For the breastfeeding woman, lactation may present an issue that needs to be addressed at the woman's job upon her return to work after the birth of a baby.

There is a huge range of maternity-based rights and privileges, depending on the country and work setting (Alewell & Pull, 2005). Whether the region has a developed or developing economy, or the government provides some (or all) health care under ministry regulation, or the mother is in an entry-level or executive position—all that will have a bearing on what benefits may accrue. In a large company, the human resources department customarily will be well versed in what benefits the employee of the company is entitled to access, because the infinite variability of birth experiences renders infinite variations on access to benefits. IBCLCs around the world should be familiar, at least in passing, with the sorts of benefits to which a working breastfeeding mother may be entitled. Let us review some of material discussed in the earlier chapter about the IBCLC in the courtroom.

When Lactation Is "Homeless" in the Law

We learned in an earlier chapter that in the United States, lactation does not neatly fit into the definitions of preexisting areas of law, carved out to address the employee's rights springing from pregnancy, childbirth and maternity (also called family) leave, and equal protection of the law (civil rights). Maternity/family leave parameters are a function of what a nation's laws permit or require (see, for example, Service Canada, 2011). While breastfeeding is linked inextricably with the biologic functions of pregnancy and childbirth, it does not have easily identified start and finish dates. It doesn't end with the delivery of the baby, as do pregnancy and childbirth. Full-term, uncomplicated pregnancy for humans worldwide is 40 gestational weeks (give or take a few weeks), yet uncomplicated lactation can occur for anywhere from a few days up to several years (Dettwyler, 1995). Mothers (and their attorneys) have had to use clever thinking to "fit" lactation into preexisting doctrines; sometimes it works, and sometimes it doesn't.

The U.S. Pregnancy Discrimination Act of 1978 (PDA) is an amendment to the Civil Rights Act of 1964, written to require fair treatment for those with pregnancy-related medical conditions (including those that may temporarily "disable" the pregnant woman from performing certain work-related tasks). Courts have not been willing to define breastfeeding, lactation, and the need to express milk as medical conditions that are protections guaranteed under this federal civil rights law (Christrup, 2001; Marcus, 2011; Orozco, 2010). It would seem that, since only women can breastfeed, they ought to enjoy protection from discrimination based on their sex under Title VII of the Civil Rights Act. Unfortunately, the courts haven't gone in that direction. A fairly steady line of decisions considers breastfeeding as distinguished from pregnancy, and inherently part of child-rearing. One court opinion stated, "it is a disservice . . . to both men and women to assume that child-rearing is a function peculiar to one sex" (Christrup, 2001, p. 485, quoting 1985 federal district court opinion); another court wrote that "Title VII and the PDA do not cover breast feeding or childrearing concerns because they are not 'medical conditions related to pregnancy, childbirth or related medical conditions'" (Orozco, 2010, p. 1305, quoting 1999 federal district court opinion).

The Americans with Disabilities Act (ADA) requires employers to provide reasonable accommodation (including flexible work schedules) to their employees with disabilities, which would seem a good fit for the accommodations the breastfeeding mother seeks (Americans with Disabilities Act, 1990). However, the ADA has not been interpreted to include lactation, in part because of reluctance to characterize the transient process of breastfeeding as a permanent "disability," as could be said about a person with permanent vision or hearing loss (Christrup, 2001).

Certainly, the Family and Medical Leave Act (FMLA) in the United States covers the mother who is caring for a newborn (including breastfeeding), but it falls short in that breastfeeding can occur for months and even years after the initial guaranteed family leave time has elapsed (a matter of weeks in the United States) and the mother is back at her place of work. Similarly, other FMLA provisions allowing employees periodically to be away from work are predicated on illness or disability of the employee, or a loved one. For example, FMLA allows an employee to take unpaid, job-protected leave to care for a seriously ill family member (Family and Medical Leave Act, 1993). But breastfeeding is not an "illness" in the same way that, for example, recovery from surgery is; indeed, breastfeeding is promoted as a public health imperative for both mother and child. Some states have laws that expand FMLA, allowing for a portion of the guaranteed leave to be paid, or increasing the leave time (e.g., the California Family Temporary Disability Insurance) (California Employment Development Dept., 2010), but they don't help shoe-horn the breastfeeding mother into the application of the law.

Civil rights in the United States (specifically, freedom from discrimination based on sex) is another area of law that has been argued on behalf of breastfeeding women. In the United States, sexual harassment, a workplace-based violation of civil rights based on sex discrimination, requires unwelcome verbal, visual, or physical conduct of a sexual nature; it must be offensive and severe or pervasive enough that it affects working conditions or creates a hostile work environment (U.S. Equal Employment Opportunity Commission, n.d.). Other countries also recognize causes of action for sexual or violent harassment in the workplace (Cowling & Sinclair, 2007). But these protections are predicated on *harassment*. The breastfeeding mother who seeks breaks to express her milk or directly feed her infant may find no help under these laws, unless her co-workers have also made crude, lewd comments about her breasts.

These inconsistencies in the United States may reflect an accurate description of how the U.S. courts have interpreted federal cases as of early 2012, but they defy common sense understanding by the mothers and their employers who are expected to comply with the law. Legislation has been introduced in recent Congressional sessions to make clear, once and for all, that a woman who is breastfeeding enjoys protections against discrimination in the workplace, and as a civil right (U.S. Breastfeeding Committee, 2011a) but the bills had not progressed to the hearings stage as of March 2012.

When Lactation Is Not "Homeless" in the Law

In 2000, the International Labour Organization (ILO) revised its maternity, pregnancy, and breastfeeding "Convention No. 183,"[2] also called the Maternity Protection

---

[2] A "convention" (vs. a "recommendation") is a policy statement adopted by the International Labour Conference; thereafter, governments may ratify it (allowing the provisions to be made a part of international treaties) but serving, regardless of ratification status, as an international labor standard (International Labour Organization, 1972).

Convention 2000, as part of a major effort to provide its member organizations (governments, employers, and workers' organizations) a toolkit of "key documents and materials on promoting equality between women and men in the world of work" (International Labour Organization, 2006). The Maternity Protection Convention 2000 is an international labor standard that applies to all employed women, "including those in atypical forms of dependent work" (Convention No. 183, Article 2, Section 1; International Labour Organization, 2006), and provides for not less than 14 weeks of maternity leave (6 weeks of which may be designated compulsory leave after childbirth) (International Labour Organization, 2006). Women are to receive cash benefits (Convention No. 183, Article 6, Section 1) during their leave (in accordance with their national laws and regulations), are guaranteed their jobs back, and may not have their employment terminated because of pregnancy/maternity leave (Convention No. 183, Article 8, Section 1). Convention No. 183 also contains language specific to the needs and rights of breastfeeding women:

Breastfeeding Mothers [Article 10].

1. A woman shall be provided with the right to one or more daily breaks or a daily reduction of hours of work to breastfeed her child.
2. The period during which nursing breaks or the reduction of daily hours or work are allowed, their number, the duration of nursing breaks and the procedures for the reduction of daily hours of work shall be determined by national law and practice. These breaks or the reduction of daily hours of work shall be counted as working time and remunerated accordingly. (International Labour Organization, 2006, p. 4 of section entitled "Convention No. 183")

This language, and the protections described by the Maternity Protection Convention 2000, go right to the heart of working conditions for the breastfeeding mother returning to her job (which should be waiting for her) after her paid leave of 14 weeks (if her national law mandates as much) under conditions in which she has paid break time to feed her baby or express her milk.

Federal regulations enacted in 2010 in the United States align with the breastfeeding-specific language suggested a decade earlier by the ILO. Healthcare reform included an amendment to the Fair Labor Standards Act, providing for unpaid but guaranteed break time, up to 1 year after the birth of the child, for a mother to express her breastmilk (U.S. Breastfeeding Committee 2011b; U.S. Dept. of Labor Wage and Hour Division, 2010). The law covers hourly wage workers; salaried (often management) workers are not covered, but their (usually more generous) benefits package may provide for workplace accommodations to express milk (U.S. Breastfeeding Committee, 2010). Employers of fewer than 50 employees can claim exemption from the law *if* they can first establish that it would be a hardship to provide "a place, other than a bathroom, that is shielded from view and free from intrusion from coworkers and the public, which may be used by an employee to express breast milk" (Patient Protection and Affordable Care Act, 29 U.S.C.

§ 207 (r)(1)(B), 2010; U.S. Breastfeeding Committee, 2011b, 2011c). With passage of this legislation, the United States "[joined] 120 other countries whose employed women enjoy protection for lactation breaks at work" (U.S. Breastfeeding Committee, 2010, p. 12). Earlier, mothers had to depend on state laws to protect their rights, and those statutes differed from state to state (Mothering.com, 2010).

Civil Rights Actions (Generally)

Civil rights law in the United States is not always a guaranteed means of protection, as of early 2012, for a breastfeeding mother in the workplace. And, there has been unwillingness to accord breastfeeding the constitutionally protected privacy rights that parenting choices customarily enjoy. Thus, the federal position offers rather halfhearted support to a breastfeeding mother: it has ruled that while states cannot specifically infringe upon a woman's right to breastfeed, neither are the states required to "legislate, enforce, or mandate any laws specifically protecting that right" (Christrup, 2001, p. 493).

In the absence of a strong federal legal precedent, many states and municipalities in the United States have taken it upon themselves to pass laws designed to protect breastfeeding as a civil right in various situations. By mid 2011, different jurisdictions had laws addressing a woman's right to breastfeed in public or in private; to exempt breastfeeding from public indecency laws; to protect breastfeeding in the workplace, to exempt a breastfeeding mother from jury duty; and to prevent discrimination by child-care providers and to ensure safe handling of breastmilk in such places (National Conference of State Legislatures, 2011).

An IBCLC in the United States should expect a patient/client to ask, "What is the law in our state?" The IBCLC (and the mother) can find state-specific information at the breastfeeding laws page at the National Conference of State Legislatures (www. ncsl.org), which maintains a frequently updated compilation of state breastfeeding bills and statutes, along with links to the bills and laws themselves, and several policy and advocacy documents the mother may also find helpful. There is also a general discussion of breastfeeding law and the mother's rights at Breastfeedinglaw.com, a website specifically covering this topic (Marcus, 2012).

Breastfeeding in Public

The most unfortunate aspect of mothers being harassed for breastfeeding in public is that it is the mothers who invariably are complying with the law. It is the harasser who is violating the mother's (or the child's) rights by scolding, lecturing, or yelling. Yet, the mother is the one put in the embarrassing situation of shielding her child(ren) from agitated and accusatory adults, having to leave a place she had every right to be, and to be left tossing and turning at night as she relives the vituperative scenario. News stories even in 2012 report of mothers who have been asked to stop breastfeeding their babies in the restaurants, museums, and airplanes where they had every right to be. The experience can be traumatizing, leaving the mother feeling ashamed when she was the only one who was acting in accordance with the law.

But, sadly, the mother who has a right to breastfeed in public, and has that right erroneously infringed by another, may not be in a position to do much about it after the fact. For:

> A basic maxim of American law is that a right without a remedy is no right at all. [Footnote omitted.] In plain terms, this means that although you may have a "right" to do anything not otherwise forbidden by law, if you do not also have a legal protection against someone interfering with that right, your ability to exercise it may be limited. (Marcus, 2007, para. 3)

IBCLCs may find themselves pulled into this fray if the mother and her allies seek redress through public awareness campaigns. Whether and how an IBCLC chooses to participate in such activities as "nurse-ins" or letter-writing campaigns depends on how comfortable she is in publicly advocating for breastfeeding mothers, breastfeeding children, and breastfeeding itself; those who opt not to participate have made as ethical and legal a decision as those who do.

Air Travel
Mothers who travel with their breastfeeding children, and/or are transporting expressed breastmilk should be encouraged to "be proactive" in their planning. Air travel in the 2010s with its heightened security measures is difficult enough. Imagine how irritating and maddening it is to be faced with airplane staff who are unaware of a woman's right to breastfeed in the waiting area or plane, or a screening agent who is ready to dump those precious ounces of expressed milk because "they are liquids."

The IBCLC can offer some suggestions to the mother. Check the website or customer service lines of the air carrier. Security rules vary from country to country, and the carriers will be the most familiar with what is permitted. If possible, print out the pages (or note the names of the customer service agents) who provide details on requirements for the safe transport of expressed breastmilk.

Consider checking luggage with expressed milk carefully packed in the suitcase. There is no restriction on the fluid ounce amount when items are in checked baggage. The mother would be wise to label her containers as holding expressed breastmilk (in case a random search of her suitcase by some zealous agent causes concern about what those bottles might contain). Depending on the length of the anticipated flight, and the facilities available to her before she travels, the mother can freeze her milk in nonbreakable containers, and pack them in a cooler or box or suitcase along with lots of scrunched-up newspaper (which is a very effective insulator). Even if she cannot freeze her milk ahead of time, packing cooled milk with ice or gel packs and insulation will allow for several hours of travel. The Academy of Breastfeeding Medicine's (ABM) Protocol for storing and handling milk for full-term infants indicates that "milk may be stored in an insulated cooler bag with ice packs for 24 hours," much longer than any plane trip (ABM, Eglash, Chantry & Howard, 2010). A mother carrying her own expressed milk, for her own healthy baby, will be the best judge of whether the milk has spoiled.

Plan extra time (on top of the extra time it already takes) to make it through security if traveling in the United States. Print out and carry the pages from the U.S. Transportation Security Administration (TSA) explaining the rule that allows mothers, whether they are traveling alone or with their children, to take expressed milk through the security and screening checkpoints in quantities over the customary 3.0 fluid ounce limit, so long as it is declared to the TSA agent before screening and X-ray starts (U.S. Transportation Security Administration, n.d.). Not every TSA agent at every X-ray machine at every airport will be aware of this rule. Thus, the mother should practice sweetly and calmly asking to be referred to the TSA supervisor if the first agent is balking about letting her items through. This is when that extra time will be a comfort.

Jury Duty

Women called to jury duty who wish to be excused from that civic obligation may find different levels of legal authority upon which they may rely. Rules will vary from court to court, but customarily those called to jury duty must spend several hours of several days as part of the pool of potential jurors. Courthouses are rich with tradition, custom, and procedure—none of which are particularly accommodating to the needs of mothers with young children. Keeping the potential jurors segregated from lawyers, witnesses, litigants, and defendants is an important prerequisite to trial, so mothers cannot freely take breaks from and leave their area (for example, to nurse a baby or express breastmilk). For this reason, many mothers will ask to be excused from jury duty until their child has weaned, or has reached an age where long separations are feasible.

Check the Law First, Then Court Rules, Then Politely Ask
There may be a law or rule that allows the mother to get out of jury service without even addressing lactation issues. Some jurisdictions will allow one to opt out of jury duty "by right": if one is a full-time student, a teacher or professor, or a practicing doctor, veterinarian, midwife, or nurse (Citizens Information Board-Ireland, 2011; Law Reform Commission of Western Australia, 2009). In Australia, one recognized ground for excuse by right, pertinent to the breastfeeding mother who is also a full-time caregiver for her children, is for "persons residing with and having full-time care of children under the age of 14 years" (Law Reform Commission of Western Australia, 2009, p. 110). Excuse from jury service may also be given "for good cause shown": the potential juror is ill, or must tend to an ill family member, or the person who has served as a juror in the last 12 months (Law Reform Commission of Western Australia, 2009).

Some jurisdictions have enacted laws specifically covering breastfeeding women and jury duty. In the United States, 12 states have such laws (Vance, 2007), and the options vary among those 12 (such as: one state allows postponement; one state requires a doctor's certification; one provides exemption for lactating women for 1 year) (Family Friendly Jury Duty, 2007). All jurisdictions will have some means by which jurors may be excused from service (Citizens Information Board–Ireland, 2011 [Ireland]; National

Association of Citizens Advice Bureaux, 2012 [Scotland]). The mother should be encouraged to check with the court that issued her the summons to serve; invariably, those documents will indicate who issued the summons, and how the called-juror may respond with legitimate objections to service.

If there are no formal means to seek excuse from service, the mother should be encouraged to simply write a letter to the office that summoned her, and ask to be excused on the grounds that breastfeeding requires her to be near her child throughout the day. Excuse from jury duty is not sought for the mother's convenience, but rather to permit her to meet the needs of the children in her care. She should be realistic about her request: if she regularly works outside the home, and away from her breastfeeding baby, for 8–10 hours per day, the court will be unimpressed with her argument that she must now be near her baby. In that case, the mother might argue that she needs the same accommodations she has in her workplace (such as frequent breaks, and access to a clean and private place to express and store her milk, or opportunity to breastfeed her child).

Several suggestions will assist the mother in her cause:

- Write sooner than later. Typically jury notice is given weeks or even months in advance. The mother should write as soon as she can assemble her information, and not wait until the week before duty is to commence.
- Most citizens dread jury service, and the courts are hardened to requests to be excused from this civic obligation because they come from every sector, not just breastfeeding women. The mother should demonstrate that she would be happy to serve once she has weaned.
- Where possible, append supporting documents, such as a letter from the pediatrician indicating that this baby requires his mothers' milk, or a letter from the midwife describing how regular emptying of the breasts is important for this mother to prevent recurrent mastitis.
- Court officials may not have any idea, whatsoever, about the biologic and physiologic functions of breastfeeding (or milk expression), and may benefit from a very short (one paragraph) description of how lactation works, and why regular access to the baby (or pump) is needed. Unlike many medical or biologic conditions, this one happens all day every day, and it takes longer to express milk than to make a customary restroom visit.
- Distinguish the difference between the need to generally care for the baby from the need to breastfeed the baby. Many courts provide compensation for (or actual) babysitting services (National Association of Citizens Advice Bureaux, 2012). The breastfed child is not customarily breastfed by the non-mother caregiver, and the court will need to see that this is an entirely different issue than that of finding a competent caregiver during jury service.
- Compare (politely) this excuse to some others that are regularly honored by the court. If a prearranged vacation (holiday) is allowed as a valid excuse from jury service, suggest that surely the mother's preexisting need to attend to her child's health and welfare is as compelling as missing some time at the beach.

Donor Human Milk

Giving the baby milk from another mother—it has been happening since the dawn of mammalian time. Now that we are in the modern age, living in societies with laws, liabilities, and efficient technology, the use of donor human milk has been accorded scrutiny (and suspicion) that medical use of other body parts and fluids seem not to be (Akre, Gribble, & Minchin, 2011). And what a shame that is. While expressing breastmilk is a fairly time-consuming commitment on the part of the woman who is doing it on a regular basis, lactating women can be found in every corner of the planet. Lots of them. Breastmilk is the ultimate renewable resource: easy to find, easy to access (not even requiring machinery, if one remembers that hand expression of breastmilk was happening for thousands of years before pumps and electricity were invented), available immediately without prior processing or cooking, cheap and fairly easy to store, readily and nearly universally consumable by those in need. What's not to like? Apparently a lot, if you ask some outside (and even within) lactation circles who have not educated themselves about the collection, storage, and use of donor human breastmilk. Mothers will turn to IBCLCs to ask about breastmilk donation, whether they are on the giving or receiving end. What better person from whom to seek evidence-based information and support? Those who are seeking such information from an IBCLC, the allied healthcare provider who is the recognized expert in breastfeeding and human lactation, deserve, at the very least, honest answers to their questions and directions of where to learn more.

Human Milk Is the Preferred Substitute for Mother's Own Milk

While this statement is stunningly obvious to IBCLCs (and perhaps some healthcare providers working in neonatology, where use of donor human milk for premature patients is well known if not prevalent), it is simply not well understood "in the real world" that there *are* options besides going to the grocery store and buying infant formula off the shelf. The definitive world public health resource describes it this way:

> The vast majority of mothers can and should breastfeed, just as the vast majority of infants can and should be breastfed. Only under exceptional circumstances can a mother's milk be considered unsuitable for her infant. For those few health situations where infants cannot, or should not, be breastfed, the choice of the best alternative, expressed breast milk from an infant's own mother, breast milk from a healthy wet-nurse or a human-milk bank, or a breast-milk substitute fed with a cup, which is a safer method than a feeding bottle and teat, depends on individual circumstances. (WHO, 2003, p. 10)

This advice is echoed by the Emergency Nutrition Network (ENN) whose relief workers assist in the aftermath of natural and man-made disasters. For breastfeeding mothers and children, the goals are fairly simple: any relief activities are to be conducted in compliance with the *International Code of Marketing of Breast-milk Substitutes*, no small feat when well-meaning but misguided donors from around the world try to rush powdered infant formula donations to the site, in a language that cannot be read by the population, and where clean water, electricity, and fuel for heating and cooking are unavailable. Emergency relief workers on the ground are to be trained in how to provide optimal feeding after the onset of the emergency, including support for and protection of breastfeeding (Gribble & Berry, 2011). They assess the affected population (how many mothers, young children, pregnant women?) and their nutritional needs; support is to be offered to

> maintain, enhance or reestablish breastfeeding using relactation. [I]f breastfeeding by the natural mother is impossible, make appropriate choices from among alternatives (wet-nursing, breastmilk from milk bank, unbranded [generic] infant formula, locally purchased commercial infant formula). (Infant and Young Child Feeding in Emergencies Core Group, 2007, Part 5.2 at p. 11)

Human milk *is* the elixir of life for premature and low or very low birth weight babies, dramatically lowering morbidity and mortality for infants who receive it rather than formula (Lawrence & Lawrence, 2011; Wight, Morton, & Kim, 2008). Its use in neonatal intensive care units (NICUs) is considered best practice (Wight, Rhine, et al., 2008). Research and technological advancements have advanced considerably since the early 1990s, including improved understanding of the use of "fortifiers" to add nutritional elements to breastmilk (for tiny babies who were supposed to still be in the womb and not eating by mouth at all), and "lactoengineering" (manipulation of breastmilk components, such as centrifuging expressed human milk to separate out the calorie-rich fatty hindmilk) (Wight, Morton, & Kim, 2008).

Human Milk from Milk Banks

The main difficulty in the 21st century with the use of donor human milk is the small number of milk banks. In the 1980s virtually every hospital NICU in the United States had access to human milk. However, inconsistent practices in pasteurization, usage, and handling led to some bacterial outbreaks. Later, concern that viral pathogens like the human immunodeficiency virus (HIV) could be transmitted in human milk virtually shuttered the milk bank network in North America (Wight, Morton, & Kim, 2008). The non-profit Human Milk Banking Association of North America (HMBANA) was established in 1985 to promulgate safe standards for the collection, screening, pasteurization, and distribution of human milk, and their stringent standards formed the basis for other milk banks opened worldwide (Jones, 2003).

Milk banks can be found all over the world: Australia, Brazil, Bulgaria, the Czech Republic, Denmark, Finland, France, Germany, Greece, India, Japan, Norway, Poland, South Africa, Sweden, Switzerland, and the United Kingdom all have milk banks, and each operates a bit differently although adhering to strict quality control standards (Arnold 2000, 2006b; Nash & Amir, n.d.; Penc, 1996; South African Breastmilk Reserve, 2011; Thorley, 2009). In March 2012, there were 11 nonprofit milk banks operating in North America (the United States and Canada; none yet in Mexico), with 5 in development (Human Milk Banking Association of North America, n.d.c). Donors are carefully screened for health behaviors and communicable diseases, using more conservative standards than those used by blood banks to screen their donors. Then, at HMBANA banks:

> Milk is transported to the milk bank frozen. The milk from several donors is pooled after thawing, and then heat-treated to kill any bacteria or viruses. The milk is processed and then refrozen. It is only dispensed after a sample is cultured and shows no bacteria growth. Milk is shipped frozen by overnight express to hospitals and to individual recipients at home. The milk is dispensed by physician prescription or by hospital purchase order only. There is a processing fee charged to cover the expense of collecting, pasteurizing, and dispensing the milk. (Human Milk Banking Association of North America, n.d.d)

While the milk coming from a nonprofit HMBANA bank is free to the recipient, the costs to process, pasteurize, and ship it are charged, and that can add up considering how much milk a baby consumes. Because of the scarcity of donor human milk, it will only be dispensed by prescription or hospital order: it is reserved for premature or critically ill (e.g., adult cancer) patients, which may come as a surprise to mothers who contact a bank to meet a temporary need for milk to give to a full-term healthy exclusively breastfed baby.

In recent years, a for-profit human milk research company "set up a network of affiliated milk collection organizations [that can be] found in hospitals, birthing centers, or associated with charities. Depending on the organization, they share the responsibilities [with the for-profit entity] of qualifying the donors and collecting the milk" (Prolacta Bioscience, 2012). That milk is then used to create products, primarily human-milk-based fortifiers for use by NICU patients (versus fortifier made by formula companies that are customarily based on cow's milk), which are then sold to hospitals at prices that reflect substantially more than the cost to process, pasteurize, and ship (Prolacta Bioscience, 2012). The screening and functioning of donors is very similar to that for the nonprofit milk banks (Prolacta Bioscience, 2012); the difference is that one organization is formed and operating under nonprofit requirements (Human Milk Banking Association of North America, n.d.e); the other is a profit-driven company (Prolacta Bioscience, 2012).

Does that make one entity "better" or "more ethical" than the other? Not at all: while each collects and processes donor human milk, they are simply operating under separate organizational frameworks and fiduciary obligations. Legal and bioethical scholars have explored the notion of the commodification of breastfeeding human milk, offering sound arguments for women to be empowered to sell and make a profit on any extra milk they can produce (Fentiman, 2009; Waldeck, 2002). Nonetheless, there are those who fear that selling human organs, tissue, and fluids might exploit vulnerable women and generate a dangerous black market.

Human Milk from a Relative or Friend

Life and lactation have a way of not always working out as planned, sometimes with heartbreaking result. Some mothers may have insufficient supply (or no supply) due to a health history they did not realize may affect lactation, or circumstances that occurred after birth (West & Marasco, 2009). Some may have a condition considered incompatible with breastfeeding (HIV; see American Academy of Pediatrics, 2012) or require treatment that precludes breastfeeding (cancer therapy) (Lawrence & Lawrence, 2011). Mothers may die in childbirth, or sometime thereafter when the infant or child is still breastfeeding. Sometimes a happy event is at play: a family adopts a child, and the adoptive mother either cannot (or chose not to) induce lactation. Whatever the reason for an early end to a mother's breastfeeding relationship, the compassionate reaction of friends and relatives of the affected family may be to offer their own breastmilk for the baby's use.

It is not up to the IBCLC to determine whether or not this is a good idea, but she will undoubtedly be asked if she was part of the healthcare team serving the family experiencing the lactation crisis. Recall the opening paragraphs of this chapter: the IBCLC's primary role and responsibility is to provide evidence-based information, so the family can make an informed decision. There are benefits, and risks, to such an arrangement of human milk donation, and the family should be apprised of them all.

One recognized expert on donor human milk and milk banking discourages the practice of personal milk sharing in lieu of a donor bank:

> Donor milk banks have put several safeguards into place to prevent the possibility of disease transmission. First, all donors are carefully screened for diseases of various kinds before their milk is accepted. In the informal sharing situation this safeguard is usually absent. Additionally, donor milk banks pasteurize all milk prior to distribution and check it for bacterial content. This safeguard is also not present when women share milk with each other informally. Because some individuals may have a viral or bacterial infection but remain asymptomatic (without symptoms), they may never know that they are infecting another party. For this reason, "knowing someone well" would be inadequate protection against disease transmission because the carrier is unaware she is infected. In the case of sexually transmitted diseases or illegal drug use, people may go to extremes to protect discovery of the behavior that led to the infection. [I]magine the strain on a family relationship and dynamic, not to mention the guilt, if a child should become ill because of a disease that was transmitted via the shared milk of a relative. (Arnold, 2000, paras. 3–6)

HMBANA's position is similar:

> The practice of casual sharing of milk or procuring milk from any source other than an established donor milk bank operating under HMBANA Guidelines, or similar guidelines established in other countries, has potential risks for both the recipient and the donor or her child. HMBANA does not endorse the practice of selling or purchasing human milk, human milk components, or human milk by-products. (Human Milk Banking Association of North America, n.d.a, p. 1)

These cautions are valid. In the compassionate rush by family and friends to "get some breastmilk to that baby!" the IBCLC may be the first person who will gently raise the notion that breastmilk is a human bodily fluid, which means it may carry pathogens. Not all viruses and bacteria are deadly; after all, we live in an unsterile world. But a grieving or traumatized family deserves a chance to "take a deep breath" and consider all the ramifications, good and bad, of relying on friends and relatives to do the job that the mother cannot now do herself. The arrangement can be hugely emotionally charged, but it can only be assessed case by case, person by person, by the family in question, after consideration of all the available evidenced-based information.

In addition to the strain and guilt if the donor passes on a disease, there is also the scenario where the donor(s) do an absolutely fantastic job of providing milk for the baby whose own mother could not. That mother may be grateful, and she may also come to resent all those family members and friends whom she feels "out-mothered" her by supplying bounteous volumes of expressed milk. To repeat: the IBCLC does not (and should not) serve as the counselor helping the affected family to work through these emotional potholes, but she can use her likely position as "first responder" to send the family to credible resources like HMBANA to learn about donor human milk.

There are options besides "No, thanks" that the family can weigh regarding the use of donor milk. The donating family/friends could agree to have a HMBANA-level screening done at their own cost and initiative, to reduce risks associated with the use of their milk. The California Perinatal Quality Care Collaborative (a consortium of NICU practitioners who develop evidence-based best practices) has forms to be used by nonmother human milk donors to take to their own healthcare providers, for screening and testing to assure their milk can be safely used by a premature infant (Wight, Rhine, et al., 2008, Appendix 4-C). The individual milk banks often have their screening and testing requirements right online; they may be reached by links at the HMBANA site (www.hmbana.org). If an independent laboratory does the screening/blood-testing, the results are kept confidential: the potential donor who learns she is not a good candidate need not share with the affected family *why* her donations won't be suitable, but she will be able to indicate that her donations aren't suitable. Since HMBANA screening and testing is so conservative, there are many innocuous reasons why a lactating woman is not a good donor candidate (for example, if she has been ingesting certain herbs to boost her own milk supply).

The affected family can decide to pool and pasteurize the milk provided by their prescreened group of donors: Holder pasteurization (heating glass bottles of pooled breastmilk in a 62.5°C [145°F] water bath for 30 minutes) is an effective means to remove bacteria from breastmilk (Landers & Updegrove, 2010). Flash heating (place a covered glass jar of milk into a pan of water; heat both until water boils and remove jar of milk to cool) and Pretoria pasteurization (place a covered glass jar of milk into a pan of water that has just been boiled, but removed from the heat; cover the pot for 15–20 minutes, remove jar of milk and allow it to cool before feeding) removes *E. coli* and *S. aureus* bacteria and destroys the HIV virus, while retaining significant nutritional aspects of the milk (Israel-Ballard et al., 2008; Morrison, 2003).

The family also needs to consider the short- and long-term health risks to the child of not receiving any breastmilk and having to rely exclusively on infant formula (ILCA, Spatz, & Lessen, 2011; Ip et al., 2007). The IBCLC can guide the affected family to consider all of these options, and their benefits and risks.

Human Milk Through Informal Sharing Networks

As mentioned earlier, the concept of a baby receiving breastmilk from someone other than her mother is hardly new. Mothers have been doing this since the dawn of time. Wet-nursing was once a well-respected form of employment, but did not involve a concept of reciprocity: the wet nurse was paid to feed the baby directly at breast. More recently, when health and altruistic motives drive a mother's desire to ensure that her child is exclusively breastfed, she may craft a reciprocal arrangement with sisters or friends who are simultaneously lactating: you feed mine when you are watching her, and I'll feed yours. Hence, the terms cross-nursing, cross-feeding, and co-feeding have been coined in the modern age (Thorley, 2009). For all of the reasons suggested in the paragraphs above, mothers engaging in informal milk sharing should consider the risks and benefits of such an arrangement.

It should not be a surprise, in 2012, that mothers have taken this one step further, and have developed informal networks to share breastmilk that go beyond the circle of immediate family and friends. Social media allows women across the globe to have instant access to one another. Given the scarcity of milk (generally) from donor human milk banks, and its preferential use for premature or ill recipients, many mothers who are "sold" on the importance of exclusive breastfeeding may be stymied when they try to find a place to procure milk for their full-term, healthy baby who cannot receive milk from his mother right now. Perhaps the mother will be away for a few days, weeks, or months, and she cannot or will not try to express milk beforehand, or express and ship her milk back home. Perhaps she is undergoing treatment that is incompatible, on a short-term basis, with breastfeeding. Maybe she has had an unexpected plunge in milk supply, and she needs to feed the baby while she figures out what happened. The great irony is that our science and culture tell us that exclusive breastfeeding is the biologic norm for human infants, designed to build everything from the baby's brain to its immune system to its mental health and well-being, and yet if the mother is unable to provide milk to her baby for even a brief period, easy and affordable alternatives to infant formula are not readily available (Arnold, 2006a).

And so, informal milk sharing networks have sprung up: on email lists, social networking sites, blogs, and online shopping or classified ad venues, where seekers of milk can match themselves with providers. Attempts to curb the advertisements may come from the Internet host (Ryan, 2010); governmental agencies may issue warnings cautioning against informal milk sharing (Health Canada, 2010; U.S. Food and Drug Administration, 2010). But the networks persist. The element of trust is heightened in such situations: it is one matter for a mother to ask her sister to get screened and tested, and to take comfort in the results that come back; it is another to rely on assurances made in an email from someone the mother has never met. Verification in the first instance is a bit easier than in the second.

IBCLCs may be asked by mothers to recommend reliable milk sharing sites for acquiring or peddling human milk. Recalling the legal and ethical sphere of our professional responsibility (described at the start of this chapter), the IBCLC can never go wrong in providing evidence-based information and support about the benefits and risks of the use of donor human milk, generally. But once the IBCLC steers a mother to one site over another, she runs the risk of appearing to be a broker, or of offering an "implied endorsement" of the source of the donor human milk.

Summary

IBCLC's may suspect that a mother's breastfeeding rights are being infringed, or the mother may come directly to the IBCLC seeking assistance to resolve nonlactation issues. *The IBCLC's legal and ethical responsibility is to provide evidence-based information and support, so the mother can make an informed decision about lactation.* The IBCLC does not serve as a legal advisor or counselor to the mother for nonlactation matters, but she can serve as a resource, steering the mother to find websites, printed materials, offices or programs that provide competent and expert help to address her specific needs.

REFERENCES

Academy of Breastfeeding Medicine, Eglash, A., Chantry, C., & Howard, C. (2010, March). *Human milk storage information for home use for healthy full-term infants, rev. 1* (Protocol No. 8). Retrieved from http://www.bfmed.org/Resources/Protocols.aspx

Akre, J., Gribble, K., & Minchin, M. (2011). Milk sharing: From private practice to public pursuit. *International Breastfeeding Journal, 6*(8). Retrieved from http://www.internationalbreastfeedingjournal.com/content/pdf/1746-4358-6-8.pdf

Alewell, D., & Pull, K. (2005, October). An international comparison and assessment of maternity leave legislation. *Comparative labor law and policy journal, 22*(2), 297–326. Retrieved from http://www.law.uiuc.edu/publications/cll%26pj/archive/vol_22/issue_2/PullArticle22-2-3.pdf

American Academy of Pediatrics. (2012, March 1). American Academy of Pediatrics policy on breastfeeding and use of human milk. *Pediatrics, 129*(3), e827–e841. Retrieved from http://pediatrics.aappublications.org/content/early/2012/02/22/peds.2011-3552.full.pdf

Americans with Disabilities Act, as amended, 42 U.S.C. § 12101 et seq. (1990), http://www.ada.gov/pubs/adastatute08.htm.

Arnold, L. D. (2000, April/May). Becoming a donor to a human milk bank. *Leaven, 36*(2), 19–23. Retrieved from http://www.llli.org/lllleaderweb/LV/LVAprMay00p19.html

Arnold, L. D. (2006a). The ethics of donor human milk banking. *Breastfeeding Medicine, 1*(1), 3–13. Retrieved from http://www.liebertonline.com/doi/pdf/10.1089/bfm.2006.1.3

Arnold, L. D. (2006b, December 12). Global health policies that support the use of banked donor human milk: A human rights issue. *International Breastfeeding Journal, 1*(26), 1–8. Retrieved from http://www.ncbi.nlm.nih.gov/pmc/articles/PMC1766344/pdf/1746-4358-1-26.pdf

Baby-Friendly USA. (2010). *Info for breastfeeding advocates/health care professionals.* Retrieved from http://www.babyfriendlyusa.org/eng/06.html

California Employment Development Department. (2010). *FAQ—Relation of the paid family insurance program to the family and medical leave act (FMLA) and the California family rights act (CFRA).* Retrieved from http://www.edd.ca.gov/disability/FAQs_for_Paid_Family_Leave.htm

Christrup, S. (2001). Breastfeeding in the American workplace. *Journal of Gender, Social Policy & the Law, 9*(3), 471–503. Retrieved from http://www.iiav.nl/ezines/web/AmericanUniversityJournal/1999-2003/american/9-3christrup.pdf

Citizens Information Board-Ireland. (2011, November 14). *Eligibility for jury service [Ireland].* Retrieved from http://www.citizensinformation.ie/en/justice/courtroom/eligibility_and_selection.html

Cowling, M., & Sinclair, A. (2007, February). *Danger! UK at work!* (Monograph No. WP10). Retrieved from http://www.employment-studies.co.uk/pdflibrary/wp10.pdf

Dettwyler, K. A. (1995). A time to wean: The hominid blueprint for the natural age of weaning in modern human populations. In P. Stuart-Macadam & K. A. Dettwyler, *Breastfeeding: Biocultural Perspectives* (pp. 39–74). New York, NY: Aldine De Gruyter.

Family and Medical Leave Act, 29 U.S.C. § 2601 et seq. (1993), http://codes.lp.findlaw.com/uscode/29/28/2601.

Family Friendly Jury Duty. (2007, March 26). *States and U.S. territories with family friendly jury duty.* Retrieved from http://www.familyfriendlyjuryduty.org/JuryStates/JuryStates.htm

Family Law Courts of Australia. (n.d.). *Family dispute resolution: Alternatives to going to court.* Retrieved from http://www.familylawcourts.gov.au/wps/wcm/connect/FLC/Home/About+Going+to+Court/Family+dispute+resolution/

Fentiman, L. (2009). Marketing mothers' milk: The commodification of breastfeeding and the new markets in human milk and infant formula. *Nevada Law Review, 10*, 1–72. Retrieved from http://papers.ssrn.com/sol3/papers.cfm?abstract_id=1370425

Gribble, K., & Berry, N. (2011). Emergency preparedness for those who care for infants in developed country contexts. *International Breastfeeding Journal, 6*(16). Retrieved from http://www.internationalbreastfeedingjournal.com/content/pdf/1746-4358-6-16.pdf

Health Canada. (2010, November 25). *Health Canada raises concerns about the use of unprocessed human milk.* Retrieved from http://www.hc-sc.gc.ca/ahc-asc/media/advisories-avis/_2010/2010_202-eng.php

Human Milk Banking Association of North America. (n.d.a). *Donor human milk: Ensuring safety and ethical allocation* [Position paper]. Retrieved from http://hmbana.org/downloads/position-paper-safety-ethical.pdf

Human Milk Banking Association of North America. (n.d.b). *Frequently asked questions.* Retrieved from https://www.hmbana.org/faq#how

Human Milk Banking Association of North America. (n.d.c). *HMBANA milk bank locations.* Retrieved from https://www.hmbana.org/milk-bank-locations

Human Milk Banking Association of North America. (n.d.d). *Processing.* Retrieved from https://www.hmbana.org/processing

Human Milk Banking Association of North America. (n.d.e). *Welcome* [Home page]. Retrieved from https://www.hmbana.org

Infant and Young Child Feeding in Emergencies (IFE) Core Group. (2007, February). *Operational guidance for emergency relief staff and programme managers* (Version No. 2.1). Retrieved from http://www.ennonline.net/pool/files/ife/ops-guidance-2-1-english-010307-with-addendum.pdf

International Board of Lactation Consultant Examiners. (2008, March 8). *Scope of practice for international board certified lactation consultants.* Retrieved from http://www.iblce.org/upload/downloads/ScopeOfPractice.pdf

International Board of Lactation Consultant Examiners. (2011, November 1). *Code of professional conduct for IBCLCs.* Retrieved from http://iblce.org/upload/downloads/CodeOfProfessionalConduct.pdf

International Code Documentation Centre (Ed.). (2007, May). *International code of marketing of breastmilk substitutes and relevant WHA resolutions (annotated)* (2nd updated edition). Penang, Malaysia: IBFAN Penang.

International Labour Organization. (1972). Chapter II Article 19. In *International labour organization constitution (as amended 1972).* Retrieved from http://www.ilo.org/ilolex/english/constq.htm

International Labour Organization (Ed.). (2006). *ILO gender network handbook.* Retrieved from http://www .ilo.org/public/libdoc/ilo/2006/106B09_302_engl.pdf

International Lactation Consultant Association. (2006). *Standards of practice for international board certified lactation consultants.* Retrieved from http://www.ilca.org/files/resources/Standards-of-Practice-web.pdf

International Lactation Consultant Association, Spatz, D., & Lessen, R. (2011). *Risks of not breastfeeding* [Monograph]. Morrisville, NC: International Lactation Consultant Association.

Ip, S., Chung, M., Raman, G., Chew, P., Magula, N., DeVine, D., . . . Lau, J. (2007, April). *Breastfeeding and maternal and infant health outcomes in developed countries* (Rep. No. 153). Rockville, MD: U.S. Agency for Healthcare Research and Quality.

Israel-Ballard, K., Coutsoudis, A., Chantry, C. J., Sturm, A. W., Karim, F., Sibeko, L., . . . Sukirtha, T. H. (2008, September). Flash-heated and pretoria pasteurized destroys HIV in breast milk and preserves nutrients! *Advanced Biotechnology,* 32–35. Retrieved from http://www.advancedbiotech.in/51%20Flash%20 heated.pdf

Jones, F. (2003, October). *The history of milk banking.* Retrieved from http://hmbana.org/index/history

La Leche League International. (2011). *Breastfeeding and family law.* Retrieved from http://www.llli.org/Law /LawUS.html?m=0,1,0

Landers, S., & Updegrove, K. (2010, June). Bacteriological screening of donor human milk before and after Holder pasteurization. *Breastfeeding Medicine, 5*(3), 117–121. Retrieved from http://www.liebertonline .com/doi/pdf/10.1089/bfm.2009.0032

Law Reform Commission of Western Australia. (2009, October). *Selection, eligibility and exemption of jurors: Discussion paper* (Monograph No. 99). Retrieved from http://www.lrc.justice.wa.gov.au/2publications /reports/P99-DP/Ch06-Jurors.pdf

Lawrence, R., & Lawrence, R. (2011). *Breastfeeding: A guide for the medical profession* (7th ed.). Maryland Heights, MO: Elsevier Mosby.

Legal Information Institute, Cornell University Law School. (n.d.a). *Divorce laws.* Retrieved from http:// topics.law.cornell.edu/wex/table_divorce

Legal Information Institute, Cornell University Law School. (n.d.b). *Family law—State statutes.* Retrieved from http://topics.law.cornell.edu/wex/table_family

Marcus, J. A. (2007, July/August). Lactation and the law. *Mothering, 143.* Retrieved from http://mothering.com /breastfeeding/lactation-and-the-law

Marcus, J. A. (2011, August 11). *Lactation and the law revisited.* Retrieved from http://mothering.com /breastfeeding/lactation-and-law-revisited

Marcus, J. A. (2012). *Think you know what your breastfeeding rights are?* Retrieved from http://breastfeeding law.com

Morrison, P. (2003). *Pasteurized breastmilk as a replacement feed for babies of HIV-infected mothers.* Retrieved from http://www.pronutrition.org/pubview.php/61

Mothering.com. (2010, December 15). *Workplace pumping and the law.* Retrieved from http://www .mothering.com/sites/resources/map.pdf

Nash, C., & Amir, L. (n.d.). *Human milk banking: A review*. Retrieved from http://www.breastfeedingindia
.com/breastfeeding/human_milk_banks.html

National Association of Citizens Advice Bureaux. (2012). *Legal system—In Scotland—Jury service* [Jury
service rights]. Retrieved from http://www.adviceguide.org.uk/scotland/your_rights/legal_system_index
_scotland/jury_service_scotland.htm

National Coalition Against Domestic Violence. (2011a). *National coalition against domestic violence* [Home
page]. Retrieved from http://www.ncadv.org

National Coalition Against Domestic Violence. (2011b). *International organization resources*. Retrieved from
http://www.ncadv.org/resources/InternationalOrganizationResources.php

National Conference of State Legislatures. (2011, May). *Breastfeeding state laws*. Retrieved from http://www
.ncsl.org/default.aspx?tabid=14389

Orozco, N. K. (2010). Pumping at work: Protection from lactation discrimination in the workplace.
Ohio State Law Journal, 71(6), 1281–1316. Retrieved from http://moritzlaw.osu.edu/lawjournal/issues
/volume71/number6/orozco.pdf

Patient Protection and Affordable Care Act [Health Care Reform] amending the Fair Labor Standards
Act, 29 U.S.C. § 207 (2010), http://www.usbreastfeeding.org/Portals/0/Workplace/HR3590-Sec4207
-Nursing-Mothers.pdf.

Penc, B. (1996). Organization and activity of a human milk bank in Poland. *Journal of Human Lactation,
12*(3), 243–246. Retrieved from http://jhl.sagepub.com/content/12/3/243.full.pdf+html

Prolacta Bioscience. (2012). *Frequently asked questions*. Retrieved from http://www.prolacta.com/faq.php

Ryan, D. (2010, November 30). Mom booted from Craigslist for offering breast milk for sale. *The Vancouver
Sun*. Retrieved from http://www.vancouversun.com/life/Spring+Preview+Anything+goes+this+spring
+your+style/2686124/booted+from+Craigslist+offering+breast+milk+sale/3908429/story.html

Service Canada. (2011, August 9). *Employment insurance maternity and parental benefits*. Retrieved from
http://www.servicecanada.gc.ca/eng/sc/ei/benefits/maternityparental.shtml

South African Breastmilk Reserve. (2011). *Keeping it real—Our footprint 2012*. Retrieved from http://www
.sabr.org.za

Thorley, V. (2009). Mothers' experiences of sharing breastfeeding or breastmilk: Co-feeding in Australia
1978–2008. *Breastfeeding Review, 17*(1), 9–18. Retrieved from http://www.waba.org.my/pdf/BFR
_Mar_09_Thorley.pdf

UNICEF. (2012, March 21). *The baby-friendly hospital initiative*. Retrieved from http://www.unicef.org
/programme/breastfeeding/baby.htm

U.S. Breastfeeding Committee. (2010). *Workplace accommodations to support and protect breastfeeding*. Retrieved
from http://www.usbreastfeeding.org/Portals/0/Publications/Workplace-Background-2010-USBC.pdf

U.S. Breastfeeding Committee. (2011a). *Breastfeeding Promotion Act of 2011*. Retrieved from http://
www.usbreastfeeding.org/LegislationPolicy/BreastfeedingAdvocacyHQ/BreastfeedingPromotionAct
/tabid/115/Default.aspx

U.S. Breastfeeding Committee. (2011b). *FAQs: Break time for nursing mothers*. Retrieved from http://www
.usbreastfeeding.org/Default.aspx?TabId=188

U.S. Breastfeeding Committee. (2011c). *Workplace support in federal law*. Retrieved from http://www
.usbreastfeeding.org/Employment/WorkplaceSupport/WorkplaceSupportinFederalLaw/tabid/175
/Default.aspx

U.S. Dept. of Labor Wage and Hour Division. (2010, December). *Fact sheet #73: Break time for nursing
mothers under the FLSA*. Retrieved from http://www.dol.gov/whd/regs/compliance/whdfs73.htm

U.S. Equal Employment Opportunity Commission. (n.d.). *Sexual harassment*. Retrieved from http://www
.eeoc.gov/laws/types/sexual_harassment.cfm

U.S. Food and Drug Administration. (2010, November 30). *Use of donor human milk.* Retrieved from http://www.fda.gov/ScienceResearch/SpecialTopics/PediatricTherapeuticsResearch/ucm235203.htm

U.S. Transportation Security Administration. (n.d.). *Important information on traveling with formula, breast milk, and juice.* Retrieved from http://www.tsa.gov/travelers/airtravel/children/formula.shtm

Vance, M. (2007, October). *Breastfeeding and jury duty.* Retrieved from http://www.llli.org/Law/LawJury.html

Waldeck, S. (2002). Encouraging a market in human milk: Research paper no. 2007-005. *Columbia Journal of Gender and Law, 11,* 361–406. Retrieved from http://papers.ssrn.com/sol3/papers.cfm?abstract_id=1024759##

West, D., & Marasco, L. (2009). *The breastfeeding mother's guide to making more milk.* New York, NY: McGraw Hill.

Wight, N., Rhine, W., Durand, D., Wirtschafter, D., Kim, J., Murphy, B., & Nisbet, C. (2008). *Nutritional support of the very low birth weight infant* (Revised Toolkit). Retrieved from http://www.cpqcc.org/quality_improvement/qi_toolkits/nutritional_support_of_the_vlbw_infant_rev_december_2008

Wight, N. E., Morton, J. A., & Kim, J. H. (2008). *Best medicine: Human milk in the NICU.* Amarillo, TX: Hale.

World Health Organization. (2003). *Global strategy for infant and young child feeding* [Monograph]. Geneva, Switzerland: Author.

Chapter 11

The IBCLC and the Internet

W̱e started with a discussion of Millennial Mom—our mythical mother, home with a new baby and a breastfeeding problem, who turns for a solution to her trusty computer (or cell phone, smartphone, or tablet computer). She reaches out to her circle of friends and search-engine-provided experts. So let us end on a similar note: The International Board Certified Lactation Consultant (IBCLC) in cyberspace. For, if mothers are looking for us "on the Web" or "in the cloud," then IBCLCs had better be there to be found. Mothers seek help from within their social networks, and the IBCLC can become a part of that trusted circle, so long as she keeps her legal and ethical responsibilities in mind.

To state the obvious: The Internet has utterly transformed how we communicate, professionally and socially. It has revolutionized research and writing; search engines (like Google, Bing, or Yahoo!) allow the curious mind, within the blink of an eye, to find thousands of websites and documents containing key terms. This reach and accessibility for scholars is nearly incomprehensible, compared to the days when one had to slog to a large library (if there was one nearby), know which indexes or sources to peruse, hope the facility carried the titles, and be willing to wait for interlibrary loans (sometimes for weeks) to receive a treasured few items requested, as one did not have the luxury of asking for it all. Online publication shortens the lag time between submission and release, speeding up the dissemination of information, and the implementation of new treatments and care plan options (Montgomery, 2002). Social networking sites, designed to promote personal or professional networking, allow for instantaneous reach using varied media. Commercial sites are available for every kind of product or service. Critiques are offered (and read) by users, readers, buyers, consumers, and sellers—and their detractors, nay-sayers, and competitors.

And IBCLCs, too, use this hugely influential and fast-paced realm, whether to gather information, do a little research, or market their services. IBCLCs using the Internet need to be savvy about how they allow their professional presence to be shared or presented, because once something is posted (on a website, in a discussion forum, or within a social network), it can be there in perpetuity. This chapter will explore the legal and ethical issues for the IBCLC who chooses to have a presence, as an IBCLC, in cyberspace. It is up to the IBCLC to learn—elsewhere, or through self-mastery—the best means for such a presence. An entire industry of website designers, software writers, and marketing experts has been born to meet the needs of computer and Internet users.

Can an IBCLC Even Do This?

Can an IBCLC conduct her profession of assisting mothers with breastfeeding and lactation issues on the Internet? Of course she can. The Internet is, after all, nothing more than a near universal form of communication, and effective communication is one of the cornerstones of an excellent IBCLC practice. There are some common sense limitations to this form of communication that must be kept in mind, especially for healthcare providers (HCPs) such as IBCLCs. The following are relevant sections of the IBCLC's practice-guiding documents that address IBCLC clinical practice, and general information sharing, using the Internet.

International Board of Lactation Consultant Examiners (IBLCE) Code of Professional Conduct (CPC)

The IBLCE CPC is a *must* document, describing mandatory professional behaviors for the IBCLC. For the practitioner who is thinking about going online for the educational or consultative aspects of her practice, the pertinent guiding principles are as follows:

Principle 1.1

> Every IBCLC shall:
>
> 1.1 Fulfill professional commitments by working with mothers to meet their breast-feeding goals. (IBLCE, 2011, CPC p. 2)

This simple statement is so profoundly obvious that it is a wonder why there was no corollary to it in the original IBLCE Code of Ethics (IBLCE, 2003), replaced in November 2011 by the Code of Professional Conduct (IBLCE, 2011). What better way to help a mother meet her breastfeeding goals than to provide her evidence-based information, even if you don't know her? The Internet allows IBCLCs easily to provide information of general interest to breastfeeding families, and of specific interest to clients/patients with whom there is a clinical relationship.

Principles 1.2 and 1.3

> 1.2 Provide care to meet clients' individual needs that is culturally appropriate and informed by the best available evidence. (IBLCE, 2011, CPC p. 2)
>
> 1.3 Supply sufficient and accurate information to enable clients to make informed decisions. (IBLCE, 2011, CPC p. 2)

Lactation consultants should be cognizant that the Internet is largely a written-and-read resource. Yes, there are videos and sound clips that can be made a part of a website or communication, but for the most part, information will be read (or more likely, skimmed). The reader will not have the benefit of context, body language, voice intonation, and facial expression, all of which are as critical in conveying meaning as the words themselves (Hall, n.d.).

Supplying "sufficient and accurate information" so the reader is adequately informed, as IBLCE CPC Principle 1.3 requires, means the person who is receiving the communication must recognize it as objective. This can be more challenging than it seems, particularly when, as IBCLCs, we are working with mothers who are attempting to master this "natural" biologic function through a filter of cultural and societal and self-imposed expectations. As an example: try writing a passage about the use of expressed breastmilk, in a bottle, by the mother who must be separated from her baby to work outside the home. The IBCLC runs the risk of appearing judgmental (nonobjective) and thus "turning off" (or worse, offending) those who:

- Stay at home and breastfeed at breast
- Those who "must" return to work outside the home (versus those who "choose" to do so)
- Those who cannot make enough breastmilk
- Those who believe the act of breastfeeding is more important to development than the breastmilk itself
- Those who believe marketing messages about the use of gadgets (like pumps and bottles) dilutes the message of breastfeeding itself

You must choose your words carefully.

Principles 1.4, 5.1 and 5.2

1.4 Convey accurate, complete and objective information about commercial products (see Principle [5.1]). (IBLCE, 2011, CPC p. 2)

5.1 Disclose any actual or apparent conflict of interest, including a financial interest in relevant goods or services, or in organizations which provide relevant goods or services. (IBLCE, 2011, CPC p. 3)

5.2 Ensure that commercial considerations do not influence professional judgment. (IBLCE, 2011, CPC p. 3)

Depending on what venue you use for your Web-based communication, you may find your work appearing on a website that accepts advertising. IBCLCs are often asked to write short articles, or answer questions about lactation. And that is fitting: IBCLCs are the internationally accredited professionals in breastfeeding and human lactation. Ad revenues generated on a website are no crime; they provide money for the website owner to continue to run the site and to allow your words of wisdom to be searched and found from all points of the globe. However, unless you are running your own website, you will not have much control over which ads appear with your article. If your column is cheek-to-jowl with an ad for a product, you (as an IBCLC) may have a real or perceived conflict of interest, because the very placement of the ad suggests your support and endorsement of the product.

Those of us outside the world of computer-based, networked advertising and programming are usually astounded to realize that ads can be tailor-made to suit Millennial Mom's perceived interests. If she is searching the Internet for information about babies and breastfeeding, the site to which she is sent may contain ads for bottles and formula. The advertising programs can be configured to connect the Internet search term "breastfeed" with a resultant ad for "bottle" (Richmond, 2010). As the IBCLC writing the article, be as protective as you can of how your materials are published in cyberspace. You must choose your words (and venue) carefully.

Principle 1.5

1.5 Present information without personal bias. (IBLCE, 2011, CPC p. 3)

There is the obvious edict: Discrimination has no place in lactation consultancy. But there is the less obvious admonition: We serve to help the mother meet *her* breastfeeding goals, even if they differ from the customary IBCLC script delivered from a soapbox. The easiest place to find a "difference of opinion" on lactation is the Internet. When discussing any issue, respectful and considerate language is your goal, and sometimes even that doesn't work, as the comments in reply will quickly reveal. You will more likely win the war (if not the battle) by using diplomacy, strong evidence, and articulate advocacy to present your thoughts. If nothing else has convinced you, Principle 1.5 should: Choose your words carefully.

Principle 2.1

2.1 Operate within the limits of the scope of practice. (IBLCE, 2011, CPC p. 3)

You do not want to appear to overstate your expertise or training while being certain to clearly explain how your particular background and experience make you a viable authority. You must choose your words carefully.

Principle 2.3

2.3 Be responsible and accountable for personal conduct and practice. (IBLCE, 2011, CPC p. 3)

Know your evidence base; respect and honor the families with whom you consult or provide general information. If you are going to put yourself and your wisdom in the very public forum that is the Internet, take care not to appear inept by sharing out-dated information. Stay on top of breastfeeding and human lactation research. Keep up with online trends to find out what mothers are talking about. Review blogs or trusted websites to see what policy issues are brewing. You must choose your words (and sources) carefully.

Principles 3.1 and 3.2

> 3.1 Refrain from revealing any information acquired in the course of the professional relationship, except to another member of a client's healthcare team, or to other persons or entities for which the client has granted express permission, except only as provided in the Definitions and Interpretations to the CPC. (IBLCE, 2011, CPC p. 3)

> 3.2 Refrain from photographing, recording, or taping (audio or video) a mother or her child for any purpose unless the mother has given advance written consent on her behalf and that of her child. (IBLCE, 2011, CPC p. 3)

This is one of the most important elements of our clinical relationship with mothers, and one of the easiest principles to be violated when using computer-based communication, even without a website. See the more detailed discussion on this subject later in this chapter. Suffice to say, for now: You must choose your words carefully, and be protective of how your materials are published (or sent) on the Internet.

Principle 4.1

> 4.1 Receive a client's consent, before initiating a consultation, to share clinical information with other members of the client's healthcare team. (IBLCE, 2011, CPC p. 3)

While conducting an entire lactation consultation online presents logistical problems, it is not impossible. Indeed, combined Web camera and Internet phone services on one computer (such as Skype, Paltalk, iChat, IM, and Google chat) allow an IBCLC to have a discreet conversation, complete with live pictures, with a mother and baby who could be halfway around the world! IBCLCs who have attained specialized expertise in rare or hard to assess clinical situations may find this is a feasible means of assisting breastfeeding families. But, all the regular rules of face-to-face consultations apply, including the need to obtain proper consents, communicate with other HCPs if needed, and obtaining payment for services rendered. The IBCLC will be careful to use whatever charting and administrative requirements are appropriate to her geopolitical and work setting, and she will choose her words carefully.

Principle 6.1

> 6.1 Behave honestly and fairly as a health professional. (IBLCE, 2011, CPC p. 4)

It is obvious, but so important it bears repeating: IBCLCs cannot say or promise more than they can deliver. Our bottom-line ethical and legal responsibility is to *provide evidence-based information and support, so the mother can make an informed decision about lactation.* However, we also know that every mother is different: her baby, her breasts, her family, her work and home situation; all of this has an "impact" on human lactation, because a breastfeeding mother's responsibility occurs every day, and often all day, until she weans. It is difficult to state something in a way that can apply to all mothers everywhere. You must choose your words carefully.

Principles 7.2, 7.3, and 7.4

7.2 Provide only accurate information to the public and colleagues concerning lactation consultant services offered. (IBLCE, 2011, CPC p. 4)

7.3 Permit use of the IBCLC's name for the purpose of certifying that lactation consultant services have been rendered only when the IBCLC provided those services. (IBLCE, 2011, CPC p. 4)

7.4 Use the acronyms "IBCLC" and "RLC" or the titles "International Board Certified Lactation Consultant" and "Registered Lactation Consultant" only when certification is current and in the manner in which IBLCE authorizes their use. (IBLCE, 2011, CPC p. 4)

These principles go to what the mother thinks she is getting when she communicates with, or visits the website of, an IBCLC. If the mother thinks she is communicating with, or reading something written by, an IBCLC, that had better be the case. If the IBCLC is using a website to advertise her lactation clinic, she should also clearly indicate the fee and insurance reimbursement arrangements. Hours and services provided (classes, retail, etc.) should be plainly and truthfully stated. And to review: the IBCLC should not make promises she cannot keep. A blanket claim in an ad that "all babies leave the office breastfeeding" simply cannot be made; some babies will not be feeding at breast yet, or perhaps ever.

These principles are designed to protect the integrity of the IBCLC certification, by asking that only those who have earned it use it. On the Internet, communication does not occur face to face, and the potential for abuse is huge. The public relies on the information provided on a website if it purports to be written by an expert, and yet, there is no easy way to verify authorship. The IBCLC may only use those initials if her certification is current, and, as there is no means to designate the retired or aspiring IBCLC, only current IBCLCs may use those initials. The practitioner who lets her certification lapse, yet continues to represent herself as an IBCLC, does her former profession and the public at large a great disservice by such misrepresentation. Is the next phrase starting to sound familiar? You must choose your words (and state your truthful certification) carefully.

Introduction, Paragraph 3

> A crucial part of an IBCLC's duty to protect mothers and children is adherence to the principles and aim of the International Code of Marketing of Breast-milk Substitutes and subsequent relevant World Health [Assembly] resolutions. (IBLCE, 2011, CPC p. 1)

The *International Code of Marketing of Breast-Milk Substitutes* (WHO Code or International Code) is a model public health policy statement about ethical marketing of four categories of products: infant formula, bottles, teats, and foods intended to be given to babies in lieu of breastfeeding at breast. The WHO Code is a *should* that may be turned into a *must* for the IBCLC, if she works in an institution that requires it be followed (Baby-Friendly USA, 2010), or she practices in a country that has enacted the International Code with enforceable legislation (WHO, 1981). Any IBCLC with an Internet presence will have to be especially mindful that her materials are not seen to be "sponsored" by one of the companies that market in violation of the WHO Code. This can be particularly difficult since the manner by which ads are selected to be shown are tailored to perceived interests of individual viewers, and many Internet search programs equate babies with bottles and formula (Richmond, 2010). It may be difficult or impossible for the IBCLC to avoid being displayed next to these ads, especially if she is a guest commentator or columnist for a Web-based resource. Making declarations of WHO Code support in the body of the article is one option, though such material may be edited out once it leaves the writer's hands. The IBCLC should not only choose her words carefully, but her Internet-based partners and presence as well.

The IBLCE Scope of Practice (SOP) for IBCLCs

The IBLCE SOP is another *must* document. It describes the professional "territory" within which an IBCLC may ethically and professional practice. All IBCLCs everywhere must practice within the confines of the IBLCE SOP; some of the duties described therein encompass the activities in which an IBCLC with an Internet presence will participate.

Preamble

> International Board Certified Lactation Consultants (IBCLCs) have demonstrated specialized knowledge and clinical expertise in breastfeeding and human lactation and are certified by the International Board of Lactation Consultant Examiners (IBLCE).

> This Scope of Practice encompasses the activities for which IBCLCs are educated and in which they are authorized to engage. The aim of the Scope of Practice is to protect the public by ensuring that all IBCLCs provide safe, competent and evidence-based care. As this is an international credential, the Scope of Practice is applicable in any country or setting where IBCLCs practice. (IBLCE, 2008, SOP paras. 1 & 2)

These two introductory paragraphs identify the IBCLC as having special knowledge in lactation, and explain that this scope of practice defines her boundaries of clinical practice. And, it is international in scope. This IBLCE SOP provides validation for the IBCLC's right, as a member of the healthcare team, to assess and care for the breast-feeding dyad. The IBLCE SOP enumerates several major duties that all IBCLCs, everywhere, must fulfill. We'll explore those for the IBCLC who chooses to use the Internet to share her expertise.

Duty to Uphold the Standards of the IBCLC Profession

The IBCLC will work within the legal framework of her geopolitical setting, and her practice-guiding documents. She will integrate knowledge and evidence in providing her specialized lactation care. Similar to the responsibilities described in the IBLCE CPC, the IBCLC with an Internet presence must uphold her own, and her profession's, standards of excellence (IBLCE, 2008, SOP para. 3). Thus, she must choose her words carefully.

Duty to Protect, Promote, and Support Breastfeeding

This duty is accomplished by "educating women, families, health professionals, and the community;" acting as an advocate for breastfeeding; using language that assists the learner; and by complying with the WHO Code (IBLCE, 2008, SOP para. 4). The IBCLC in cyberspace must choose her words carefully, and be protective of overt or subtle conflicts of interest due to ad placement.

Duty to Provide Competent Services

If the IBCLC will be promoting her own lactation consultancy over the Internet, or providing one-on-one care using such electronic or computer-based methods, she will be held to the same standards of competence and propriety required of a face-to-face encounter. This includes her duties to perform a comprehensive assessment, to develop individualized care plans with the mother's input, to offer evidence-based information regarding lactation-impacting therapies and drugs, and to offer support and encourage-ment (IBLCE, 2008, SOP para. 5). All of these clinical and educational actions will have limitations when offered over a communication system that prevents face-to-face assessment and discussion. The IBCLC will have to choose her words carefully.

Duty to Report Truthfully and Fully; Duty to Preserve Client Confidence

This one is fairly straightforward: follow the laws of the land to record, chart, and maintain your clinical contacts (IBLCE, 2008, SOP para. 6). For the IBCLC on the Internet, the challenge is in doing so in a manner that protects the confidentiality of the client/patient (IBLCE, 2008, SOP para. 7), as materials can much more easily be erroneously disseminated when computers and mobile phones are at play. This begs the question of what is considered a "clinical contact" when it happens over the computer. The IBCLC will choose her words carefully.

Duty to Act with Reasonable Diligence

The IBCLC will provide evidence-based, conflict-free information to families, make necessary referrals to other experts as needed, and work collaboratively with the rest of the mother's and baby's healthcare team (IBLCE, 2008, SOP para. 8). Failure to do so will be grounds for a disciplinary action filed with IBLCE. You will want to choose your words carefully.

The International Lactation Consultant Association (ILCA) Standards of Practice

The ILCA Standards of Practice for International Board Certified Lactation Consultants (ILCA Standards) is a model document that is a compendium of best professional practices in which the IBCLC *should* engage. While no sanctions attach for failure to follow the ILCA Standards, they lay out an easy-to-follow roadmap of best practices for the IBCLC, and all of the sections have relevance to the IBCLC using the Internet to communicate, educate, and advertise. The major elements are discussed in the following sections.

Standard 1. Professional Responsibilities

> The IBCLC has a responsibility to maintain professional conduct and to practice in an ethical manner, accountable for professional actions and legal responsibilities. (ILCA, 2006, Standard 1)

The IBCLC will support the IBLCE CPC and WHO Code, and be mindful of conflicts of interest while communicating on the Internet just as when she is in face-to-face consultations. While the publication of the ILCA Standards predates the publication of the IBLCE SOP, the latter is *must* document for IBCLCs, and they will honor its requirements.

Standard 2. Legal Considerations

> The IBCLC is obligated to practice within the laws of the geopolitical region and setting in which she/he works. The IBCLC must practice with consideration for rights of privacy and with respect for matters of a confidential nature. (ILCA, 2006, Standard 2)

Maintaining records according to the laws of the land or workplace; respecting client/patient confidentiality; obtaining necessary consents; all are familiar concepts in real-life practice that must translate to computer-based media.

Standard 3. Clinical Practice

The clinical practice of the IBCLC focuses on providing clinical lactation care and management. This is best accomplished by promoting optimal health, through collaboration and problem solving with the client and other members of the healthcare team. The role of the IBCLC includes:

- Assessment, planning, intervention, and evaluation of care in a variety of situations
- Anticipatory guidance and prevention of problems
- Complete, accurate, and timely documentation of care
- Communication and collaboration with other healthcare professionals (ILCA, 2006, Standard 3)

The IBCLC using social media will need to accomplish her full range of services and education just as conscientiously as if she were working with a mother face to face, and had to share concerns with another HCP down the hall.

Standard 3. Clinical Practice

Breastfeeding education and counseling are integral parts of the care provided by the IBCLC. (ILCA, 2006, Standard 3)

Education and counseling can be offered over the Internet. To comply with *any* aspect of the ILCA Standards of Practice, the IBCLC will want to choose her words carefully.

What Is Out in Cyberspace?

There are many ways to communicate using networked media on the Internet. Some modes are openly available for public access; some allow only pre-designated individuals to have access; some are intended for private communication only. The most basic (and self-protective) notion that the IBCLC will want to keep in mind, whether she is using the Internet for personal or professional messages, is that using a computer, phone or tablet means *the communication can be permanent, and might be seen by anyone.* That is why the suggestion has been made, *ad nauseum*: **The IBCLC must choose her words carefully**.

The surge of social media and networking (where participants post messages and pictures on websites accessible by others) allows for increased visibility of the IBCLC and her message, but it can also blur the lines between one's professional and personal life. Do you really want your clients to know that you had dinner with your in-laws yesterday? Do you really want your cousin to read your pontifications on sore nipples? Only you can answer that. One consideration that never had to be made "back in the day" (when conversations evaporated into thin air as soon as one got up from the coffee klatsch table) is that social networking sites allow for permanence. Recognize your audience and choose your language, because it will be available for others to see for a very long time.

Websites

Most of us are familiar with the concept of turning on the computer and visiting a website. Just the "address" or domain name can give the IBCLC a clue about her use of the Internet as a resource for research, and to evaluate the reliability of the information. A website that ends in *.com* was originally used only by *com*mercial enterprises. Enough noncommercial entities began using the *.com* domain address, however, that *.biz* was created to identify websites that are truly businesses (Verio Communications Co., 2012). Such a site is being run by a business, with the business's interest the first and foremost objective. Other common domains:

.edu   Restricted for use by accredited educational institutions (and recall just how difficult it is to actually become accredited as an educational institution).

.gov   Restricted for use by the United States government.

.org   Not restricted; customarily used by organizations such as not-for-profit entities.

.name   Restricted for use by individuals who want to register their own name as a domain name. This permits for a personal website (and is one means of effective branding for IBCLCs who want to market their services).

.info   Not restricted; used by organizations that provide useful reference information (Verio Communications Co., 2012).

Besides these generic domains, a growing number of country code domain names will identify websites from a particular country or political union, such as ".au" for Australia or ".eu" for the European Union (Wikipedia, 2012). This might be important to a company that does extensive business in another country. To the IBCLC, it is a clue into the source of origin for the material she is accessing, and the IBCLC or lactation support practices in that part of the world. One's ability to register a company and domain name will vary from country to country.

The mechanics of getting a website up and running are not all that difficult (to those who understand these matters). You can use a do-it-yourself template or spend hundreds of thousands of dollars for a website design, development, and marketing agency. While it is possible to create a website and make it operational for virtually no cost, the IBCLC who is planning to use a website as her professional platform should approach this matter as thoughtfully as any professional or business decision. Most IBCLCs do not have training in graphics and marketing and computer programming, even if they are savvy about the need to be accessible on the Internet by mothers and other healthcare providers. It will be well worth the time and effort to learn what elements are needed for a well-designed and user-friendly website. It is far more than the content (all those carefully chosen words): everything from color to font to graphics to ease of navigation must be considered. A poorly designed website is instantly passed over, and its operator (our well-intentioned, excellent IBCLC) may be deemed unprofessional in the mind of the Web surfer. Not exactly the message that was intended.

At the very least, a website allows the visitor to see the information the website owners have chosen to display. It may be content that has been (carefully) written. It may be material from another source; permission for such use must be granted, in keeping with copyright law requirements mandated by the IBLCE CPC (IBLCE, 2011, CPC Principle 2.5; Pennsylvania Bar Institute, 2010). Customarily, a website is meant for one-way communication: The website owners decide what goes on the site, and the Web surfer can poke around to her heart's content. There is usually a Contact Us page on a website, so an inquiry can be made of the website operator. Or, there may be a comments page where you can share your thoughts on a page that will, subsequently, be viewed by every new visitor to the webpage. But for the most part, if it is on a website, it is content put there by the website owner to be accessed and viewed by the public.

Social Media or Social Networks

"Web 2.0" is parlance—already considered gimmicky in 2012—that describes the phenomenon of social media, or social networking, that has exploded in the last decade. The premise is that Web-based services provide a platform that allows users to establish a personal (or professional/business) profile. That profile allows contact with other individuals for the purpose of communicating, collaborating, and/or *sharing* content (such sharing being the primary objective for social media users). Most services allow members to restrict the visibility of their profile information to registered members only (those people on an established list of contacts or particular groups of service users). However, these privacy safeguards can be circumvented by savvy users, and the hosting platform may change the parameters without much notice. Yet the reach of social networks is phenomenal and undeniable. One well-known social media network is Facebook; opened to the public in 2007, it had 500,000,000+ members by 2010 (Ellis, 2011), and was up to 845,000,000 "monthly active users" as of December 2011 (Facebook, 2012d).

While a website's content is controlled by its owner/manager, the user does not have much control in a social networking site, even where safety and privacy controls have been applied. Let's imagine you have a professional presence on such a site, as an IBCLC. You were careful to create a business page account.[1] Your interactions from a business page account are more limited compared to your individual account: while you can create a message or ad campaign, you cannot view the profiles of users (visitors),

---

[1] Facebook was originally designed for *individual* account holders only, who by agreement with the Terms of Service had only one account (Facebook, 2012e). As Facebook has become an increasingly popular social media platform, Facebook account holders with a "profile" who also seek a presence as a business, organization, or cause have been allowed to create a "page" (Facebook, 2012c): "Profiles (timelines) represent individuals and must be held under an individual name, while Pages allow an organization, business, celebrity, or band to maintain a professional presence on Facebook. You may only create Facebook Pages to represent real organizations of which you are an authorized representative" (Facebook, 2012a, para. 2).

and business accounts cannot be "searched" nor send and receive "friend requests" (Facebook, 2012a). Thus, some IBCLC professionals decide to stick with opening a personal account/profile, but confining their own posts to professional or business matters. There can be risks to this practice, however. Imagine that one of your business associates (whom you have designated as a "friend" on your profile page, with appropriate access to it) now responds to your blurb about sore nipples using language that you (or others) find uncomfortable (or demeaning, or profane). The entire discourse is happening on your page that has been created to give you a professional identity. Is this the image that you want to project to clients or colleagues who visit? If you want someone to hear your words alone, you invite her over for coffee, one at a time (as with a website, where the information flow is one-way). If you want many to hear the conversations you have, you invite them to your backyard barbecue party (more akin to a social media page, where two-way communication dominates).

Because social media networks are platforms constructed and operated by their owners, often at no cost to the individual user, those who establish accounts may find they are subject to the whims of the platform owners. Personal Facebook profiles, operated by mothers who were proud to show images of themselves nursing their children, found their pages shut down (Arthur, 2012; Sweney, 2008). One IBCLC who had built a business page with over 3500 contacts, and who used the page to conduct and schedule many facets of her educational and consultative services, found her page summarily shut down because of a posted photograph of a breastfeeding mother that was deemed outside Facebook's guidelines (CBS Los Angeles, 2012).

Another popular social network is Twitter, whose distinction is that no commentary may be longer than 140 characters (Twitter, 2012), hence its description as "microblogging." It can be easily accessed and used from Web-enabled cell phones. Messages (called "tweets") are charged against your text limit; you may consider revisiting your data usage plan for your mobile/cell phone account if you will send and receive many tweets from Twitter. For real social media fans out there, Facebook and Twitter can be linked to one another and to other platforms, allowing you to post once and be "seen" in all places.

One can choose to merely "follow" other Twitter account holders, and this may actually be a soft entry for an IBCLC seeking to learn more about social media. The account holder is not compelled to post or initiate conversations; she can just read what others have to say (in 140 characters or less). This platform can also be a fairly reliable barometer of hot-button issues about which the "thought leaders" in any particular field are interested.

There are many different social media sites. LinkedIn is another option; its reputation is as a professional referral resource (Ellis, 2011). Facebook and Twitter are known to proudly mix personal and business interests. While this can have drawbacks, as we mentioned above, it is also true that an IBCLC hoping to reach the vast mothers-with-babies audience is more likely to find them on platforms that have a mix of personal and professional networking.

Some Cautions About Social Networks

When you open an account with a social medial network, you agree to their policies and terms of use (Facebook, 2011). But as we mentioned above: *If it is on the Internet, it can be permanent, and someone can find it.* The privacy policy for Facebook users cautions how to protect personal information and posts (Facebook, 2012b). Be judicious when you fashion your social media presence. Do you really want your professional email address or log-on name to be "sparkleponyunicorn"? Pictures, whether posted as a profile picture, or added as a photo album that your friends can access from your page, can be a land mine of unforeseen embarrassment or offense. Something you post as a joke, even for a day, can be quickly captured (and forwarded) by anyone with legitimate access to your page. Then, someone else's circle of friends, whom you've never met, has your embarrassing picture in front of them. It is nearly impossible to secure against that sort of unknown redistribution, so the best tactic is to think very long and hard about what you post *before* you post it.

Web Logs or Blogs

"Blogs" (short for Web logs) are another means of having a permanent Internet presence. They allow for frequent continuing publication of comments on a specific topic or subject (broad or narrow in scope). The process of maintaining a Web log is known as *blogging* (Weblog, 2010).

Think of a blog as your very own magazine: you pick the topics, you write the articles (making you the "blogger"), and you add the links, pictures, or videos. People interested in the same topic will enjoy reading your articles, just as car lovers buy automobile magazines and gardeners read publications about growing flowers and vegetables. You can ask someone to do a "guest blog" to add to your site, but you are the editor-in-chief. There are programs and websites available to create do-it-yourself blog sites; experts are also happy to take your money and set up and administer the site for which you provide the content. The same considerations of looking professional and polished are as important for a blog as they are for a website. A blog permits for immediate publication of thoughtful discourse on topics, and they are searchable on the Internet. Opinion pieces that might never have been printed in a paper journal or magazine now have a voice on the Internet. With some clever cross-posts on your social media sites, interest in your writing can be generated, and those who read and like your posts can encourage others (using the Internet, of course) to read them, too. Blogs often have a section for comments about an article to be posted; these can be viewed by subsequent readers. This immediate feedback from readers can be positive or negative and may offer very thought-provoking commentary. Note, though, that blogs must be frequently updated (new material added every few weeks) or they are quickly considered out of date. Go back to our magazine analogy: When you pick up a publication in the grocery store checkout line, you expect the articles to be recent, not 10 months old.

Texts, Email, Phones, and Faxes

Even if venturing into cyberspace does not appeal to the IBCLC, she is no doubt answering a phone (whether on a landline, fiber-optic, or cell system) and sending and receiving emails, whether at home or work. While landline telephones are being supplanted by some customers with exclusive mobile/cell phone use, hospitals and businesses still rely primarily on landline or fiber-optic systems for telecommunications. For the IBCLC, there are some legal and ethical considerations to keep in mind, even for something as seemingly simple as using a phone.

Text Messaging

In recent years, text messages sent and received by cell/mobile phones have become a predominant means of communication, especially by younger users, and are preferred over regular phone calls or recorded messages (Gahran, 2011). Some breastfeeding support programs are built entirely around the concept of sending informational texts to the mothers who have agreed to receive them (Perrin, 2012). Texts can be a wonderful way for a private practice IBCLC to do quick follow-up with a client seen earlier. However, the mother should first consent to such exchanges (as texts and cell phone use are not as private as traditional landlines). The IBCLC must also consider how she will methodically capture and record such exchanges in her own charting for the client/patient, as they are certainly germane to the care plan and follow-up that is occurring.

Privacy and Courtesy

The obvious consideration: the IBCLC's requirement to maintain confidentiality when discussing a patient/client's clinical situation (IBLCE, 2011, CPC Principles 3.1 & 4.1; IBLCE, 2008, SOP paras. 6 & 7; ILCA, 2006, Standards 2 [introduction], 2.3, & 2.4). Where conversations occur in public places (the office; the clinic) the IBCLC will know to keep patient charts covered so straying eyes cannot view them, to avoid use of the mother's name or identifying information when discussing matters where she might be overheard, and to keep her voice low. But think of the last time you sat on a train or in a restaurant, and the person nearby was on a mobile/cell phone. Did it seem like he was shouting? He might well have been. Many people with customarily quiet voices will raise them while on a handheld phone. And technology is advancing faster than we are able to fashion rules of etiquette for its use (McCluggage, 2009). Whenever you need to use technology to discuss a lactation case, whether it be with the mother or another HCP, have consideration to protect the patient's privacy rights.

Oops, I Hit the Wrong Button

We have all done it, because we are all human: we misdialed the telephone; we sent to the wrong fax machine; we hit "reply all" on an email when we really intended to hit "reply sender." Mistakes happen, but when a client/patient's privacy is at stake, the mistake can have serious consequences. Not only is it a breach of professional responsibility, in some countries there are overlaying statutory or regulatory requirements to maintain patient privacy (such as the Health Insurance Portability and Accountability Act of 1996 [HIPAA] in the United States).

Whenever you have made such a mistake, do your best immediately to mitigate the damage. Once you realize the mistake, call the office that received the faxed report of your lactation consultation in error, apologize, and ask them to destroy the report. Often we are unaware that we misdialed. So, the IBCLC should consider adding a paragraph on the fax cover sheet (and on the signature lines for professional emails) indicating that the content may be protected, and if received in error to please let the sender know immediately. One example of language for a fax cover sheet sent is:

> The attached pages are a report of a recent lactation consultation.
>
> Consent has been obtained from the mother involved to transmit this report to her healthcare provider(s), as required by the International Board of Lactation Consultant Examiners (IBLCE) Code of Professional Conduct, the IBLCE Scope of Practice for International Board Certified Lactation Consultants (IBCLCs), and the International Lactation Consultant Association (ILCA) Standards of Practice.
>
> If you received this fax in error, please respect the privacy of the people involved:
>
> (1) Contact the sender at [phone number] or via fax at [fax number] to say the fax went to the wrong number, and
>
> (2) Destroy the report you received by mistake.

A practitioner in the United States would also add the following as the third paragraph:

> This report contains personal information that falls under the privacy sections of the Health Insurance Portability and Accountability Act of 1996 (HIPAA).

Most healthcare facilities, clinics, and physician practices will have similar language as a standard section in any messages sent as part of patient care. The irony of using similar language in an email is that it usually appears at the end, with the signature line. Thus, the reader who receives the message in error is being told *after* the fact that the content may be privileged, and should not be read. The alert would probably make more sense as the standard *opening* paragraph of any email containing private content (though anyone who gets an email hinting that personal information is to follow will no doubt keep right on reading). Nonetheless, institutions do often insist on them, as a means of demonstrating that they are really, truly trying to keep private matters private. They are probably not enforceable (Shafer, 2004). Recalling the IBCLC's obligation to practice under the policies and procedures of her workplace (even if self-employed) (IBLCE, 2011, CPC Principle 2.4; IBLCE, 2008, SOP para. 3; ILCA, 2006, Standard

2), if the IBCLC is asked or intends to use disclaimer language on all outgoing emails, she should always do so.

Stream of Consciousness Posting

Emails, text messages, social network postings, and tweets are modes of communication so informal that misspellings and abbreviations have become common parlance. Compare the way you draft a report that will be presented at a meeting with the manner in which you draft an email or text message. The report is probably carefully crafted, rewritten, test-driven in front of a spouse or colleague, and then tweaked yet again. Too bad emails are not so thoughtfully drafted. Just because you can type it fast and send it instantly doesn't mean the reader wants to plow through your stream of consciousness. Consider drafting and rewriting *before* posting.

Consultation, Education, or Both?

The IBCLC who plans to have an Internet presence needs to make the penultimate decision: offer education and information only, or enter into one-on-one lactation consultations? There are some variations in-between, such as the website about an IBCLC's service that offers contact information for the visitor to schedule an in-person visit. *The greatest legal and ethical risk for the IBCLC is to inadvertently slide back and forth between these very different professional roles.*

Offering Online Consults

Having a secure and private means to conduct a consultation over the computer or telephone (and to be reimbursed for the professional healthcare that is being provided) can be accomplished. Our responsibilities as allied healthcare providers who specialize in breastfeeding and human lactation do not change one whit because the mother is across the ether rather than across the room. Indeed, some aspects of the consultation will be lost altogether: the IBCLC does not have the ability to make a physical assessment of the mother and child (IBLCE, 2008, SOP para. 5; ILCA, 2006, Standard 3) or employ some "principles of adult education" (that may require demonstrations by the IBCLC) (IBLCE, 2008, SOP para. 4). It may be problematic offering effective counseling (IBLCE, 2008, SOP para. 5; ILCA, 2006, Standards 3 & 4) when the important elements of eye contact, body language, or gentle touch cannot be employed. Maintaining appropriate privacy and confidentiality (IBLCE, 2011, CPC Principle 3.1; IBLCE, 2008, SOP para. 7; ILCA, 2006, Standard 2) is as important during the computer-based consult as with any clinical visit, charting and reporting. U.S.-based IBCLCs who have a website that describes their consultation services, even if the consultations do not occur over the Internet, are required to include a Web page with a copy of their Notice of Privacy Practices posted, as required by HIPAA privacy regulations, in addition to providing a copy to the patient/client (HIPAA, 45 CFR § 164.520(c)(3) and 45 CFR § 164.520(c)(2)(ii)).

Avoid the Consult Masquerading as a Question or Comment

As mentioned above, the greatest risk for the IBCLC is to slide from offering information of general interest to all, to offering advice that is specific to one. When you engage in the latter, you are now acting as the mother's very own IBCLC, and all of the formalities associated with a consultation must occur: obtaining consent, taking a history and making an assessment, preparing a chart and possibly a report for others members of the healthcare team, and being compensated for all of that professional time.

How might this unintentional consultation happen? Imagine you post a general, evidence-based article about common causes of low milk supply on your website. Now, a mother posts in your comment section, or sends you an email via the Contact Us page, and asks a question specific to her situation, prompted by your excellent article. Millennial Mom writes, "Thank you for that great column! I've been timing my baby's feeds since we got home two weeks ago. Here he is [photo attached]! Your article says I may have low supply because of the training I've been doing. Do you think that's true for me?"

It is very easy, and very tempting, for the IBCLC to dash off a quick reply, either on the website, or via email. You may see this as a great way to build up a "following" for the site. You might reply by saying something like, "Thank you so much for your positive feedback. Yes, timed feeds are often the culprit. That picture of your baby is gorgeous! Visit my site again; I have new articles all the time."

Remember what we discussed in earlier chapters about the different hats the IBCLC wears, and how they bring with them different sets of legal and ethical responsibilities. You may think you are simply putting on your Website Owner hat, building enthusiasm for your Internet website and presence. But what matters is the *mother's* view of your role. Here is how *she* might view this "innocent" exchange: "I'm worried about my low supply, so I am surfing the Web for answers. I read this intriguing article, and I have confirmed with the IBCLC that it was the timed feeds. Phew. I knew she'd love to see the picture of my son; I think he is special, too."

But is this all that is going on? There can be dozens of reasons for low milk supply, and if "feed the baby" is rule 1, then anything that might compromise that is cause for grave concern and swift action. The mother mentioned "training." Is she trying to put a newborn on some sort of schedule? Perhaps trying to get him to sleep through the night? The IBCLC has no idea. Does mom have a history of infertility or breast surgery that may impact supply? IBCLC doesn't know. How far along was baby when he was born? Is poor or sleepy feeding (because the baby was a late preterm, born at 37 weeks adjusted gestational age) resulting in poor milk transfer? There could be any number of reasons that the mother has low milk supply, including timed feeds.

And what happens if the IBCLC was wrong? And Millennial Mom goes into the pediatrician's office a few weeks later, and discovers to her horror that the baby is barely above birth weight? An unlikely and yet conceivable scenario is that Millennial Mom will sue the IBCLC for not fulfilling her professional obligations as an allied healthcare professional. The more likely scenario is the mother will now be "soured" on IBCLCs, will say as much to the pediatrician, will tell all her friends what a "waste" it is to use an IBCLC, and so on. A public relations nightmare for the IBCLC and her website and another unearned bad review for the entire profession of lactation consultation.

Webinars or Real-Time Q&A Sessions

One popular means of generating interest in, and traffic to, an Internet site is to offer a "live" class or webinar, or a real-time question and answer session, with the website owner or other expert. This is an excellent idea if the expert is a chef, or craftsman, or artist, with no professional obligations for the health, safety, and welfare of clients/patients. This form of outreach to mothers and breastfeeding babies is fraught with risk for the IBCLC. If a mother poses a 1–2 paragraph question, or a 1–2 minute verbal question, the IBCLC cannot possibly know all of the history and circumstances needed to adequately address the lactation issue. Even if we assume the mother is willing to discuss her case in a nonprivate manner, there is no consent between the mother and her allied healthcare provider for the lactation consultation, no consent to share clinical information with the rest of the healthcare team, no means to receive payment or seek reimbursement. The mother will no doubt act upon whatever suggestions are offered; after all, it is why she participated in the webinar. And, it is entirely possible the Internet conversation can be captured through computer forensics (Gubanov, 2011), making the mother's potential lawsuit for failure to provide appropriate care and follow-up reasonably actionable.

A Few Easy Precautions

Thankfully, this unhappy result can be fairly easily avoided. The IBCLC with a website should have a disclaimer that states information is provided for educational purposes only, and should not be considered a replacement for assessment or treatment by a healthcare provider. You'll see something like this on just about any website offering healthcare information. Popular consumer-oriented website WebMD.com simply states, at the bottom of every single Web page on the site, "WebMD does not provide medical advice, diagnosis, or treatment. See additional information" (WebMD.com, 2012b). The second sentence may be clicked, to bring the reader to the Web page with the fuller disclaimer, rather remarkable for its scope:

> The contents of the WebMD Site, such as text, graphics, images, and other material contained on the WebMD Site ("Content") are for informational purposes only. The Content is not intended to be a substitute for professional medical advice, diagnosis, or treatment. Always seek the advice of your physician or other qualified health provider with any questions you may have regarding a medical condition. Never disregard professional medical advice or delay in seeking it because of something you have read on the WebMD Site!

If you think you may have a medical emergency, call your doctor or 911 immediately. WebMD does not recommend or endorse any specific tests, physicians, products, procedures, opinions, or other information that may be mentioned on the Site. Reliance on any information provided by WebMD, WebMD employees, others appearing on the Site at the invitation of WebMD, or other visitors to the Site is solely at your own risk.

The Site may contain health- or medical-related materials that are sexually explicit. If you find these materials offensive, you may not want to use our Site. The Site and the Content are provided on an "as is" basis. (WebMD.com, 2012a)

If the IBCLC gets a direct email seeking individualized lactation advice, she can use a standard reply to make clear the limitations of an online consultation. The author's is as follows:

Thank you for your email regarding your breastfeeding issue. The ethics of my profession, and my business practices as a private practitioner, require that you be a client of mine before I discuss your specific situation.

Mothers I see as an International Board Certified Lactation Consultant (IBCLC) sign a consent form, to show they understand that I will send a report to their healthcare provider after the visit, and that they will pay me for the time I spend in consultation and follow-up.

I live just outside Philadelphia [Pennsylvania, USA]. If you live near here, call me at [phone number]. We can discuss beforehand the fees for a home visit, and insurance coverage (if any), and schedule a consult.

If you live elsewhere, visit the International Lactation Consultant Association website at www.ilca.org, and click the button for "Find a Lactation Consultant."

If you feel your needs can be met by a mother-to-mother counselor, you can find a La Leche League Leader near you by visiting www.llli.org, and searching by location.

Good luck to you and your baby.

This sets out parameters, expectations, and options right up front (IBLCE, 2011, CPC Principles 7.2, 7.3, & 7.4), and allows the mother to decide how she wants to proceed.

Telephone Consults

Email and telephone exchanges with a client/patient certainly make a great deal of sense *for follow-up* to an in-person consultation. The IBCLC can picture the mother and her baby (and her breasts); she will have a chart she can consult detailing the in-person visit; and she will be familiar with the care plan options that are now being fine-tuned (IBLCE, 2008, SOP paras. 5, 6, & 8; ILCA, 2006, Standards 3 & 4).

It is more prickly when you are having a conversation—even a well-constructed lactation consultation—with a mother whom you have never seen. Long before the

Internet came along, the telephone was a primary means of communication. But it presented back in the landline days just as many issues for HCPs as discussions on today's cell phones. Nothing can compare with a face-to-face assessment and consultation. It is hard for a dermatologist to diagnose a skin disorder over the phone; it is difficult for the pediatrician to know how "swollen" that limb is; it is impossible for the physical therapist to see range of motion.

Nonetheless, a telephone conversation at least allows the HCP to ask questions "in real time," and listen to the patient's voice, to try to narrow down what might be occurring. Many medical practices have scheduled "telephone hours" so that patients can have a quick conversation to answer nagging but nonemergency questions. If an office visit is deemed necessary, the appointment can be made right then and there.

The IBCLC can certainly use this model for first-time inquiries. The IBCLC should lay out the ground rules at the start of the exploratory conversation. Explain that any consultation over the phone must be conducted with all the formalities of an in-person visit (including consents, charting, reports, payment and follow-up). Some suggestions:

- Explain that a consultation over the phone has limitations that do not occur with face-to-face assessment, and the mother must agree to an assessment with that limitation.
- Any clinical conversation that takes longer than 5 or 10 minutes is indicative of a complex problem that probably requires an in-person visit.
- The IBCLC has the right to decide, at any time, that the situation cannot be adequately addressed with a phone conversation and requires an in-person visit. The mother can be encouraged to make that appointment with anyone, but this ground rule puts the IBCLC in control of the conversation, and avoids a verbal tug of war with a client who may want to continue eking a consult out of a phone call the IBCLC realizes is not sufficient.

If a mother is willing to agree to these conditions, the next step will be to get the formalities out of the way: obtain verbal consent, and note as much on the chart. Obtain a pertinent history. Find out who the other HCPs are. Discuss payment (or reimbursement) arrangements. Then plunge into the consult.

Using a Little Bit of Everything

Internet-based communication allows for flexibility so that a little bit here and a little bit there can allow the IBCLC to effectively market her expertise, provide a safe and secure environment to assist clients, and save time in her own professional responsibilities. Information can be offered on a website. The Contact Us page can be used by mothers seeking to arrange an appointment. The visit can be confirmed with text or email messages. The IBCLC might consider putting blank consent and history forms on her website, available for download. When she does "meet" with her client, the mother will (with any luck) have read the forms, and even filled them out and returned them via email attachment to the IBCLC. This will speed things along administratively. Online payment systems (credit cards or PayPal) allow for global financial transactions if the IBCLC's fees are not reimbursed by a third-party payer or government program. Email exchanges can be (silently) made 24 hours a day; questions often arise at 3:00 a.m. when mothers are pacing the floors with their fussy babies. The old fax machine (or, the newer fax programs on the computer), along with emails and attachments, allow an IBCLC to provide pertinent information to other HCPs privately and immediately, if the situation warrants. Digital pictures of short frenula, or damaged nipples, and even diaper contents have been known to be taken and sent by anxious parents to the IBCLC; these may prove very helpful to assessment as the conversation or email conversation unfolds.

The bottom line: there are limitations and cautions inherent in any nonpersonal consultation, but it is not impossible. The IBCLC should devise practices that protect herself, and the mother, from expectations that cannot be met.

Information Only, Please

If the IBCLC seeks to provide information and education only, on whatever platform will best suit her needs, some considerations will save her from stepping into legal and ethical potholes. Just as an Internet-based consultation must be conducted with all the formality of an in-person visit, the IBCLC sharing information or opinion pieces via cyberspace needs to be every bit as professional.

- Use (every) opportunity to explain what an I-B-C-L-C does, both to educate and protect the public, and to market the credential and profession (ILCA & Henderson, 2011; IBLCE, 2011, CPC Principles 7 & 8; IBLCE, 2008, SOP paras. 2, 4, 5, & 8; ILCA, 2006, Standards 1, 2, 3, & 4).
- Information must be evidence-based, and up-to-date (IBLCE, 2011, CPC Principles 1.2 & 1.3; IBLCE, 2008, SOP paras. 4 & 5; ILCA, 2006, Standards 1.8 & 4.5).
- The site should avoid real or perceived conflicts of interest if it accepts or is presented alongside advertisements (IBLCE, 2011, CPC Principles 1.4, 5.1, & 5.2; IBLCE, 2008, SOP para. 8; ILCA, 2006, Standard 1.3). The IBCLC must be especially cognizant of advertising of products that fall under the scope of the *International Code of Marketing of Breast-milk Substitutes* (WHO, 1981, Preamble and Articles 4, 5, & 7).
- Copyright law applies to works accessed or shared over the Internet. Materials you create should be appropriately labeled by you (if you wish to retain copyright protection), and materials you share must be offered only with appropriate permission (IBLCE, 2011, CPC Principle 2.5). If copyrighted materials are erroneously published on the Internet, they are immediately accessible around the world. The original copyright laws were enacted in an era when printing

was accomplished one character at a time. Penalties were built around how many erroneous publications occurred. It is impossible to make such calculations in cyberspace. In the United States, amendments to the law in 1998 allow for mitigation of damages for such erroneous publication but do not excuse the copyright violation itself (Digital Millennium Copyright Act, 1998).

- Offering links to other excellent sources of Web-based information is helpful, but those sites may change, or the information that was once there may be removed. It will make *your* site seem outdated and incompetent if you link to other sites suffering from those fatal flaws. One way to avoid this is simply to explain, on your page of links, the limitations (Smith, n.d.).
- Your website or blog must be current and up to date. The Internet thrives on immediacy. If your materials appear dated (even if they are still evidence-based and correct), it will make the entire site seem amateurish and hopelessly out of touch. You don't want your lead article to be about an issue that was on everyone's mind a year ago. Deciding to operate a website or blog means you should commit to providing constant updates.

Summary

The Internet is becoming a dominant means of communication and information sharing. The IBCLC may ethically and legally choose to have a presence on the World Wide Web, but she should conduct herself with all the same attention to professionalism and propriety as in a face-to-face visit. Caution must be used to learn the pitfalls, and practicalities, of being on the Internet. Mistakes are easily made and nearly impossible to erase. And the IBCLC should choose her words carefully.

REFERENCES

Arthur, C. (2012, February 21). Facebook's nudity and violence guidelines are laid bare. *Guardian*. Retrieved from http://www.guardian.co.uk/media/2008/dec/30/facebook-breastfeeding-ban

Baby-Friendly USA. (2010). *The ten steps to successful breastfeeding*. Retrieved from http://www.babyfriendlyusa.org/eng/10steps.html

CBS Los Angeles. (2012, March 23). *Facebook backpedals after deleting account over photo of breastfeeding mother*. Retrieved from http://losangeles.cbslocal.com/2012/03/23/facebook-backpedals-after-deleting-account-over-photo-of-breastfeeding-mother

Digital Millennium Copyright Act: Limitations on liability relating to material online, 17 U.S.C. § 512 (1998), http://www.copyright.gov/title17/92chap5.html#512.

Ellis, J. (2011, February 8). *A practical guide to social media*. Lecture presented at Pennsylvania Bar Institute, Philadelphia, PA.

Facebook. (2011, April 26). *Statement of rights and responsibilities*. Retrieved from https://m.facebook.com/terms.php?_rdr

Facebook. (2012a). *About Facebook pages*. Retrieved from https://www.facebook.com/help ?page=262355163822084

Facebook. (2012b). *Basic privacy controls*. Retrieved from https://www.facebook.com/help/privacy /basic-controls

Facebook. (2012c). *Facebook pages*. Retrieved from https://www.facebook.com/FacebookPages

Facebook. (2012d). *Newsroom factsheet*. Retrieved from http://newsroom.fb.com/content/default.aspx ?NewsAreaId=22

Facebook. (2012e). *Overview*. Retrieved from http://newsroom.fb.com/content/default.aspx?NewsAreaId=21

Gahran, A. (2011, October 22). One-third of Americans prefer texts to voice calls. *CNN Tech*. Retrieved from http://articles.cnn.com/2011-09-22/tech/tech_mobile_americans-prefer-text -messages_1_text-messaging-cell-voice?_s=PM:TECH

Gubanov, Y. (2011, October 21). *Retrieving Internet chat history with the same ease as a squirrel cracks nuts*. Conference presentation presented at SANS Forensic Summit [slides available online at http:// computer-forensics.sans.org/summit-archives/2011/files/1-instant-messangers-investigations.pdf], London, Great Britain.

Hall, L. M. (n.d.). The 7%, 38%, 55% myth, by C. E. "Buzz" Johnson [orig. published 1994]. In *About non-verbal dominance: Blasting away an old NLP myth* (pars. 3 et seq.). Retrieved from http://www .inteligenciadinamica.com.br/php/conteudos/textos/non_verbal.php

Health Insurance Portability and Accountability Act of 1996 [HIPAA], 45 C.F.R. § Parts 160, 162 & 164 (1996), http://www.access.gpo.gov/nara/cfr/waisidx_07/45cfr164_07.html.

International Board of Lactation Consultant Examiners. (2003). *Code of ethics for international board certified lactation consultants*. Retrieved from http://www.iblce.org/upload/downloads/CodeOfEthics.pdf

International Board of Lactation Consultant Examiners. (2008, March 8). *Scope of practice for international board certified lactation consultants*. Retrieved from http://www.iblce.org/upload/downloads/Scope OfPractice.pdf

International Board of Lactation Consultant Examiners. (2011, November 1). *Code of professional conduct for IBCLCs*. Retrieved from http://iblce.org/upload/downloads/CodeOfProfessionalConduct.pdf

International Lactation Consultant Association. (2006). *Standards of practice for international board certified lactation consultants*. Retrieved from http://www.ilca.org/files/resources/Standards-of-Practice-web.pdf

International Lactation Consultant Association, & Henderson, S. (2011, June). *Position paper on the role and impact of the IBCLC* (Monograph). Retrieved from http://www.ilca.org/files/resources/ilca_publications /Role%20%20Impact%20of%20the%20IBCLC-webFINAL_08-15-11.pdf

McCluggage, D. (2009). Basic rules of cell phone etiquette. *Road & Travel*. Retrieved from http://www .roadandtravel.com/yougogirl/cellphone2.htm

Montgomery, S. L. (2002). The online world: Using the Internet. In *The Chicago guide to communicating science* (pp. 183–198). Retrieved from http://www.press.uchicago.edu/Misc/Chicago/534855.html

Pennsylvania Bar Institute (Ed.). (2010, September). *Intellectual property defense in an age of social media* (PBI No. 2010-6581). Mechanicsburg, PA: Pennsylvania Bar Institute.

Perrin, M. (2012, April 3). *Using text messaging to support breastfeeding in WIC* [Web log post]. Retrieved from http://lactationmatters.org/2012/04/03/using-text-messaging-to-support-breastfeeding-in-wic

Richmond, R. (2010, November 10). Resisting the online tracking programs. *The New York Times*.

Shafer, J. (2004, June 1). Who's afraid of Time Inc.'s legal disclaimer? *Slate*, 1–4.

Smith, L. J. (n.d.). *Links to sites related to breastfeeding*. Retrieved from http://www.bflrc.com/links.htm

Sweney, M. (2008, December 30). Mums furious as facebook removes breastfeeding photos. *Guardian*. Retrieved from http://www.guardian.co.uk/media/2008/dec/30/facebook-breastfeeding-ban

Twitter. (2012). *The fastest, simplest way to stay close to everything you care about*. Retrieved from https://twitter.com/about

Verio Communications Co. (2012). *Domain names explained*. Retrieved from http://www.verio.com/resource-center/business-guides/domain-explained/

Weblog. (2010). In J. Reitz (Ed.), *ODLIS: Online dictionary for library and information science*. Retrieved from http://lu.com/odlis/odlis_w.cfm

WebMD.com. (2012a). *Additional information*. Retrieved from http://www.webmd.com/about-webmd-policies/additional-info?ss=ftr

WebMD.com. (2012b). *WebMD home* [Home page]. Retrieved from http://www.webmd.com/default.htm

Wikipedia. (2012, April 6). *List of Internet top-level domains*. Retrieved from http://en.wikipedia.org/wiki/List_of_Internet_top-level_domains#Country_code_top-level_domains

World Health Organization. (1981). *International code of marketing of breast-milk substitutes*. Retrieved from http://www.who.int/nutrition/publications/code_english.pdf

Chapter 12

Quiz Time! What Would You Do?

Let's try to put this all together. Reading about legal and ethical principles, in the abstract, will appeal to few outside the fields of law and ethics. Practicing International Board Certified Lactation Consultants (IBCLCs) want pragmatic and practical answers to their questions, "How do I stay out of trouble? What *should* I do? What do I *have* to do?"

What follow are some scenarios that have occurred to your IBCLC colleagues. Facts may have been tweaked a bit to make the questions tidier, but all of these fact patterns contain ethical and legal tensions that a real, live, IBCLC practitioner has faced in her lactation consultancy. See which answer you think best addresses the problem presented.

Don't jump to the answers right away. While the author's suggestion at an answer is offered, recall what has been discussed throughout this book: ethics and the law are filled with gray areas, and very rarely is there a single correct answer. As facts change, so do the options, and hence the conclusions. Analyzing legal and ethical tensions is a process of discerning: what is really going on, what parts can I ignore, what parts require my IBCLC attention, and how can I justify my decision? It is easy and safe and absolutely without consequence, here, to ponder the "what-ifs" and take a stab at an answer. You're simply reading a book (thank you), and this is the time to imagine how you might react in a sticky situation.

Go through these questions, and ask yourself, "What would I do?" Your gut instinct is often correct, even if you can't put your finger on the exact principle or edict that would back you up. To really be on top of your game, keep the appendices and tables dog-eared. The appendices have two of our major practice-guiding documents: the voluntary International Lactation Consultant Association Standards of Practice for IBCLCs (ILCA Standards, 2006) and the voluntary-unless-it-is-mandatory *International Code of Marketing of Breast-milk Substitutes* (WHO Code or International Code) (International Baby Food Action Network [IBFAN], n.d.; World Health Organization [WHO], 1981). The mandatory International Board of Lactation Consultant Examiners Code of Professional Conduct (IBLCE CPC, 2011a) can be found online at http://www.iblce.org/upload/downloads/CodeOfProfessionalConduct.pdf. The mandatory IBLCE Scope of Practice for IBCLCs (IBLCE SOP, 2008) can be found online at http://www.iblce.org/upload/downloads/ScopeOfPractice.pdf. Table 2-2 will remind you of the IBCLC's core responsibilities; Table 3-1 compares key concepts in our four major practice-guiding documents; Figure 4-1 will give you a decision-steps pathway for analyzing whether you should take action; and Table 5-1 will put you in the right frame of mind by showing how conflicts of interest are analyzed, and how the conclusions change as the facts change.

All in the Family

Question: Mother has a baby in the neonatal intensive care unit (NICU); 37-weeker, born at 34 weeks. Mom has been pumping for 3 weeks, but her supply is very low. Her sister (the new Auntie) has a 7-month-old. Auntie has offered to provide milk for the NICU baby. The IBCLC should:

a. Inform mother about donor human milk banks, but only nonprofit ones.
b. Ignore the offer. Wet nursing has been around for centuries; there is no issue.
c. Inform mother about the risks and benefits associated with the use of donor human milk.

The answer is (c). Mother has turned to the IBCLC, asking about something involving breastfeeding, lactation, and the use of human milk. Who *better* to discuss these sensitive matters with mother than the IBCLC? Information and support may always be given to the mother, so she can make an informed feeding decision about her baby. Given this baby's NICU status, the doctors and nurses also need to be apprised of Auntie's offer, and mother's request for more information; the IBCLC may be the first person to whom the mother raises this possibility, and the IBCLC should tell the mother that as a part of the healthcare team, she will make sure the other healthcare providers (HCPs) know about mother's inquiry. Remember: the IBCLC does not tell mother what to do; IBCLCs provide information and support so the mother can make an informed decision about her own and her child's health care, in consultation with all her HCPs.

Option (a) is not a good choice because the IBCLC should not limit the clinical information she shares with mother based on what is primarily a political issue. Whether the milk bank operates to enrich corporate shareholders or to provide revenues to plow back into the nonprofit operation is irrelevant. How donors are found and screened, and how the milk is pasteurized, spot-checked, and distributed, are far more relevant to the NICU mother's analysis of her options. Option (b) comes up short because, while it is true that wet nursing has been around for centuries, some pathogens carried in body fluids are fairly new to the biologic scene, and caution has been suggested by public health agencies. Any HCP must be sensitive to legal-based liability issues; failing to alert the mother of health risks is an almost blatant disregard for professional self-protection.

Support for option (c): IBLCE, 2011a, CPC Principles 1.1, 1.2, 1.3, 1.5, 2.2, and 4.1; IBLCE, 2008, SOP paras. 2, 3, 4, 5, 7, and 8; ILCA, 2006, Standards 1.4, 1.5, 1.8, 3.1.3, 3.3.1, 3.3.4, 4.1, 4.2, 4.3, 4.4, and 4.5; WHO, 2003, strategy 18.

Like It? Buy It!

Question: An IBCLC has written a chapter that was included in a recently published book about lactation. She has been asked to speak at her ILCA chapter meeting about this topic. As part of her presentation, she would like to tell the attendees about the book, and maybe even have some at the venue for sale. Which is *most* accurate?

  a. It is a conflict of interest for the IBCLC to mention the book during the education session.
  b. It is a declaration of interest to mention the book as a part of the education session.
  c. The publication can be mentioned, but it may not be offered for sale at the meeting.

Answer (b) is probably the most accurate, but (a) is likely to fly as a "correct" answer too. Remember our COINs: it *is* a technical conflict of interest (or could be perceived as one) for the speaker to mention her book during the talk, because a commercial product is being mentioned in an educational session, and its sale will enrich the author. However, if the speaker merely mentions the book as part of the disclosure/declaration of interest slide (that any self-respecting speaker uses in a conference setting), she is *curing* that conflict of interest by her *full and prior disclosure* that she is an author of a chapter of a book on the topic about which she is about to present.

By declaring her interest at the start of the talk, it allows the audience to better evaluate the IBCLC's talk. They will know up front just where she is coming from, and can decide for themselves whether the presentation is an evidence-based discussion of the topic or merely an infomercial for the book itself.

A note of caution. As for option (c), sales are fine regardless of what the speaker says from the podium, *so long as* the conference host (an ILCA chapter in this quiz question) does not endanger its application for continuing education recognition points (CERPs) from the International Board of Lactation Consultant Examiners (IBLCE, 2011c). There are strict guidelines requiring that any commercial activities be kept separate and distinct from the educational sessions (IBLCE, 2011b). It is not "wrong" for a speaker/publisher to want to encourage sales of the book; it is not "wrong" for the hosts to feature a speaker who has a demonstrated track record of expertise through publishing; it is not "wrong" for those who attended the session to decide they want to buy the book. But out-and-out promotion or sale of the book should take place someplace away from the teaching session itself.

Support for options (b) and (a) both: IBLCE, 2011a, CPC Principles 1.4, 5.1, and 5.2; IBLCE, 2008, SOP para. 8; ILCA, 2006, Standard 1.3.

Glossy Handouts Look Better

Question: Your IBCLC colleague just gave a handout to a mother about breastfeeding and nutrition for her premature baby, who is receiving doctor-ordered fortifiers (made by a formula manufacturer) along with mother's expressed breastmilk. The glossy handout was produced and published by the formula company. Your best option in this situation:

a. Tell your colleague you want to "pick her brain" over lunch about working with mothers with NICU babies.
b. This is not an issue so long as the handout discusses *organic* formula, clearly identified with the brand's logo.
c. Fire off a complaint to IBLCE immediately; sever all ties with this IBCLC, and tell all your other colleagues about what she did.

The answer is (a). And then *do* it.

Option (b) will never be a viable practice option for the practitioner: the use of a formula-company-written educational handout is a violation of the International Code, no matter how glossy the brochure or how wonderful the manufacturer makes it all seem (WHO, 1981, Articles 4.2, 4.3, 6.3, 6.8, & 7). Under the IBLCE CPC, "a crucial part of an IBCLC's duty to protect mothers and children is adherence to the principles and aim of the [International Code]" (IBLCE, 2011a, CPC Introduction, p. 1). Under the IBLCE SOP, "IBCLCs have the duty to protect, promote and support breastfeeding by complying with the [International Code]" (IBLCE, 2008, SOP para. 4). It hardly achieves the public health goals envisioned by the WHO Code, and professional demeanor envisioned by the IBLCE Code of Professional Conduct, to have IBCLCs using option (c)—the most punitive form of redress (filing a complaint with the IBLCE Ethics & Discipline Committee pursuant to Principle 8.1 of the IBLCE CPC)—as their first course of action when they see a colleague's misstep. Even IBLCE has recognized this: The primary goal if an IBCLC sees another IBCLC acting outside the ethical code is to prevent repetition of the error (Scott, 2005).

And so, option (a) is best. It is unlikely the IBCLC would take kindly and listen openly to you if you march up and bark at her, "You're a violator of the WHO Code! *And* our practice-guiding documents!" But if you can pull her aside, or talk to her at lunch, you may be able to gently raise the notion that her clinical actions do not meet professional standards. Be open-minded; your colleague may not be aware that using materials produced by the manufacturer is an (unpaid and implied) endorsement of that product, and a violation of the WHO Code. Yes, she should know, but since IBCLCs are drawn from the human race, they are prone to the foibles and errors of human beings, including not knowing everything. Don't be accusatory; simply say something like, "As IBCLCs, we are supposed to be supporting the International Code. I saw we have some handouts from Formula Company up in the NICU. We should not be using them at all. What do you think?" That may open the door to discussion, without putting your colleague on the spot (and on the defensive).

Support for option (a): IBLCE, 2011a, CPC Principles 1.2, 1.3, 1.4, 2.3, 5.1, 5.2, 6.1, and 8; IBLCE, 2008, SOP paras. 4, 5, and 8; ILCA, 2006, Standards 1.2, 3 (Introduction), 3.3.1, 3.3.7, 4.2, 4.4, and 4.5; WHO, 1981, Preamble, Articles 1, 2, 4, 5, 6, 7, and 9.

Covert Community-Based Lactation Support?

Question: IBCLC used to work at a hospital where she had frequent struggles with a mean supervisor who played favorites. After leaving the hospital, she opened a small private practice with a partner, offering breastfeeding support group meetings, some retail offerings, and lactation consultations. IBCLC wants the hospital to list her new office on the handout it gives to discharging mothers of community-based lactation support. She calls former supervisor, who refuses to do so, claiming it violates the anti-compete clause the IBCLC had with the hospital when she was employed there. IBCLC should exercise which option:

a. Throw in the towel for this facility. Anti-compete clauses sound scary.
b. Write to the ex-supervisor, with a copy to the department head(s) for patient education, community outreach, and/or public relations, asking that the hospital please include the IBCLC's private practice in its packet of discharge information so that it accurately reflects community-based lactation support, and to provide continuity of care to its patients.
c. Throw in the towel for this facility. It is a conflict of interest for you to be on the list of community-based lactation support.

The answer is (b). This is a variation on a quiz question posed previously in the conflicts of interest (COI) chapter, where the IBCLC was still employed at the hospital. Here, all of the current-hospital-employee issues are moot: the IBCLC has left her hospital job, and started up her storefront private practice. Option (b) is the best because IBCLC is simply doing what private practitioners have to do: get word out in the local community of their services. She should contact all the local hospitals and birth centers, and all the local doctors' offices that serve mothers and families, and post ads in local parent-centered publications. She has "history" with one person at her former hospital, who may present a roadblock for her. For that reason, it is wise to simultaneously contact other decision makers at the facility who want to show their patients (the customers) that they support breastfeeding by providing community-based information. After all, helping mothers who want to breastfeed to get the support they need has been identified as a key public health objective (U.S. Dept. of Health and Human Services, Office of the Surgeon General, 2011) and IBCLCs are an appropriate allied healthcare provider to fulfill this support role (ILCA & Henderson, 2011).

Option (a) is a "red herring" roadblock the ex-supervisor has raised: anti-compete (or non-compete) clauses in employment contracts are customarily restricted to specialized situations where the former employee may have unique insider information (think researcher or scientist at a high-technology firm, or a professional with access to exclusive client/patient lists or information). It is highly unlikely an allied healthcare provider hired by a hospital would have such a clause in her contract. Even assuming she did, it is probably unenforceable: unless the IBCLC is opening a brand new hospital across the street, her private practice could hardly be seen as "competing" with the former employer in a way that compromises their ability to run their hospital, especially if the hospital offered no outpatient IBCLC services (Harris, 2009).

Option (c) is not a viable answer: The decision rests with the hospital as to whom it shall include on its handout. The hospital is providing continuity of care by having a discharge sheet with local resources listed; the IBCLC is merely seeking to promote her new office by also being included in the list. There are no conflict of interest tensions because the IBCLC is an outsider, entirely.

Support for option (b): IBLCE, 2011a, CPC Principles 1.1, 2.3, 5.2, 6.1, 7.2, and 7.4; IBLCE, 2008, SOP paras. 4, 5, and 8; ILCA, 2006, Standards at Preface, 1.3, Standard 2 (Introduction), 2.1, and 4.5. And it wouldn't hurt to mention the Ten Steps to Successful Breastfeeding; even if this hospital is not officially designated as Baby-Friendly, it helps their overall public image if they can demonstrate they already comply with Step Ten by letting mother know of community-based support groups like those offered by our IBCLC's private practice (Baby-Friendly USA, 2010a, 2010b; UNICEF, 2012; WHO, 1998).

Are Baby Fairs Fair?

Question: A "baby fair" is being hugely promoted in your area: expectant parents and new families are the target audience. IBCLC is considering renting booth space to promote breastfeeding and to share information about the local breastfeeding coalition's efforts to pass lactation-friendly legislation in the state. Other booths will promote various items and services for families with young children (toys, classes, baby gear, clothing, etc.). The fair is being cosponsored by a local grocery store chain and a leading formula manufacturer. Which is your best option?

a. The International Code forbids the IBCLC and her breastfeeding coalition from marketing breastfeeding or IBCLC services.
b. The IBCLC and breastfeeding coalition may rent a booth, but may only provide "scientific and factual matters" in their handouts or poster displays.
c. The IBCLC and breastfeeding coalition can rent a booth, have handouts of any kind, offer freebies such as pens and notepads with the coalition's website on it, and even have a contest to give away one future lactation consultation to any pregnant woman who is willing to put her contact information on the game ticket.

The answer is (c). This is not a WHO Code problem! Yes, the fair is cosponsored by a formula manufacturer, but the IBCLC and her breastfeeding coalition are paying the going, advertised rate to rent their booth space, just like any other vendor at the fair. They are not accepting any freebies from the formula manufacturer (which *would* represent a violation of the International Code, under Article 7). This breastfeeding-friendly booth may be one of the very few in the baby fair offering any information about breastfeeding—a message families need to hear.

Option (a) is not a good answer choice. The International Code restricts marketing of specific product types, but IBCLCs may market breastfeeding and IBCLC services everywhere they go. Indeed, with breastfeeding seen as a public health imperative, alerting families to the availability of IBCLC services could be characterized as required marketing (ILCA & Henderson, 2011; U.S. Dept. of Health and Human Services, 2011). Adhere to common-sense rules of truthfulness (IBLCE, 2011a, CPC Principles 7.2 & 7.4).

Option (b) does not apply to IBCLCs; if that phrase about "scientific and factual matters" sounds familiar, it should: it comes from Article 7.2 of the WHO Code, and describes restrictions in informational offerings made *by* WHO-Code-covered marketers *to* healthcare providers.

Support for option (c): IBLCE, 2011a, CPC Introduction at para. 3 and principles 1.1, 7.2, 7.4, and 24; IBLCE, 2008, SOP paras. 4, 5, and 8; ILCA, 2006, Standards 1.2, 3 (Introduction), and 4.1; WHO, 1981, Preamble and Articles 1, 2, 4, 5, 6, and 7.

Warm Line Hot Seat?

Question: Hospital offers a "warm line" for discharged mothers to call if they have a question about breastfeeding. It is staffed during daylight hours, by whomever happens to answer the phone. The nice auxiliary volunteer sitting at the desk gave caller-mother non-evidence-based information about lactogenesis II. Which option is best?

a. This is the volunteer's problem, not the IBCLC's. IBCLC didn't answer the call.
b. This is the hospital's problem, not the IBCLC's. IBCLC didn't answer the call.
c. IBCLC should offer to develop a protocol for answering (and charting) warm line calls.

The answer is (c), although the hospital had better sit up and take notice, because they have allowed a problematic situation to happen.

Options (a) and (b) are not best answers because, like it or not, this *is* the IBCLC's problem. The reputation of the IBCLC profession may be impugned if someone who is not certified is looking, acting, or sounding like an IBCLC. If a mother has been seen by an IBCLC in the hospital, and has been told she can call a special number once she gets home if she has any other questions, she is surely going to assume that the person answering the warm line knows what she is talking about. Some facilities are eager to advertise they have "A-to-Z services" for their patients, but if they cannot deliver quality, evidence-based care, it is worse than not having the extra service at all. The hospital should not be overstating what it is offering in outpatient services unless those services can be competently provided. Just ask the fellows in the risk management office.

Option (c) is the best option for an IBCLC working at the hospital, for several reasons. The protocol need not be complex: the facility can keep a simple spiral notebook next to the phone to record brief notes from warm line phone conversations. Make several columns; enter the date and time of the call, person answering the call, the caller's name and phone number, a brief description of her problem, and the response given. The calls should be handled by IBCLCs, as they are the HCPs at the facility who are the recognized experts on breastfeeding and lactation. IBCLCs can "triage" incoming calls and messages: answering the query outright, referring mothers who need encouragement more than clinical help to breastfeeding support groups, or suggesting follow-up with an IBCLC and/or other HCP as the mother's clinical situation warrants. Tracking how many calls come in, and the nature of the concerns raised, can help the hospital to determine whether it is meeting its goals in health care and patient satisfaction. It may also help the lactation department demonstrate the value of the services IBCLCs provide come budget time.

Support for option (c): IBLCE, 2011a, CPC Principles 1.1, 1.2, 2.3, 3.1, 6.1, 7.2, 7.3, and 7.4; IBLCE, 2008, SOP paras. 2, 3, 4, 5, 6, 7, and 8; ILCA, 2006, Standards 2 (Introduction), 2.1, 2.3, 2.4, 2.5, 3 (Introduction), 3.1, 3.2, 3.3, 3.4, 4.2, and 4.5.

Be Careful What You Wish For

Question: A mother you saw as an IBCLC at the public health office was thrilled with your help. She has started to drag her friends to the office to see you. They are all pregnant, and confirmed formula-feeders. The mother wants you to convince her friends to switch to breastfeeding. Options:

   a. A privacy problem! Your confidentiality requirements with the first mother forbid you from discussing similar matters with all of the friends: they will know what you told her.
   b. Not an ethics problem. This is what breastfeeding education and support are all about.
   c. Not an ethics problem. This is a time management issue.

The answer is (b), with a little bit of (c) thrown in. This is the real world! Not every mother wants to breastfeed her baby as much as *you* want her to breastfeed her baby. But part of our mission as IBCLCs is to provide education about breastfeeding, especially when we work in an office dedicated to public health and education. Part of the process of making breastfeeding culturally acceptable at all ages of a child's life, in all places that mothers and children happen to be, is slogging away with an "audience" that may initially be resistant and negative. Over time, with repeated messages offered in a nonjudgmental and supportive manner, some women who were confirmed formula-feeders may be willing to see breastfeeding as an option (U.S. Dept. of Health and Human Services, 2011).

Option (a) misstates the privacy requirement. General breastfeeding information can be provided to anyone in a public health office. Privacy rights are for the mother's protection: if she chooses to tell all her friends every little detail about her lactation consultation, that is her right. As the IBCLC, you will not share specific private information about one client or patient with outsiders. But if you are teaching about the importance of skin-to-skin contact between mother and baby, it is perfectly okay if the friends figure out you must have said the same thing to the mother, because she won't stop talking about skin-to-skin. This is what education is all about!

Support for option (b): IBLCE, 2011a, CPC Principles 1.1, 1.2, 1.3, 1.5, 3.1, 6.1, and 6.3; IBLCE, 2008, SOP paras. 4, 5, 7, and 8; ILCA, 2006, Standards at Preface, Standards 1.4, 2.4, and 4.

Nipple Shield Frisbees

Question: Lately, you've arrived at the birthing center in the morning to find nipple shields on nearly every bedside table, as though they were wrist-flicked Frisbee-style inside every new mother's room. The mothers tell you "the nurse last night" offered it, to treat . . . and here, various "problems" are mentioned (flat nipples, large nipples, small nipples, big babies, small babies, sleepy babies, etc.). Now, the mother is frustrated and demoralized because the baby won't latch without it. The IBCLC should:

a.   Schedule an in-service training session to discuss evidence-based nipple shield use.
b.   Lock up the nipple shields with the drugs; to be distributed only by IBCLCs.
c.   Write up the offending nurse if you can figure out which one did this; be sure to say she knows absolutely nothing about breastfeeding!

The answer is (a). Look at the bright side: The other HCPs on the floor are paying attention to solutions they have seen the IBCLC use, and are now trying to emulate the procedure. What is needed here is to capture and focus the willingness to learn, and to teach evidence-based means to assess and document clinical need for nipple shields (when they are appropriate, nipple shield sizing, cleaning, and transition off their use). Option (b) is limiting; it perpetuates the notion that only IBCLCs can address all breastfeeding issues. Yes, we can certainly do that, but most of the concerns raised on the postpartum floor (sleepy baby, mum on pain medications, baby who "won't latch," mum who "has no milk") can be reassuringly handled by the bedside caregiver. IBCLCs are needed for the more complicated lactation histories or breastfeeding challenges. Option (c) will only earn you a reputation as a know-it-all smarty-pants who likely will be ridiculed or ignored whenever she tries to offer "education" in the future.

Support for option (a): IBLCE, 2011a, CPC Principles 1.1, 1.2, 1.3, 1.4, and 2.2; IBLCE, 2008, SOP paras. 4, 5, and 8; ILCA, 2006, Standards 3.3.6 and 4.5.

This Is the Thanks I Get?

Question: IBCLC got up from her holiday dinner table to hand over a rental pump to a desperate father, whose wife and 35-weeker were being discharged that day. He didn't have his credit card with him that day; IBCLC agreed to send him a bill. He hasn't paid the rental and it has been 2 months. Meanwhile, IBCLC has formed a close relationship with the mother, talking her through very low supply and sluggish feeds over the phone. This private practice lactation consultant's (LCinPP) options are:

a. Stop talking to the mother until she gets paid.
b. Stop talking to the mother because rental agents cannot also serve as lactation consultants.
c. Add a hefty penalty charge to the next bill, for late payment.

The answer is (c), and even that is a lousy option. Remember those different hats we wear! This LCinPP has gotten herself into a tangled professional mess. This "simple rental" when all the other retail centers were closed for the holiday has transmogrified into a lactation consultation, given all the client-specific advice the IBCLC has been offering the mother over the phone. The IBCLC has now taken on this mother as a client, with all of the attendant professional responsibilities. Yet, no consents have been signed, no reports have been sent to HCPs, no payment for the lactation consultant has been discussed, and they still owe the IBCLC for the pump rental!

Option (a) is not practical; the LCinPP cannot now simply drop a client who is in the middle of her lactation care. By now, the mother surely feels she has had a consultation, and it is the mother's viewpoint that counts when assessing whether or not a professional relationship has commenced. Option (b) is simply untrue; LCinPPs who rent or sell breastfeeding equipment may also consult with mothers. But the rules and responsibilities need to be carefully spelled out from the outset, to avoid an appearance of a conflict of interest.

Thus, option (c) is the best of three unsavory options. Wearing her rental agent hat, this small business owner is certainly within her rights to charge a late fee or a penalty for a customer who is not paying on time, in keeping with the rental contract. But in this case, that will probably sour the relationship with the mother: it is awfully hard to be the hard-nosed bill collector one minute, and the compassionate IBCLC the next.

This LCinPP hopefully has learned a professional practice lesson the hard way from this case. In future, if she gets a pump customer who starts to ask questions about her lactation situation (and what sensible mother would not, knowing she is renting from a LCinPP?) the IBCLC should be prepared to explain that while she is happy to provide (and charge for) IBCLC services, she does not give clinical advice when renting a pump, only technical information about the use and cleaning of the pump. Or, she may ask if the mother is interested in a mini-consult on pump use (only). When the IBCLC has on her retail hat, she should be providing no more nor less than any store clerk who stands behind a counter: prompt and courteous customer service, explanation of the product being rented or purchased, and the financial transaction for that rental/sale. If she does engage in a professional relationship with a customer to provide IBCLC services, then all of her IBCLC duties and responsibilities kick into gear, as if the rental transaction had never happened.

Support for option (c) : IBLCE, 2011a, CPC Principles 1.1, 1.4, 2.3, 4.1, 5.1, 5.2, 7.1, 7.2, and 7.4; IBLCE, 2008, SOP paras. 4, 5, 6, 7, and 8; ILCA, 2006, Standards 1.3, 2 (Introduction), 2.2, 2.3, 2.4, 3.1, 3.2, 3.3.1, 3.3.4, 3.3.6. 3.3.7, and 4.5.

Just One Quick Question

Question: IBCLC is in private practice, trying to build business. A mother calls, and wants to "ask a quick question." IBCLC agrees, and spends 45 minutes on the phone with mother until IBCLC concludes an in-person consultation is necessary. Mother declines the opportunity to schedule a consultation. LCinPP options:

a. Bill mother for the phone consult, if she agreed at the start.
b. Practice saying, when you answer the phone, "It sounds like you'd like to schedule a consult. My fees are . . ."
c. Phone consults are unethical, period.

The answer is (a) or (b). Phone consults (and computer-based or email consults) are perfectly legal and ethical, although they limit the IBCLC's consultative care. As discussed in the question above, once an IBCLC is "in a professional relationship" with the mother, she has taken on all the responsibilities of an IBCLC, including obtaining consents, charting appropriately, writing a report if need be to other HCPs, and collecting a fee (or submitting for reimbursement to the appropriate authority). IBCLCs have developed various means to avoid being sucked into a consultative relationship before each party's responsibilities are clearly explained and agreed to. IBCLCs may certainly include in their list of services fees for phone, email or even camera-based online consultations, with the proviso that if the IBCLC determines in the course of the call that an in-person consultation is really needed, that the mother must be willing to schedule one. IBCLCs frequently use phone, text or email as follow-up after an in-person consult.

Support for options (a) and (b): IBLCE, 2011a, CPC Principles 1.1, 1.3, 2.1, 2.2, 2.3, 3.1, 4.1, and 7.1; IBLCE, 2008, SOP paras. 3, 4, 5, 6, 7, and 8; ILCA, 2006, Standards 1.5, 2 (Introduction), 2.2, 2.3, 2.4, 2.5, 3.1, 3.3.1, 3.3.4, 3.3.7, and 4.5.

What He Doesn't Know Won't Hurt Him

Question: The head of pediatrics has had standing orders for 25 years: top off all breastfeeding babies with 1 ounce formula at each feed. The nurses, however, have seen the light. They routinely ignore this order, to encourage skin-to-skin and exclusive breastfeeding. The IBCLC who learns of this should:

a. Ignore. This is a doctor-nurse issue, not an IBCLC matter.
b. Advise the nurses to *chart* that they have followed orders, even if they didn't.
c. Ask to meet with the nurse manager, or raise the issue at the next Breastfeeding Task Force meeting (if the facility has one).

The answer is (c). Option (a) is not viable; the IBCLC can't ignore this situation any more than she could ignore the reverse situation: learning that a baby who is "exclusively breastfed" was given formula bottles by the grandmother when the mother was in the shower. It is entirely relevant to the care of and charting about breastfeeding babies: if they are receiving nonmedically indicated formula, it may have an impact on mother's milk supply, and baby's suckling behaviors at breast. Indeed, these will be issues that must be addressed even if the supplementation is medically warranted.

Option (b) is not a choice. It encourages out-and-out fraud on the part of the nurses (to enter into the chart wholly false information), for which the hypothetical IBCLC (and nurses) by all rights should be sanctioned.

Having now been made aware of a very alarming situation, this is one of those scenarios where the IBCLC should take action. There are lots of "layers" that need to be considered here, not the least of which is the 25-year history and seniority of an old-school pediatrician who had never even heard of IBCLCs during his training, because the profession had not yet been invented. The nurse manager can help "run interference" as an administrator. Even if the pediatrician is a curmudgeon, the evidence-base for support of exclusive breastfeeding is so overwhelming (American Academy of Pediatrics, 2012; ILCA, Spatz, & Lessen, 2011; Ip et al., 2007), and the risks associated with standard orders for unwarranted medical intervention (e.g., supplementation) so tangible (Colorado Dept. of Public Health and Environment, 2007), that it is time for someone (or some group) to stand up to the HCP who is not using best practices. His standing order requires changing. Nudging him into better support for breastfeeding babies will take tact, and time, and probably more than one IBCLC voice.

Support for option (c): IBLCE, 2011a, CPC Principles 1.1, 1.2, 1.3, 1.5, 2.1, 2.2, 2.3, 4.1, 4.2, 6.1, and 7.1; IBLCE, 2008, SOP paras. 2, 3, 4, 5, 6, and 8; ILCA, 2006, Standards 1.8, 2 (Introduction), 2.1, 2.5, 3 (Introduction), 3.2, 3.3.1, 3.3.3, 3.3.7, 4.2, and 4.5; WHO, 1981, Preamble, Articles 1, 2, 4, 5, 6, 7, 10, and 11.

Whose Fight Is This?

Question: You learn from an email list that social workers for the mother of a 6-month-old breastfed baby have threatened to take the baby and put him into protective custody because the family bed-shares. A campaign by family-bed and breastfeeding advocates is underway to show the judge the evidence base favoring frequent nighttime breastfeeding in a safe sleeping environment. The email asks everyone to send a letter to the judge. Which is the *most* accurate?

a. IBCLC may write only if she attaches copies of the research papers; citations aren't enough.
b. IBCLC may offer her opinion on this case if she is subpoenaed to appear by the court.
c. IBCLC may not appear or write, since she did not consult with the mother.

Of the three options, (b) is the *most* accurate. Any IBCLC will obey a valid subpoena issued by a court, seeking her expert or fact witness testimony. Option (a) is unrealistic and limiting; if the IBCLC is in a position to write a report to the judge, the court will want citations to support assertions and claims made, but the physical document need not be attached. Indeed, most legal opinions are written using frequent citations to prior court cases with precedential rulings without attaching a copy. Option (c) is also too limiting; courts may seek expert opinions from nonclinical experts on any aspect of a fact in question.

And yet, such displays of vast public support are common, and easy to muster using social media and Internet communication. There are political ramifications to take into consideration: an intensive letter-writing campaign may actually backfire, if the judge resents having all these unsworn outsiders, with no connection to the parties or the facts in the case, suddenly weighing in on the matter. Sometimes, however, public pressure has successfully been brought to bear, with more thoughtful jurisprudence as the happy result. But the sensitivities and privacy requirements of each case must be considered.

Support for option (b): IBLCE, 2011a, CPC Principles 1.5, 2.3, 7.1, 7.2, 7.3, and 7.4; IBLCE, 2008, SOP paras. 3, 4, 5, and 8; ILCA, 2006, Standards at Preface, 1 (Introduction), 1.4, 1.5, 2 (Introduction), 2.5, and 4.4.

Summary

An IBCLC's practice changes every single day, depending on the mothers that come before her and the work environment in which she practices. It is helpful to review mock situations, when nothing truly is at stake, to test how the IBCLC might respond in the situation, and how she might resolve the ethical and legal tensions.

REFERENCES

American Academy of Pediatrics. (2012, March 1). American Academy of Pediatrics policy on breastfeeding and use of human milk. *Pediatrics, 129*(3), e827–e841. Retrieved from http://pediatrics.aappublications .org/content/early/2012/02/22/peds.2011-3552.full.pdf

Baby-Friendly USA. (2010a). *Info for breastfeeding advocates/health care professionals*. Retrieved from http:// www.babyfriendlyusa.org/eng/06.html

Baby-Friendly USA. (2010b). *The ten steps to successful breastfeeding*. Retrieved from http://www .babyfriendlyusa.org/eng/10steps.html

Colorado Dept. of Public Health and Environment. (2007, August). *Getting it right after delivery: Five hospital practices that support breastfeeding* (Monograph). Retrieved from http://www.cdphe.state.co.us /ps/mch/gettingitright.pdf

Harris, S. (2009, February 16). Non-compete clause may not restrict you. *American Medical News*. Retrieved from http://www.ama-assn.org/amednews/2009/02/16/bica0216.htm

International Baby Food Action Network. (n.d.). *The full code and subsequent WHA resolutions*. Retrieved from http://www.ibfan.org/issue-international_code-full.html

International Board of Lactation Consultant Examiners. (2008, March 8). *Scope of practice for international board certified lactation consultants*. Retrieved from http://www.iblce.org/upload/downloads/Scope OfPractice.pdf

International Board of Lactation Consultant Examiners. (2011a, November 1). *Code of professional conduct for IBCLCs*. Retrieved from http://iblce.org/upload/downloads/CodeOfProfessionalConduct.pdf

International Board of Lactation Consultant Examiners. (2011b, November 1). *Minimizing commercial influence on education policy*. Retrieved from http://www.iblce.org/upload/downloads/Commercial InfluenceOnEducation.pdf

International Board of Lactation Consultant Examiners. (2011c, December 9). *Guide for shortterm providers of CERP approved education*. Retrieved from http://www.iblce.org/upload/downloads/Short TermProviderGuide.pdf

International Lactation Consultant Association. (2006). *Standards of practice for international board certified lactation consultants*. Retrieved from http://www.ilca.org/files/resources/Standards-of-Practice-web.pdf

International Lactation Consultant Association (ILCA) & Henderson, S. (2011, June). *Position paper on the role and impact of the IBCLC* [Monograph]. Retrieved from http://www.ilca.org/files/resources /ilca_publications/Role%20%20Impact%20of%20the%20IBCLC-webFINAL_08-15-11.pdf

International Lactation Consultant Association (ILCA), Spatz, D., & Lessen, R. (2011). *Risks of not breastfeeding* [Monograph]. Morrisville, NC: International Lactation Consultant Association.

Ip, S., Chung, M., Raman, G., Chew, P., Magula, N., DeVine, D., . . . Lau, J. (2007, April). *Breastfeeding and maternal and infant health outcomes in developed countries* (Rep. No. 153). Rockville, MD: U.S. Agency for Healthcare Research and Quality.

Scott, J. W. (Speaker). (2005, July 5). *From code to consultation: Applying IBCLC ethics to practice* [MP3]. ProLibraries.com, for La Leche League International. Retrieved from http://www.prolibraries.com

UNICEF. (2012, March 21). *The baby-friendly hospital initiative*. Retrieved from http://www.unicef.org /programme/breastfeeding/baby.htm

U.S. Dept. of Health and Human Services, Office of the Surgeon General. (2011, January). *The surgeon general's call to action to support breastfeeding*. Washington, DC: Author.

World Health Organization. (1981). *International code of marketing of breast-milk substitutes*. Retrieved from http://www.who.int/nutrition/publications/code_english.pdf

World Health Organization. (1998). *Evidence for the ten steps to successful breastfeeding (revised)*. Geneva, Switzerland: Author.

World Health Organization. (2003). *Global strategy for infant and young child feeding* [Monograph]. Geneva, Switzerland: Author.

ILCA Standards of Practice for International Board Certified Lactation Consultants

Preface

This is the third edition of *Standards of Practice for International Board Certified Lactation Consultants* (IBCLCs) published by the International Lactation Consultant Association (ILCA).

All individuals practicing as a currently certified IBCLC should adhere to ILCA's *Standards of Practice* and the International Board of Lactation Consultant Examiners (IBLCE) *Code of Ethics for International Board Certified Lactation Consultants* in all interactions with clients, families and other health care professionals. ILCA recognizes the certification conferred by the IBLCE as the worldwide professional credential for lactation consultants.

Quality practice and service are the core responsibilities of a profession to the public. Standards of practice are stated measures or levels of quality that are models for the conduct and evaluation of practice. Standards of practice:

- promote consistency by encouraging a common systematic approach
- are sufficiently specific in content to guide daily practice
- provide a recommended framework for the development of policies and protocols, educational programs, and quality improvement efforts
- are intended for use in diverse practice settings and cultural contexts

Standard 1. Professional Responsibilities

The IBCLC has a responsibility to maintain professional conduct and to practice in an ethical manner, accountable for professional actions and legal responsibilities.

1.1 Adhere to these ILCA *Standards of Practice* and the IBLCE *Code of Ethics*
1.2 Practice within the scope of the *International Code of Marketing of Breast-milk Substitutes* and all subsequent World Health Assembly resolutions
1.3 Maintain an awareness of conflict of interest in all aspects of work, especially when profiting from the rental or sale of breastfeeding equipment and services

1.4 Act as an advocate for breastfeeding women, infants, and children

1.5 Assist the mother in maintaining a breastfeeding relationship with her child

1.6 Maintain and expand knowledge and skills for lactation consultant practice by participating in continuing education

1.7 Undertake periodic and systematic evaluation of one's clinical practice

1.8 Support and promote well-designed research in human lactation and breast-feeding, and base clinical practice, whenever possible, on such research

Standard 2. Legal Considerations

The IBCLC is obligated to practice within the laws of the geopolitical region and setting in which she/he works. The IBCLC must practice with consideration for rights of privacy and with respect for matters of a confidential nature.

2.1 Work within the policies and procedures of the institution where employed, or if self-employed, have identifiable policies and procedures to follow

2.2 Clearly state applicable fees prior to providing care

2.3 Obtain informed consent from all clients prior to:
- assessing or intervening
- reporting relevant information to other health care professional(s)
- taking photographs for any purpose
- seeking publication of information associated with the consultation

2.4 Protect client confidentiality at all times

2.5 Maintain records according to legal and ethical practices within the work setting

Standard 3. Clinical Practice

The clinical practice of the IBCLC focuses on providing clinical lactation care and management. This is best accomplished by promoting optimal health, through collaboration and problem-solving with the client and other members of the health care team. The role of the IBCLC includes:

- assessment, planning, intervention, and evaluation of care in a variety of situations
- anticipatory guidance and prevention of problems
- complete, accurate, and timely documentation of care
- communication and collaboration with other health care professionals

3.1 Assessment

3.1.1 Obtain and document an appropriate history of the breastfeeding mother and child

3.1.2 Systematically collect objective and subjective information

3.1.3 Discuss with the mother and document as appropriate all assessment information

3.2 Plan

3.2.1 Analyze assessment information to identify issues and/or problems

3.2.2 Develop a plan of care based on identified issues

3.2.3 Arrange for follow-up evaluation where indicated

3.3 Implementation

3.3.1 Implement the plan of care in a manner appropriate to the situation and acceptable to the mother

3.3.2 Utilize translators as needed

3.3.3 Exercise principles of optimal health, safety and universal precautions

3.3.4 Provide appropriate oral and written instructions and/or demonstration of interventions, procedures and techniques

3.3.5 Facilitate referral to other health care professionals, community services and support groups as needed

3.3.6 Use equipment appropriately:
- refrain from unnecessary or excessive use
- assure cleanliness and good operating condition
- discuss the risks and benefits of recommended equipment including financial considerations
- demonstrate the correct use and care of equipment
- evaluate safety and effectiveness of use

3.3.7 Document and communicate to health care providers as appropriate:
- assessment information
- suggested interventions
- instructions provided
- evaluations of outcomes
- modifications of the plan of care
- follow-up strategies

3.4 Evaluation

3.4.1 Evaluate outcomes of planned interventions

3.4.2 Modify the care plan based on the evaluation of outcomes

Standard 4. Breastfeeding Education and Counseling

Breastfeeding education and counseling are integral parts of the care provided by the IBCLC

4.1 Educate parents and families to encourage informed decision-making about infant and child feeding

4.2 Utilize a pragmatic problem-solving approach, sensitive to the learner's culture, questions and concerns

4.3 Provide anticipatory guidance (teaching) to:
- promote optimal breastfeeding practices
- minimize the potential for breastfeeding problems or complications

4.4 Provide positive feedback and emotional support for continued breastfeeding, especially in difficult or complicated circumstances

4.5 Share current evidence-based information and clinical skills in collaboration with other health care providers

International Code of Marketing of Breast-milk Substitutes

This text is from the original 1981 World Health Organization (WHO) publication intro-ducing and explaining the International Code. Approximately every 2 years since then, the World Health Assembly (the governing arm of WHO) has adopted resolutions expanding or clarifying elements of the International Code. These 17 resolutions are most easily accessed at www.ibfan.org, and should be read in conjunction with this original text for a complete understanding of "the International Code."

Introduction

The World Health Organization (WHO) and the United Nations Children's Fund (UNICEF) have for many years emphasized the importance of maintaining the practice of breast-feeding—and of reviving the practice where it is in decline—as a way to improve the health and nutrition of infants and young children. Efforts to promote breast-feeding and to overcome problems that might discourage it are a part of the overall nutrition and maternal and child health programmes of both organizations and are a key element of primary health care as a means of achieving health for all by the year 2000.

A variety of factors influence the prevalence and duration of breast-feeding. The Twenty-seventh World Health Assembly, in 1974, noted the general decline in breast-feeding in many parts of the world, related to sociocultural and other factors including the promotion of manufactured breast-milk substitutes, and urged "Member countries to review sales promotion activities on baby foods to introduce appropriate remedial measures, including advertisement codes and legislation where necessary".[1]

The issue was taken up again by the Thirty-first World Health Assembly in May 1978. Among its recommendations were that Member States should give priority to preventing malnutrition in infants and young children by, *inter alia*, supporting and promoting breast-feeding, taking legislative and social action to facilitate breast-feeding

---

[1] Resolution WHA27.43 (Handbook of Resolutions and Decisions of the World Health Assembly and the Executive Board, Volume II, 4th ed., Geneva, 1981, p. 58).

by working mothers, and "regulating inappropriate sales promotion of infant foods that can be used to replace breast milk".[2]

Interest in the problems connected with infant and young child feeding and emphasis on the importance of breast-feeding in helping to overcome them have, of course, extended well beyond WHO and UNICEF. Governments, nongovernmental organizations, professional associations, scientists, and manufacturers of infant foods have also called for action to be taken on a world scale as one step towards improving the health of infants and young children.

In the latter part of 1978, WHO and UNICEF announced their intention of organizing jointly a meeting on infant and young child feeding, within their existing programmes, to try to make the most effective use of this groundswell of opinion. After thorough consideration on how to ensure the fullest participation, the meeting was convened in Geneva from 9 to 12 October 1979 and was attended by some 150 representatives of governments, organizations of the United Nations system and other intergovernmental bodies, nongovernmental organizations, the infant-food industry, and experts in related disciplines. The discussions were organized on five main themes: the encouragement and support of breast-feeding; the promotion and support of appropriate and timely complementary feeding (weaning) practices with the use of local food resources; the strengthening of education, training and information on infant and young child feeding; the promotion of the health and social status of women in relation to infant and young child health and feeding; and the appropriate marketing and distribution of breast-milk substitutes.

The Thirty-third World Health Assembly, in May 1980, endorsed in their entirety the statement and recommendations agreed by consensus at this joint WHO/UNICEF meeting and made particular mention of the recommendation that "there should be an international code of marketing of infant formula and other products used as breast-milk substitutes", requesting the Director-General to prepare such a code "in close consultation with Member States and with all other parties concerned".[3]

To develop an international code of marketing of breast-milk substitutes in accordance with the Health Assembly's request, numerous and lengthy consultations were held with all interested parties. Member States of the World Health Organization and groups and individuals who had been represented at the October 1979 meeting were requested to comment on successive drafts of the code, and further meetings were held in February and March and again in August and September in 1980. WHO and UNICEF placed themselves at the disposal of all groups in an effort to foster a continuing dialogue on both the form and the content of the draft code and to maintain as a basic minimum content those points which had been agreed upon by consensus at the meeting in October 1979.

---

[2] Resolution WHA31.47 (Handbook of Resolutions and Decisions.... Volume II, 4th ed., p. 62).
[3] See resolution WHA33.32, reproduced in Annex 2.

In January 1981, the Executive Board of the World Health Organization at its sixty-seventh session, considered the fourth draft of the code, endorsed it, and unanimously recommended[4] to the Thirty-fourth World Health Assembly the text of a resolution by which it would adopt the code in the form of a recommendation rather than as a regulation.[5] In May 1981, the Health Assembly debated the issue after it had been introduced by the representative of the Executive Board.[6] It adopted the code, as proposed, on 21 May by 118 votes in favour to 1 against, with 3 abstentions.[7]

The International Code of Marketing of Breast-milk Substitutes

The Member States of the World Health Organization:

Affirming the right of every child and every pregnant and lactating woman to be adequately nourished, as a means of attaining and maintaining health;

Recognizing that infant malnutrition is part of the wider problems of lack of education, poverty, and social injustice;

Recognizing that the health of infants and young children cannot be isolated from the health and nutrition of women, their socioeconomic status and their roles as mothers;

Conscious that breast-feeding is an unequalled way of providing ideal food for the healthy growth and development of infants; that it forms a unique biological and emotional basis for the health of both mother and child; that the anti-infective properties of breast-milk help to protect infants against disease; and that there is an important relationship between breast-feeding and child-spacing;

Recognizing that the encouragement and protection of breast-feeding is an important part of the health, nutrition and other social measures required to promote healthy growth and development of infants and young children; and that breast-feeding is an important aspect of primary health care;

Considering that, when mothers do not breast-feed, or only do so partially, there is a legitimate market for infant formula and for suitable ingredients from which to prepare it; that all these products should accordingly be made accessible to those who

---

[4] See resolution EB67.R12, reproduced in Annex 1.

[5] The legal implications of the adoption of the code as a recommendation or as a regulation are discussed in a report on the code by the Director-General of WHO to the Thirty-fourth World Health Assembly; this report is contained in document WHA34/1981/REC/1, Annex 3.

[6] See Annex 3 for excerpts from the introductory statement by the representative of the Executive Board.

[7] See Annex 1 for the text of resolution WHA34.22, by which the code was adopted. For the verbatim record of the discussion at the fifteenth plenary meeting, on 21 May 1981, see document WHA34/1981/REC/2.

need them through commercial or non-commercial distribution systems; and that they should not be marketed or distributed in ways that may interfere with the protection and promotion of breast-feeding;

Recognizing further that inappropriate feeding practices lead to infant malnutrition, morbidity and mortality in all countries, and that improper practices in the marketing of breast-milk substitutes and related products can contribute to these major public health problems;

Convinced that it is important for infants to receive appropriate complementary foods, usually when they reach four to six months of age, and that every effort should be made to use locally available foods; and convinced, nevertheless, that such complementary foods should not be used as breast-milk substitutes;

Appreciating that there are a number of social and economic factors affecting breast-feeding, and that, accordingly, governments should develop social support systems to protect, facilitate and encourage it, and that they should create an environment that fosters breast-feeding, provides appropriate family and community support, and protects mothers from factors that inhibit breast-feeding;

Affirming that health care systems, and the health professionals and other health workers serving in them, have an essential role to play in guiding infant feeding practices, encouraging and facilitating breast-feeding, and providing objective and consistent advice to mothers and families about the superior value of breast-feeding, or, where needed, on the proper use of infant formula, whether manufactured industrially or home-prepared;

Affirming further that educational systems and other social services should be involved in the protection and promotion of breastfeeding, and in the appropriate use of complementary foods;

Aware that families, communities, women's organizations and other nongovernmental organizations have a special role to play in the protection and promotion of breast-feeding and in ensuring the support needed by pregnant women and mothers of infants and young children, whether breast-feeding or not;

Affirming the need for governments, organizations of the United Nations system, nongovernmental organizations, experts in various related disciplines, consumer groups and industry to cooperate in activities aimed at the improvement of maternal, infant and young child health and nutrition;

Recognizing that governments should undertake a variety of health, nutrition and other social measures to promote healthy growth and development of infants and young children, and that this Code concerns only one aspect of these measures;

Considering that manufacturers and distributors of breast-milk substitutes have an important and constructive role to play in relation to infant feeding, and in the promotion of the aim of this Code and its proper implementation;

Affirming that governments are called upon to take action appropriate to their social and legislative framework and their overall development objectives to give effect to the principles and aim of this Code, including the enactment of legislation, regulations or other suitable measures;

Believing that, in the light of the foregoing considerations, and in view of the vulnerability of infants in the early months of life and the risks involved in inappropriate feeding practices, including the unnecessary and improper use of breast-milk substitutes, the marketing of breast-milk substitutes requires special treatment, which makes usual marketing practices unsuitable for these products;

THEREFORE:

The Member States hereby agree the following articles which are recommended as a basis for action.

Article 1. Aim of the Code

The aim of this Code is to contribute to the provision of safe and adequate nutrition for infants, by the protection and promotion of breast-feeding, and by ensuring the proper use of breast-milk substitutes, when these are necessary, on the basis of adequate information and through appropriate marketing and distribution.

Article 2. Scope of the Code

The Code applies to the marketing, and practices related thereto, of the following products: breast-milk substitutes, including infant formula; other milk products, foods and beverages, including bottlefed complementary foods, when marketed or otherwise represented to be suitable, with or without modification, for use as a partial or total replacement of breast milk; feeding bottles and teasts [sic]. It also applies to their quality and availability, and to information concerning their use.

Article 3. Definitions

For the purposes of this Code:

"Breast-milk substitute"	means	any food being marketed or otherwise presented as a partial or total replacement for breast milk, whether or not suitable for that purpose.
"Complementary food"	means	any food whether manufactured or locally prepared, suitable as a complement to breast milk or to infant formula, when either become insufficient to satisfy the nutritional requirements of the infant. Such food is also commonly called "weaning food" or "breast-milk supplement".

"Container"	means	any form of packaging of products for sale as a normal retail unit, including wrappers.
"Distributor"	means	a person, corporation or any other entity in the public or private sector engaged in the business (whether directly or indirectly) of marketing at the wholesale or retail level a product within the scope of this Code. A "primary distributor" is a manufacturer's sales agent, representative, national distributor or broker.
"Health care system"	means	governmental, nongovernmental or private institutions or organizations engaged, directly or indirectly, in health care for mothers, infants and pregnant women; and nurseries or child-care institutions. It also includes health workers in private practice. For the purposes of this Code, the health care system does not include pharmacies or other established sales outlets.
"Health worker"	means	a person working in a component of such a health care system, whether professional or non-professional, including voluntary unpaid workers.
"Infant formula"	means	a breast-milk substitute formulated industrially in accordance with applicable Codex Alimentarius standards, to satisfy the normal nutritional requirements of infants up to between four and six months of age, and adapted to their physiological characteristics. Infant formula may also be prepared at home, in which case it is described as "home-prepared".
"Label"	means	any tag, brand, marks, pictorial or other descriptive matter, written, printed, stencilled, marked, embossed or impressed on, or attached to, a container (see above) of any products within the scope of this Code.
"Manufacturer"	means	a corporation of other entity in the public or private sector engaged in the business or function (whether directly or through an agent or through an entity controlled by or under contract with it) of manufacturing a product within the scope of this Code.

"Marketing"	means	product promotion, distribution, selling, advertising, product public relations, and information services.
"Marketing personnel"	means	any persons whose functions involve the marketing of a product or products coming within the scope of this Code.
"Samples"	means	single or small quantities of a product provided without cost.
"Supplies"	means	of a product provided for use over an extended period, free or at a low price, for social purposes, including those provided to families in need.

Article 4. Information and education

4.1 Governments should have the responsibility to ensure that objective and consistent information is provided on infant and young child feeding for use by families and those involved in the field of infant and young child nutrition. This responsibility should cover either the planning, provision, design and dissemination of information, or their control.

4.2 Informational and educational materials, whether written, audio, or visual, dealing with the feeding of infants and intended to reach pregnant women and mothers of infants and young children, should include clear information on all the following points: (a) the benefits and superiority of breast-feeding; (b) maternal nutrition, and the preparation for and maintenance of breast-feeding; (c) the negative effect on breast-feeding of introducing partial bottle-feeding; (d) the difficulty of reversing the decision not to breast-feed; and (e) where needed, the proper use of infant formula, whether manufactured industrially or home-prepared. When such materials contain information about the use of infant formula, they should include the social and financial implications of its use; the health hazards of inappropriate foods or feeding methods; and, in particular, the health hazards of unnecessary or improper use of infant formula and other breast-milk substitutes. Such materials should not use any pictures or text which may idealize the use of breast-milk substitutes.

4.3 Donations of informational or educational equipment or materials by manufacturers or distributors should be made only at the request and with the written approval of the appropriate government authority or within guidelines given by governments for this purpose. Such equipment or materials may bear the donating company's name or logo, but should not refer to a proprietary product that is within the scope of this Code, and should be distributed only through the health care system.

Article 5. The general public and mothers

5.1 There should be no advertising or other form of promotion to the general public of products within the scope of this Code.

5.2 Manufacturers and distributors should not provide, directly or indirectly, to pregnant women, mothers or members of their families, samples of products within the scope of this Code.

5.3 In conformity with paragraphs 1 and 2 of this Article, there should be no point-of-sale advertising, giving of samples, or any other promotion device to induce sales directly to the consumer at the retail level, such as special displays, discount coupons, premiums, special sales, loss-leaders and tie-in sales, for products within the scope of this Code. This provision should not restrict the establishment of pricing policies and practices intended to provide products at lower prices on a long-term basis.

5.4 Manufacturers and distributors should not distribute to pregnant women or mothers or infants and young children any gifts of articles or utensils which may promote the use of breast-milk substitutes or bottle-feeding.

5.5 Marketing personnel, in their business capacity, should not seek direct or indirect contact of any kind with pregnant women or with mothers of infants and young children.

Article 6. Health care systems

6.1 The health authorities in Member States should take appropriate measures to encourage and protect breast-feeding and promote the principles of this Code, and should give appropriate information and advice to health workers in regard to their responsibilities, including the information specified in Article 4.2.

6.2 No facility of a health care system should be used for the purpose of promoting infant formula or other products within the scope of this Code. This Code does not, however, preclude the dissemination of information to health professionals as provided in Article 7.2.

6.3 Facilities of health care systems should not be used for the display of products within the scope of this Code, for placards or posters concerning such products, or for the distribution of material provided by a manufacturer or distributor other than that specific it Article 4.3.

6.4 The use by the health care system of "professional service representatives", "mother-craft nurses" or similar personnel, provided or paid for by manufacturers or distributors, should not be permitted.

6.5 Feeding with infant formula, whether manufactured or home-prepared, should be demonstrated only by health workers, or other community workers if necessary; and only to the mothers or family members who need to use it; and the information given should include a clear explanation of the hazards of improper use.

6.6 Donations or low-price sales to institutions or organizations of supplies of infant formula or other products within the scope of this Code, whether for use in the institutions or for distribution outside them, may be made. Such supplies should only be used or distributed for infants who have to be fed on breast-milk substitutes. If these supplies are distributed for use outside the institutions, this should be done only by the institutions or organizations concerned. Such donations or low-price sales should not be used by manufacturers or distributors as a sales inducement.

6.7 Where donated supplies of infant formula or other products within the scope of this Code are distributed outside an institution, the institution or organization should take steps to ensure that supplies can be continued as long as the infants concerned need them. Donors, as well as institutions or organizations concerned, should bear in mind this responsibility.

6.8 Equipment and materials, in addition to those referred to in Article 4.3, donated to a health care system may bear a company's name or logo, but should not refer to any proprietary product within the scope of this Code.

Article 7. Health workers

7.1 Health workers should encourage and protect breast-feeding; and those who are concerned in particular with maternal and infant nutrition should make themselves familiar with their responsibilities under this Code, including the information specified in Article 4.2.

7.2 Information provided by manufacturers and distributors to health professionals regarding products within the scope of this Code should be restricted to scientific and factual matters, and such information should not imply or create a belief that bottle-feeding is equivalent or superior to breast-feeding. It should also include the information specified in Article 4.2.

7.3. No financial or material inducements to promote products within the scope of this Code should be offered by manufacturers or distributors to health workers or members of their families, nor should these be accepted by health workers or members of their families.

7.4 Samples of infant formula or other products within the scope of this Code, or of equipment or utensils for their preparation or use, should not be provided to health workers except when necessary for the purpose of professional evaluation or research at the institutional level. Health workers should not give samples of infant formula to pregnant women, mothers of infants and young children, or members of their families.

7.5 Manufacturers and distributors of products within the scope of this Code should disclose to the institution to which a recipient health worker is affiliated any contribution made to him or on his behalf for fellowships, study tours, research grants, attendance at professional conferences, or the like. Similar disclosures should be made by the recipient.

Article 8. Persons employed by manufacturers and distributors

8.1 In systems of sales incentives for marketing personnel, the volume of sales of products within the scope of this Code should not be included in the calculation of bonuses, nor should quotas be set specifically for sales of these products. This should not be understood to prevent the payment of bonuses based on the overall sales by a company of other products marketed by it.

8.2 Personnel employed in marketing products within the scope of this Code should not, as part of their job responsibilities, perform educational functions in relation to pregnant women or mothers of infants and young children. This should not be understood as preventing such personnel from being used for other functions by the health care system at the request and with the written approval of the appropriate authority of the government concerned.

Article 9. Labelling

9.1 Labels should be designed to provide the necessary information about the appropriate use of the product, and so as not to discourage breast-feeding.

9.2 Manufacturers and distributors of infant formula should ensure that each container as a clear, conspicuous, and easily readable and understandable message printed on it, or on a label which cannot readily become separated from it, in an appropriate language, which includes all the following points: (a) the words "Important Notice" or their equivalent; (b) a statement of the superiority of breast-feeding; (c) a statement that the product should be used only on the advice of a health worker as to the need for its use and the proper method of use; (d) instructions for appropriate preparation, and a warning against the health hazards of inappropriate preparation. Neither the container nor the label should have pictures of infants, nor should they have other pictures or text which may idealize the use of infant formula. They may, however, have graphics for easy identification of the product as a breast-milk substitute and for illustrating methods of preparation. The terms "humanized", "materialized" or similar terms should not be used. Inserts giving additional information about the product and its proper use, subject to the above conditions, may be included in the package or retail unit. When labels give instructions for modifying a product into infant formula, the above should apply.

9.3 Food products within the scope of this Code, marketed for infant feeding, which do not meet all the requirements of an infant formula, but which can be modified to do so, should carry on the label a warning that the unmodified product should not be the sole source of nourishment of an infant. Since sweetened condensed milk is not suitable for infant feeding, nor for use as a main ingredient of infant formula, its label should not contain purported instructions on how to modify it for that purpose.

9.4 The label of food products within the scope of this Code should also state all the following points: (a) the ingredients used; (b) the composition/analysis of the product; (c) the storage conditions required; and (d) the batch number and the date before which the product is to be consumed, taking into account the climatic and storage conditions of the country concerned.

Article 10. Quality

10.1 The quality of products is an essential element for the protection of the health of infants and therefore should be of a high recognized standard.

10.2 Food products within the scope of this Code should, when sold or otherwise distributed, meet applicable standards recommended by the Codex Alimentarius Commission and also the Codex Code of Hygienic Practice for Foods for Infants and Children.

Article 11. Implementation and monitoring

11.1 Governments should take action to give effect to the principles and aim of this Code, as appropriate to their social and legislative framework, including the adoption of national legislation, regulations or other suitable measures. For this purpose, governments should seek, when necessary, the cooperation of WHO, UNICEF and other agencies of the United Nations system. National policies and measures, including laws and regulations, which are adopted to give effect to the principles and aim of this Code should be publicly stated, and should apply on the same basis to all those involved in the manufacture and marketing of products within the scope of this Code.

11.2 Monitoring the application of this Code lies with governments acting individually, and collectively through the World Health Organization as provided in paragraphs 6 and 7 of this Article. The manufacturers and distributors of products within the scope of this Code, and appropriate nongovernmental organizations, professional groups, and consumer organizations should collaborate with governments to this end.

11.3 Independently of any other measures taken for implementation of this Code, manufacturers and distributors of products within the scope of this Code should regard themselves as responsible for monitoring their marketing practices according to the principles and aim of this Code, and for taking steps to ensure that their conduct at every level conforms to them.

11.4 Nongovernmental organizations, professional groups, institutions and individuals concerned should have the responsibility of drawing the attention of manufacturers or distributors to activities which are incompatible with the principles and aim of this Code, so that appropriate action can be taken. The appropriate governmental authority should also be informed.

11.5 Manufacturers and primary distributors of products within the scope of this Code should apprise each member of their marketing personnel of the Code and of their responsibilities under it.

11.6 In accordance with Article 62 of the Constitution of the World Health Organization, Member States shall communicate annually to the Director-General information on action taken to give effect to the principles and aim of this Code.

11.7 The Director-General shall report in even years to the World Health Assembly on the status of implementation of the Code; and shall, on request, provide technical support to Member States preparing national legislation or regulations, or taking other appropriate measures in implementation and furtherance of the principles and aim of this Code.

Annex 1

Resolutions of the Executive Board at its Sixty-seventh Session and of the Thirty-fourth World Health Assembly on the International Code of Marketing of Breast-milk Substitutes

Resolution EB67.R12 Draft International Code of Marketing of Breast-milk Substitutes

The Executive Board,

Having considered the report by the Director-General on the Draft International Code of Marketing of Breast-milk Substitutes;

1. ENDORSES in its entirety the Draft International Code prepared by the Director-General;
2. FORWARDS the Draft International Code to the Thirty-fourth World Health Assembly;
3. RECOMMENDS to the Thirty-fourth World Health Assembly the adoption of the following resolution:

28 January 1981

[The text recommended by the Executive Board was adopted by the Thirty-fourth World Health Assembly, on 21 May 1981, as resolution WHA34.22, reproduced overleaf.]

Resolution WHA34.22 International Code of Marketing of Breast-milk Substitutes

The Thirty-fourth World Health Assembly,

Recognizing the importance of sound infant and young child nutrition for the future health and development of the child and adult;

Recalling that breast-feeding is the only natural method of infant feeding and that it must be actively protected and promoted in all countries;

Convinced that governments of Member States have important responsibilities and a prime role to play in the protection and promotion of breast-feeding as a means of improving infant and young child health;

Aware of the direct and indirect effects of marketing practices for breast-milk substitutes on infant feeding practices;

Convinced that the protection and promotion of infant feeding, including the regulation of the marketing of breast-milk substitutes, affect infant and young child health directly and profoundly, and are a problem of direct concern to WHO;

Having considered the draft International Code of Marketing of Breast-milk Substitutes prepared by the Director-general and forwarded to it by the Executive Board;

Expressing its gratitude to the Director-General and to the Executive Director of the United Nations Children's Fund for the steps they have taken in ensuring close consultation with Member States and with all other parties concerned in the process of preparing the draft International Code;

Having considered the recommendation made thereon by the Executive Board at its sixty-seventh session;

Confirming resolution WHA33.32, including the endorsement in their entirety of the statement and recommendations made by the joint WHO/UNICEF Meeting on Infant and Young Child Feeding held from 9 to 12 October 1979;

Stressing that the adoption of and adherence to the International Code of Marketing of Breast-milk Substitutes is a minimum requirement and only one of several important actions required in order to protect health practices of infant and young child feeding;

1. ADOPTS, in the sense of Article 23 of the Constitution, the International Code of Marketing of Breast-milk Substitutes annexed to the present resolution;
2. URGES all Member States:
   (1) to give full and unanimous support to the implementation of the recommendations made by the joint WHO/UNICEF Meeting on Infant and Young Child Feeding and of the provisions of the International Code in

its entirety as an expression of the collective will of the membership of the World Health Organization;

(2) to translate the International Code into national legislation, regulations or other suitable measures;

(3) to involve all concerned social and economic sectors and all other concerned parties in the implementation of the International Code and in the observance of the provisions thereof:

(4) to monitor the compliance with the Code;

3. DECIDES that the follow-up to and review of the implementation of this resolution shall be undertaken by regional committees, the Executive Board and the Health Assembly in the spirit of resolution WHA33.17.

4. REQUESTS the FAO/WHO Codex Alimentarius Commission to give full consideration, within the framework of its operational mandate, to action it might take to improve the quality standards of infant foods, and to support and promote the implementation of the International Code;

5. REQUESTS the Director-General:

(1) to give all possible support to Member States, as and when requested, for the implementation of the International Code, and in particular in the preparation of national legislation and other measures related thereto in accordance with operative subparagraph 6(6) of resolution WHA33.32;

(2) to use his good offices for the continued cooperation with all parties concerned in the implementation and monitoring of the International Code at country, regional and global levels;

(3) to report to the Thirty-sixth World health Assembly on the status of compliance with and implementation of the Code at country, regional and global levels;

(4) based on the conclusions of the status report, to make proposals, if necessary, for revision of the text of the Code and for the measures needed for its effective application.

21 May 1981

Annex 2

Resolution of the Thirty-third World Health Assembly on Infant and Young Child Feeding

Resolution WHA 33.32 Infant and young child feeding

The Thirty-third World Health Assembly,

Recalling resolutions WHA27.43 and WHA31.47 which in particular reaffirmed that breast-feeding is ideal for the harmonious physical and psychosocial development of the child, that urgent action is called for by governments and the Director-General in order to intensity activities for the promotion of breast-feeding and development of actions related to the preparation and use of weaning foods based on local products, and that there is an urgent need for countries to review sales promotion activities on baby foods and to introduce appropriate remedial measures, including advertisement codes and legislation, as well as to take appropriate supportive social measures for mothers working away from their homes during the lactation period;

Recalling further resolutions WHA31.55 and WHA32.42 which emphasized maternal and child health as an essential component of primary health care, vital to the attainment of health for all by the year 2000;

Recognizing that there is a close interrelationship between infant and young child feeding and social and economic development, and that urgent action by governments is required to promote the health and nutrition of infants, young children and mothers, *inter alia* through education, training and information in this field;

Noting that a joint WHO/UNICEF Meeting on Infant and Young Child Feeding was held from 9 to 12 October 1979, and was attended by representatives of governments, the United Nations system and technical agencies, nongovernmental organizations active in the area, the infant-food industry and other scientists working in this field;

1. ENDORSES in their entirety the statement and recommendations made by the joint WHO/UNICEF meeting, namely on the encouragement and support of breast-feeding; the promotion and support of appropriate weaning practices; the strengthening of education, training and information; the promotion of the health and social status of women in relation to infant and young child feeding; and the appropriate marketing and distribution of breast-milk substitutes. This statement and these recommendations also make clear the responsibility in this field incumbent on the health services, health personnel, national authorities, women's and other nongovernmental organizations, the United Nations agencies and the infant-food industry, and stress the importance for countries to have a coherent food and nutrition policy and the need for pregnant and lactating women to be adequately nourished; the joint Meeting also recommended that "There should be an international code of marketing of infant formula and other products used as breast-milk substitutes. This should be supported by both exporting and importing countries and observed by all manufacturers. WHO and UNICEF are requested to organize the process for its preparation, with the involvement of all concerned parties, in order to reach a conclusion as soon as possible";

2. RECOGNIZES the important work already carried out by the World Health Organization and UNICEF with a view to implementing these recommendations and the preparatory work done on the formulation of a draft international code of marketing of breast-milk substitutes;

3. URGES countries which have not already done so to review and implement resolutions WHA27.43 and WHA32.42;

4. URGES women's organizations to organize extensive information dissemination campaigns in support of breast-feeding and healthy habits;

5. REQUESTS the Director-General;
   (1) to cooperate with Member States on request in supervising or arranging for the supervision of the quality of infant foods during their production in the country concerned, as well as during their importation and marketing;
   (2) to promote and support the exchange of information on laws, regulations, and other measures concerning marketing of breast-milk substitutes;
6. FURTHER REQUESTS the Director-General to intensify his activities for promoting the application of the recommendations of the joint WHO/UNICEF Meeting and, in particular:
   (1) to continue efforts to promote breast-feeding as well as sound supplementary feeding and weaning practices as a prerequisite to healthy child growth and development;
   (2) to intensify coordination with other international and bilateral agencies for the mobilization of the necessary resources for the promotion and support of activities related to the preparation of weaning foods based on local products in countries in need of such support and to collate and disseminate information on methods of supplementary feeding and weaning practices successfully used in different cultural settings;
   (3) to intensify activities in the field of health education, training and information on infant and young child feeding, in particular through the preparation of training and other manuals for primary health care workers in different regions and countries;
   (4) to prepare an international code on marketing of breast-milk substitutes in close consultation with Member States and with all other parties concerned including such scientific and other experts whose collaboration may be deemed appropriate, bearing in mind that:
      (a) the marketing of breast-milk substitutes and weaning foods must be viewed within the framework of the problems of infant and young child feeding as a whole;
      (b) the aim of the code should be to contribute to the provision of safe and adequate nutrition of infants and young children, and in particular to promote breast-feeding and ensure, on the basis of adequate information, the proper use of breast-milk substitutes, if necessary;
      (c) the code should be based on existing knowledge of infant nutrition;
      (d) the code should be governed *inter alia* by the following principles:
         (i) the production, storage and distribution, as well as advertising, of infant feeding products should be subject to national legislation or regulations, or other measures as appropriate to the country concerned;

(ii) relevant information on infant feeding should be provided by the health care system of the country in which the product is consumed;

(iii) products should meet international standards of quality and presentation, in particular those developed by the Codex Alimentarius Commission, and their labels should clearly inform the public of the superiority of breast-feeding;

(5) to submit the code to the Executive Board for consideration at its sixty-seventh session and for forwarding with its recommendations to the Thirty-fourth World Health Assembly, together with proposals regarding its promotion and implementation, either as a regulation in the sense of Articles 21 and 22 of the Constitution of the World Health Organization or as a recommendation in the sense of Article 23, outlining the legal and other implications of each choice;

(6) to review the existing legislation in different countries for enabling and supporting breast-feeding, especially by working mothers, and to strengthen the Organization's capacity to cooperate on the request of Member States in developing such legislation;

(7) to submit to the Thirty-fourth World Health Assembly, in 1981, and thereafter in even years, a report on the steps taken by WHO to promote breast-feeding and to improve infant and young child feeding, together with an evaluation of the effect of all measures taken by WHO and its Member States.

23 May 1980

Annex 3

Excerpts from the Introductory Statement by the Representative of the Executive Board to the Thirty-fourth World Health Assembly on the Subject of the Draft International Code of Marketing of Breast-milk Substitutes[8]

The topic "infant and young child feeding" was extensively reviewed and discussed in May 1980 at the Thirty-third World Health Assembly, and it has also been extensively

---

[8] This statement by Dr Torbjørn Mork (Director-General of Health Services, Norway), representative of the Executive Board, was delivered before Committee A on 20 May 1981. The summary records of the discussion of this topic at the thirteenth, fourteenth and fifteenth meetings of Committee A are contained in document WHA34/1981/REC/3.

discussed this morning. Delegates will recall last year's Health Assembly's resolution WHA33.32 to this effect, which was adopted unanimously and which among other things requested the Director-General "to prepare an international code of marketing of breast-milk substitutes in close consultation with Member States and with other parties concerned". The need for such a code and the principles on which it should be developed were thus unanimously agreed upon at last year's Health Assembly.[9] It should therefore not be necessary in our deliberations today to repeat this review and these discussions.

There are two issues before the Committee today: firstly, the content of the code; and secondly, the question of whether the code should be adopted as a regulation in the sense of Articles 21 and 22 of the WHO Constitution or as a recommendation in the sense of Article 23.

The proposal now before the Committee in document A34/8 is the fourth distinct draft of the code; it is the result of a long process of consultations carried out with Member States and other parties concerned, in close cooperation with UNICEF. Few, if any, issues before the Executive Board and the Health Assembly have been the object of such extensive consultations as has the draft code.

. . . . . .

During the Executive Board's discussion on this item at its sixty-seventh session, in January 1981, many members addressed themselves to the aim and the principles of the code and stressed that, as presently drafted, it constituted the minimum acceptable requirements concerning the marketing of breast-milk substitutes. Since even at this late date, as reflect in recent newspaper articles, some uncertainty persists with respect to the content of the code, particularly its scope, I believe it would be useful to make some remarks on this point. I hasten to remind delegates, however, that the scope of the code was not the source of difficulty during the Board's discussion.

The scope of the draft code is defined in Article 2. During the first four to six months of life, breast milk alone is usually adequate to sustain the normal infant's nutritional requirements. Breast milk may be replaced (substituted for) during this period by bona fide breast-milk substitutes, including infant formula. Any other food, such as cow's milk, fruit juices, cereals, vegetables, or any other fluid, solid or semisolid food intended for infants and given after this initial period, can no longer be considered as a replacement for breast milk (or as its *bona fide* substitute). Such foods only complement breast milk or breast-milk substitutes, and are thus referred to in the draft code as complementary foods. They are also commonly called weaning foods or breast-milk supplements.

Products other than *bona fide* breast-milk substitutes, including infant formula, are covered by the code only when they are "marketed or otherwise represented to be

---

[9] See document WHA33/1980/REC/1, Annex 6; document WHA33/1980/REC/2, page 327; and document WHA33/1980/REC/3, pages 67-95 and 200-204.

suitable . . . . for use as a partial or total replacement of breastmilk". Thus the code's references to products used as partial or total replacements for breast milk are not intended to apply to complementary foods unless these foods are actually marketed — as breast-milk substitutes, including infant formula, are marketed — as being suitable for the partial or total replacement of breast milk. So long as the manufacturers and distributors of the products do not promote them as being suitable for use as partial or total replacements for breast milk, the code's provisions concerning limitations on advertising and other promotional activities do not apply to these products.

The Executive Board examined the draft code very carefully.[10] Several Board members indicated that they considered introducing amendments in order to strengthen it and to make it still more precise. The Board considered, however, that the adoption of the code by the Thirty-fourth World Health Assembly was a matter of great urgency in view of the serious situation prevailing, particularly in developing countries, and that amendments introduced at the present stage might lead to a postponement of the adoption of the code. The Board therefore unanimously recommended to this Thirty-fourth World Health Assembly the adoption of the code as presently drafted, realizing that it might be desirable or even necessary to revise the code at an early date in the light of the experience obtained in the implementation of its various provisions. This is reflected in operative paragraph 5(4) of the recommended resolution contained in resolution EB67.R12.

The second [main question] before the Executive Board was whether it should recommend the adoption of the code as a recommendation or as a regulation. Some Board members expressed a clear preference for its adoption as a regulation in the sense of Articles 21 and 22 of the WHO Constitution. It became clear, however, that, although there had not been a single dissenting voice in the Board with regard either to the need for an international code or to its scope or content, opinion was divided on the question of a recommendation versus a regulation.

It was stressed that any decision concerning the form the code should take should be based on an appreciation of which alternative had the better chance of fulfilling the purpose of the code—that is, to contribute to improved infant and child nutrition and health. The Board agreed that the moral force of a unanimous recommendation could be such that it would be more persuasive than a regulation that had gained less then unanimous support from Member States. It was considered, however, that the implementation of the code should be closely monitored according to the existing WHO constitutional procedures; that future Assemblies should assess the situation in the light of reports from Member States; and that the Assembly should take any measures it judged necessary for its effective application

---

[10] The summary record of the Board's discussions is contained in document EB67/1981/REC/2, pages 306–322.

After carefully weighing the different points raised during its discussion, the Board unanimously adopted resolution EB67.R12, which contains the draft resolution recommended for adoption by the World Health Assembly. In this connexion I wish to draw the Committee's particular attention to the responsibilities outlined in the draft resolution: those of Member States, the regional committees, the Director-General, the Executive Board, and the Health Assembly itself for appropriate follow-up action once the code has been adopted.

In carrying out their responsibilities, Member States should make full use of their Organization—at global, regional and country levels—by requesting its technical support in the preparation of national legislation, regulations or other appropriate measures, and in the monitoring of the application of the code.

. . . . . .

I think that I can best reflect the sentiments of the Board by closing my introduction with a [plea] for consensus on the resolution as it was unanimously recommended to the World Health Assembly by the Board. We are not today dealing with an economic issue of particular importance only to one or a few Member States. We are dealing with a health issue of essential importance to all Member States, and particularly to developing countries, and of importance to the children of the world and thus to all future generations.

Source: World Health Organization (WHO). (1981). *International code of marketing of breast-milk substitutes.* Geneva, Switzerland: Author. Retrieved from http://www.who.int/nutrition/publications/code_english.pdf. Used with permission.

Index

Note: Italicized page locators indicate figures; tables are noted with *t*.